A SYNOPTIC KEY OF THE MATERIA MEDICA

A SYNOPTIC KEY OF THE MATERIA MEDICA

C.M. BOGER

Published by

FacsiMile Publisher
12 Pragati Market
Ashok Vihar, Ph-2
Delhi - 110052, India
Phone: 011-47034999
Email: www.facsimilepublishers.com
info@facsimilepublishers.com

Distribution Network
gyanbooks.com
India, USA, Canada, UK, Australia

ISBN: 978-93-6896-871-9 (PB)

First Published, 1916

2nd Impression 2025

Printed at: Gyan Press, Delhi.

A SYNOPTIC KEY OF THE MATERIA MEDICA
Author: C.M. BOGER

A
Synoptic Key
of the
MATERIA MEDICA

By

C. M. BOGER, M. D.

SECOND EDITION

FOREWORD

Correct prescribing is the art of carefully fitting pathogenetic to clinical symptoms, and as such at present requires a special aptness in grasping the essential points of symptom images, great drudgery in mastering a working knowledge of our large materia medica or a most skilful use of many books of reference.

It is the aim of this book to simplify and introduce method into this work, so that the truly homœopathic curative remedy may be worked out with greater ease and certainty. For this purpose a combination of the analytic and synoptic methods has been thought best, hence the *Key* and *Synopsis* have been made to interlock with and complement each other and are intended to be used conjointly. A great aid to this is found in the *Supplemental Index Table.*

The spirit of the clinical symptom picture is best obtained by *asking the patient to tell his own story,* whenever this is possible. This account is then amplified and more accurately defined by the questioner, who should first try to elicit the evident *cause and course of the sickness down to the latest symptom,* to which he will especially add all the things which *now seem to interfere* with the sufferer's comfort. Especially should the natural modifiers of sickness—*the modalities*—be very definitely ascertained. The following are the most vitally important of such influences, *Time, Temperature, Open Air, Posture, Being Alone, Motion, Sleep, Eating and Drinking, Touch, Pressure, Discharges, etc.*

A consideration of the *mental state* comes next in order of importance. Here the presence of *Irritability, Sadness* or *Fear* is the ruling factor.

The third step concerns the estimate to be put upon the patient's own description of his sensations. This is a very vital point and in order not to be misled it is always well to ascertain whether any of the following primary sensations are present: *Burning, Cramping, Cutting, Bursting, Soreness, Throbbing* and *Thirst.* There may be many others, but the presence of any one of these often overshadows them, especially such as may be due to the play of the imagination; which feature is in itself often of more importance than the particular thing imagined.

Next in order comes the *entire objective aspect or expression of the sickness*: This should especially include the *Facial Expression, Demeanor, Nervous Excitability. Sensibility, Restlessness* or *Torpor, State of the Secretions* and any abnormal coloring that may be present.

Lastly the *part affected* must be determined; which also brings the investigation in touch with diagnosis.

By going over the above rubrics in the order named the contour of the disease picture will be pretty clearly outlined and will point fairly well toward the simillimum, and the prescriber has only to keep in mind the fact that the actual *differentiating factor may belong to any rubric whatsoever* and also that the scope of these rubrics reaches far beyond the appended synoptic text.

For ready reference the following diagram has been arranged:

CAUSATION. TIME. THE MOST PECULIAR OR LATEST SYMPTOM.

REACTION TO (Modality)
- **HEAT AND COLD.** OPEN AIR.
- WEATHER. **DISCHARGES.** LIGHT.
- NOISE. TOUCH. PRESSURE.
- **POSTURE.** MOTION. EATING.
- DRINKING. COMPANY. SLEEP.

MIND
- IRRITABILITY.
- SADNESS.
- FEAR.
- PLACIDITY.

DOMINATING SENSATION
- BURNING. CRAMPING.
- CUTTING. BURSTING.
- SORENESS. THROBBING.
- THIRST.

OBJECTIVE ASPECT
- DEMEANOR. POSTURE.
- RESTLESSNESS.
- NERVOUS EXCITABILITY.
- FACIAL EXPRESSION.
- TORPOR. SECRETIONS AND DISCHARGES.
- COLOR. ODOR.

PART AFFECTED
- **Organs.**
- **Right.**
- **Left.**

THE SYNOPSIS, is intended to make clear the *general expression or genius* of each remedy, and thereby help the prescriber correct his bearings. The scope of its contents is much enlarged by bracketing the most nearly affiliated remedies after some of the more important symptoms; this also helps in making differentiations.

What often makes a cure hard is the laying of too much stress upon some particular factor at the expense of the disease picture as a whole, thus destroying its symmetry and forming a distorted conception of the natural image of the sickness. This does not however mean that all symptoms stand on the same level, for certain effects must be more prominent than others, yet be part and parcel of them. This is the sense in which we must learn to know our remedies, just as we do our friends, *by their air or personality;* an ever changing, composite effect, but always reflecting the same motive.

Whenever the chosen remedy excites little or no reaction, the selection has either been faulty, or what is just as likely, one of the fundamental miasms which calls for either Psorinum, Sulfur, Medorrhinum or Syphilinum, is present.

Whenever the general benefit derived from a single dose lags, the remedy should be repeated in the next higher potency instead of looking upon the new symptoms as indicators for some other drug; for only the most inveterately rooted dyscrasia can, by varying its expression, resist the whole scale of an indicated remedy. Sometimes we can advantageously change to another potency scale of the same remedy, before attempting to scrutinize the remaining picture for those new developments which must point toward our next choice, nor should this successor be chosen until the new symptom picture—disease phase—takes on a fairly definite or settled form.

Parkersburg. W. Va., Sept. 23, 1916.

KEY TO THE MATERIA MEDICA

PART 1

THE ANALYSIS

PERIODICALLY, in general, **Agg.**: ARS. Cact. **Caps.** Ced. CHIN. **Eupat.** Gel. **Ip.** NAT-M. **Nux-v. Pul. Sul.**

daily, Agg.: Aran. Ars. Caps. Ip. Nux-v. Pul.

twice, Agg.: Grap.

at the same hour, Agg.: Aran. Bov. **Ced. Chin-s.** Lyc. Nat-m. Saba.

alternate days, on, **Agg.**: **Ars.** Canth. CHIN. Ip. Nat-m. Nux-v. Pul. Rhus-t.

every 4th day, Agg.: Ars. Lyc. Pul. Saba.

weekly, Agg.: Ars. Canth. Gel. **Iris.** Lac-d. Lyc. Pho. **Sang.** Sil. Sul.

fourteen days, Agg.: Con.

DAYTIME, **Agg.**: Kali-c. Med. Sep.

MORNING, **Agg.**: **Am-m. Ant-t. Aur.** Bor. Bov. Bry. **Calc-c.** Carb-v. Chel. Con. Croc. Hep. Kali-bi. Kali-c. Kali-n. **Nat-m.** Nat-s. Nit-ac. NUX-V. **Pho.** Pod. Rhod. **Rhus-t.** Saba. **Scil.** Sep. Sul.

in bed, Agg.: Alo. **Amb.** Am-m. Bry. Con. **Kali-c. Lyc. Nux-v.** Pho. Sep. **Sul.**

and evening, Agg.: **Coc-c.** Lach. **Pho.** Psor. Sep. Ver-a.

one day and afternoon of next, Agg.: Eupat. Lac-c.

FORENOON, **Agg.**: Cann. **Nat-c.** Saba. Sep. Sul-ac.

10-11 a. m., Agg.: Cact. NAT-M. Sep. SUL.

NOON, **Agg.**: Arg.

AFTERNOON, **Agg.**: **Alu. Ang.** Ap. Asaf. BELL. Chin. Colo. Dig. Ign. **Kali-n. Lyc. Pul.** Rhus-t. Sep. Sil. Sul. Thu. **Zin.**

3 p. m., Agg.: **Bell.**

4 p. m., Agg.: Ap. Chel. LYC. Nat-s. Zin.

4-8 p. m., Agg.: Hell. LYC. Zin.

EVENING, **Agg.**: Alu. Amb. Am-c. Ant-c. Ant-t. Arg-n. Arn. Ars. **Bell.** Bry. Caps. **Caus.** Chin. Colch. **Cyc. Euphr.** Flu-ac. Grap. Hell. Hyo. **Kali-n.** LYC. Mag-c. **Men.** Mez. Nat-s. **Nit-ac.** Petr. Pho. **Plat.** Plb. PUL. **Ran-sc. Sep.** Stan. **Stro. Sul.** Sul-ac. Val. Zin.

NIGHT, **Agg.**: **Aco.** Arn. **Ars.** Asaf. Aur. Bar-c. Bell. Bry. Calc-c. Caus. **Cham. Chin.** Cimi. **Colch.** Con. Dulc. **Fer. Grap. Hep.** Iod. Led. **Mag-c.** Mag-m. Mang. MERC. Mez. **Nit-ac.** Nux-v. **Plb. Psor.** Saba. **Sil. Stro. Sul. Syph.**

6 p. m.-6 a. m. Agg.: Kre. Syph.

P. M., Agg.: Carb-v. Led. Lyc. PUL. **Ran-sc.** Saba.

A. M., Agg.: ARS. Dros. **Fer.** KALI-C. **Kali-n.** NUX-V. Pho. Pod. RHUS-T. Sil. Sul. **Thu.**

2-3 a. m., Agg.: **Ars. Kali-bi. Kali-c.**

2-5 a. m.: Sul.

5 a. m., Agg.: Nat-c.

AIR, **open, Agg.** Also **averse to open air, better in room, etc.: Agar.** Am-c. Anac. **Bell.** CALC-C. Cam. Carb-v. Caus. CHAM. **Chin.** COCCL. COFF. GUAI. **Hep.** IGN. Kali-bi. KALI-C. Merc. NAT-C. Nit-ac. **Nux-m.** NUX-V. PETR. Rum. Sele. SIL. Spig. Sul.

Amel.: also air hunger, wants to be fanned; worse in room, etc.: **Aesc.** ALU. Ant-t. **Ap. Arg-n.** ARS. **Ars-iod.** Asaf. AUR. Cann. CARB-V. **Cep.** Coc-c. CROC. FLU-AC. **Glo.** Grap. IOD. Ip. **Kali-io. Lach.** Laur. Lit-t. **Lyc.** MAG-C. Mag-m. **Med.** Mez. Nat-s. Pho. PUL. SABI. Sec-c. Sep. **Sul.** Tub.

draft of, Agg.: Aco. BELL. **Calc-c.** CAPS. **Chin.** Hep. Ign. **Kali-c.** Lach-def. **Nux-v.** RHUS-T. SIL. SUL.

Comp. **Weather, Windy.**

inspiring, Agg. (Cold): Am-c. Caus. **Cist.** Cor-r. Hyo. Ign. Merc. **Nux-v. Rum.** Saba. Sep.

night, Agg.: Aco. Am-c. Carb-v. **Merc.** Nat-s. Nit-ac. Sul.

uncovering, from, Amel. Warm wraps or warmth of bed, etc. **Agg.:** Ap. CHAM. DROS. **Euphor.** Fer. Flu-ac. LED. **Lyc. Men.** MERC. Mos. **Mur-ac.** Nit-ac. **Op. Pul.** SABI. **Sec-c.** SUL.

Agg., see **Cold.**

ALONE, **when, Agg.: Wants company:** Ap. Arg-n. **Ars.** Dros. **Hep.** Hyo. Kali-c. LYC. Merc. **Pho. Pul.** STRAM.

Amel.: averse to company: Amb. BAR-C. Bell. **Bry.** Carb-a. Carb-v. Gel. **Ign.** Lach. **Lyc. Nat-m.** Plb. Pul. SEP. Stram. Sul. Taren.

yet dreads being alone: Ars. Clem. Con. **Lyc.** Sep. Stram.

BED, **getting out of, when, Agg.: Bry.** Calc-c. **Carb-v. Coccl. Con. Lach.**

Comp. **Cold Becoming.**

Amel.: Aur Dulc. Ign. Pul. Sep.

after, Agg.: Am-m. Lach. Rhus-t.

BENDING. **Agg.:** Bell. **Calc-c. Ign.** Nux-v. Pul.

Amel.: Bell.

backward, Agg.: Sep.

Amel.: Alet. **Bell.** Dios. Ign.

BITING AND CHEWING, **Agg.: Am-c. Am-m. Hep. Men.** RHUS-T. Thu.

Comp. **Eating.**

BLEEDING, **Amel.:** Fer.

BLOWING NOSE, **Agg.: Aur. Hep. Merc. Pul. Spig.**

BORING INTO PART, **Amel.: Aru-t. Nat-c.**

BREATHING, **Agg.:** BRY. **Colch. Sep. Spig.**

deeply, Agg.: ACO. Ascl. BRY. Lyc. Merc. Ran-sc. **Rhus-t. Sabi.** Sul.

Inspiration, Agg.: Aco. Bry. Ip. **Rhus-t.** Rum. **Sabi. Scil. Spo.**

Amel.: Colch. Ign. Spig. Verb.
out, expiration, Agg.: CHLOR. **Colch. Pul. Spig.**
Amel.: Aco. Rhus-t. Sabi.

BURNS AND SCALDS, **Agg.: Ars.** CANTH. **Caus.**

CHILDBED, puerperal state, **Agg.: Aco. Bell. Bry.** Cham. Cimi. Nux-v. **Plat. Pul. Pyro. Rhus-t.** Sabi. Sec-c. **Sep.**

CLIMACTERIC, **Agg.: at Amy-n.** Cimi. LACH. **Sang.** SUL. Sul-ac.

CLUTCHING, **grasping, Agg.: Caus. Cham.**

COITION, **venery, and sexual excesses, Agg.: Agar. Ag-c.** Calc-c. **Calad.** Kali-br. **Kali-c. Pho-ac.** SEP. **Stap.**

COLD, **Agg.:** Also **chilled easily and lack of vital heat: Agar. Am-c.** Aran. ARS. **Aur. Bar-c.** **CALC-C. Calc-p.** Cam. **Caps.** CAUS. **Chin.** Cimi. **Cist.** Cocl. **Dulc.** Eupat. **Fer. Grap. Hell.** HEP. Hyper. **Kali-bi.** KALI-C. Lac-def. **Lyc. Mag-c. Mag-p.** Merc. Mez. MOS. **Nit-ac. Nux-m.** NUX-V. **Pho.** Pho-ac. **Psor.** Pyro. Ran-b. Rhod. RHUS-T. **Rum.** SABA. **Sep.** SIL. Spig. Stan. STRO. Sul.

Amel.: He feels too hot, etc.: Aco. Alo, Ant-t. **Ap. Arg-n. Bell. Bry. Carb-v.** Cham. Coc-c. Cycl. Dros. Euphr. **Flu-ac.** GEL. **Clo.** Guai. IOD. Kali-io. LACH. Led. Lil-t. Lyc. Med. Merc. Nit-c. NAT-M. **Nat-s.** Op. PUL. Sabi. **Sang. Sec-c. Sul.**

Comp. **Burning Sensation.**

becoming, Agg., uncovering Agg. Warmth of bed or external heat, Amel.: Ars. Bell. BRY. Caus. **Cham.** Chin. Clem. Cocl. **Dros.** Grap. HEP. Hyo. Kali-c. **Led. Lyc.** Mag-c. **Mag-p.** MERC. Nat-c. **Nux-m.** NUX-V. Rhod. RHUS-T. Rum. **Samb. Scil.** Sep. SIL. SUL. STRO. Zin.

Comp. **Undressing.**

Amel.: uncovering or cold applications, **Amel. Heat of bed, Agg.:** Aco. Calc-c. Cham. Fer. Flu-ac. Guai. IOD. **Led.** LYC. **Merc.** Mur-ac. Op. PUL. Sabi. **Sec-c.** SUL. Tab.

entering the, Agg.: Bell. Ip.

sitting or lying on ground: Ars. Calc-c. Dulc. Sil.

while hot or sweating, Agg.: Aco. Ars. **Bry.** Clem. Colch. Dulc. Kali-bi. **Rhus-t.** Sep.

Single parts, agg.: Hep. Nux-v. Rhus-t. Sep. Sil.

head, Agg.: Bell. Hep. Kali-bi. Mag-m. NUX-V. **Psor.** RHUS-T. **Sep.** SIL.

hands in water, etc., **Agg.:** Clem. Con. Ign. **Lac-d. Pho. Sep.** Sul.

feet, Agg.: Bar-c. Dulc. Lach. Nux-v. Pho. Pul. **Sil.**

on entering a cold place, Agg.: Ars. Ran-b.

and heat both, extremes, Agg.: Carb-v. Caus. **Flu-ac. Lyc.** Merc. Pho-ac. Sul. Syph.

taking, Agg.: after being chilled while hot or sweating, etc.: ACO. Ars. **Bell. Bry. Cham.** Clem. Coff. **Colch. Dulc.** Hyo. **Ip.** MERC. **NUX-V.** PHO. **Pul. RHUS-T.** Sep. **Sil. Spig. Sul.** Ver-a.

COUGHING, **Agg.**: Aco. Ars. **Bell.** BRY. Calc-c. **Dros.** Ip. NUX-V. **Pho. Pul. Rhus-t.** Sep.

DEBAUCH, dissipation, **Agg.**: **Carb-v.** NUX-V. **Op. Stram.**

DENTITION, **Agg.**: ACO. Bor. CALC-C. CALC-P. CHAM. Coff. Ip. Kre. **Merc. Pod.**

DISCHARGES, **excessive, Agg.: Depletions, Loss of vital fluids, emissions, hemorrhages, sweats,** etc.: Agar. **Calc-c. Carb-v.** CHIN. Cob. Ip. **Kali-c. Nux-v.** Pho. PHO-AC. **Pul. Sep. Stap. Ver-a.**

suppressed, scanty, etc., **Agg.: Checked sweats or eruptions;** FREE DISCHARGES, AMEL.: **Aco.** Ant-t. Ap. **Ars. Bell.** BRY. **Calc-c.** Cam. Caus. Cham. Chin. Colch. **Cup. Dulc. Grap.** Hep. **Ip. Kali-bi.** LACH. **Lyc.** Mez. NUX-V. Op. Pho. **Pho-ac. Psor.** PUL. Rhus-t. **Sep. Sil.** Spig. **Stap.** Stram. SUL. **Zin.**

DUST, **Agg.: Ars-io.** Brom.

EATING, **before,** fasting, etc., **Agg.**: CALC-C. **Croc.** FLU-AC. IOD. LAUR. NAT-C. PHO. **Stap.**

Amel.: Cham. Con. Nat-m.

while, Agg.: Bell. CARB-A. CARB-V. CON. **Fer.** Hep. Kali-c. Merc. Nat-c. NIT-AC.

Amel.: ANAC. Caps. Grap. IGN. LACH. ZIN.

after, Agg.: Alo. Anac. ARS. BRY. CALC-C. Carb-v. CAUS. Chin. **Colo.** CON. **Fer.** Ign. **Kali-bi.** KALI-C. **Lach.** LYC. NAT-M. NUX-V. Petr. PHO. **Pul.** Rum. SEP. SIL. SUL. Ver-a. Viol-t. **Zin.**

Amel.: Bov. Chel. Flu-ac. **Iod.** Kali-bi. NAT-C. **Pho.** Plb. Sep.

long, Agg.: Anac. Fer. **Kre.** Pul. Sul.

breakfast, Agg.: Cham. Nux-v. Pho.

Amel.: Calc-c. Croc. Iod. Stap.

dinner, Agg.: Bry. Grat.

a little, Agg.: Con. Kali-c. LYC. **Nux-v. Sul.**

too much, Agg.: overloading the stomach: **Aeth. Ant-c.** Calc-c. **Carb-v. Lyc.** NUX-V. Sul.

EMOTIONS, **Agg.: mental excitement,** etc.: **Aco.** Amy-n. **Arg-n.** Aur. Bell. Bry. **Cham.** Coff. Cob. COLO. **Gel. Hyo.** IGN. **Lach. Nat-m.** NUX-V. Pho. PHO-AC. PUL. STAP. Ver-a.

Comp. **Nervous Effects.**

mortification, vexation, chagrin, etc., **Agg.: Colo.** IGN. Lyc. NAT-M. **Op. Petr.** Pho-ac. Plat. STAP.

See also Mind.

ERUCTATIONS, **Agg.: Cham.**

Amel.: Ant-t. CARB-V. **Grap. Ign.** KALI-C. LYC. **Nux-v.** Sang.

EXERTION, **mental, Agg.:** Anac. Arg-n. Aur. CALC-C. **Calc-p.** IGN. LACH. Lyc. **Nat-m.** NUX-V. Pho. **Pho-ac.** Pic-ac. Nux-v. Rhe. RHUS-T. Rut. Sil. SUL. **Ver-a.**

manual, Agg.: Nat-m.

physical, Agg.: fatigue, tired feeling, etc.: Aco. ARN. ARS. BRY. Cact. **Calc-c.** Cann. **Coccl.** Croc. Hep. Lyc. Nux-v. Pic-ac. Pul. Rhe. RHUS-T. Rut. SUL. **Ver-a.**

EXHAUSTION, **nervous, see Mind, Excitement.**

EYES, **opening, Amel.: Bry. Therid.**

Comp. **Sleep.**

FEATHERBED, **Agg.: Mang.**

FEMALES, **Agg.:** BELL. **Calc-c. Caps. Cham. Coccl. Croc.** PUL. SABI. SEP. **Val. Vibur.**

FOOD, **beer, Agg.:** Kali-bi. Nux-v.

bread, Agg.: Bry. Nux-v. Pul. Sul.

and butter, Agg. Pul.

butter, Agg.: Carb-v. Pul.

cabbage, Agg.: Bry. Lyc. Petr.

cheese, bad, Agg.: Bry.

coffee, Agg.: Canth. Caus. CHAM. IGN. NUX-V. Pul.

Amel.: Cham.

cold, Agg.: Ars. Bell. Chel. **Lyc. Nux-v. Rhus-t.**

Amel.: Ap. Caus. Bell. Bry. LACH. **Pho.** Phyt. **Pul.**

water, Agg.: Canth. Cham. **Nux-v. Rhus-t. Sep.**

Amel.: Caus. Pho. Sep.

condiments, drugs, etc., **Agg.: Nux-v.**

dry, Agg.: Calc-c.

farinaceous: Lyc. Nat-s.

fat, Agg.: CARB-V. **Caus. Chin.** CYC. **Fer. Grap.** PUL. **Tarax.**

fish, Agg.: Plb.

spoiled, Agg.: Pul.

frozen, Agg.: ices, etc.: **Ars. Pul.**

fruit, Agg.: Ars. Bry. Chin. **Pul. Ver-a.**

hot cakes, Agg.: Pul.

indigestible foods, Agg.: Iod.

legumes, Agg.: Bry. Lac.

liquids, drinks, etc., after: **Agg.:** ARS. **Chin. Coccl.** Colo. Crot-t. **Fer.** Nat-m. PHO. **Rhus-t. Sil. Ver-a.**

cold, Agg.: Lyc.

meat, Agg.: Caus. Colch.

milk, Agg.: AETH. Bry. CALC-C. **Chin.** Lac-def. **Nit-ac.** Pho. **Pul.** Sul.

pork, Agg.: CARB-V. **Grap.** PUL. **Sep.**

potatoes, Agg.: Alu. Pul. Ver-a.

raw, Agg.: Pul. **Rut.** Ver-a.

rich, Agg.: Pul.

sausage, Agg.: Bell. Bry.

sour, Agg.: Ant-c. Carb-v. Pul. Sep.

sour-krout, Agg.: Bry. Petr.
spirits, Agg.: alcoholic liquors; for drunkards, etc.: **Ars.** Calc-c. Carb-v. Cimi. **Lach. Lyc.** NUX-V. **Op. Pho. Ran-b.** Sul. **Zin.**
strawberries, Agg.: Sep.
sweet, Agg.: Arg-n. Ign. Merc.
tea, Agg.: Fer. **Sele.** Thu.
tobacco, Agg.: Ars. Gel. **Ign. Pul. Spo. Stap.**
Amel.: Aran. Taren.
veal, Agg.: Ip. Kali-n.
vegetables, Agg.: Ars. Bry.
vinegar, Agg.: Ant-c. Ars. Sul.

FROZEN, **after being,** frostbite, etc., **Agg.:** AGAR. **Ars. Bry.** Carb-v. **Nit-ac. Petr. Pul.**

HAIR, **cutting, Agg.:** Bell. Pho. **Sep.**
letting it down, Amel.: Bell. Cina. Fer. Pho.
touching, Agg.: Pul. **Sele.**

HEATED, **becoming, Agg. heat of sun; sunstroke,** etc.: **Aco. Ant-c. Bell. Bry. Carb-v.** GLO. **Kali-c. Lach.** Nat-c. **Nat-m. Pho.** Pul. Sele. Thu. Ver-v. Zin.
by the fire, lamp, ironing, etc., **Agg.:** Ap. **Bry.** Glo. Kali-io. Merc. Mez. **Pul.**
Amel.: Ars. Ign.

HICCOUGH, **Agg.: Am-m.**

HOT APPLICATIONS, **Amel.:** Ars. Mag-p. Radm. **Rhus-t.**

INATTENTION, **Agg.:** Gel. **Hell.**

INJURY, wounds, etc., **Agg.:** ARN. Con. Hep. **Hyper. Led. Pul. Rhus-t.** Rut. Sul-ac.
deep: Bels.
to head, Agg.: Arn. Cic. **Hyper. Nat-s.**
incised, Agg.: Stap.
muscles, to, Agg.: Rhus-t.
punctured, Agg.: Hyper. Led. Nit-ac.
reopening of old, Agg. Pho.
soft parts, to, Agg.: Arn.

KINDNESS, **consolation and sympathy,** if **spoken to,** etc., **Agg.:** Ars. **Bell. Calc-c.** IGN. **Nat-m. Plat.** Sep. Sil.

LAUGHING, **Agg.:** Bell. **Bor.** Chin. **Pho.**

LIFTING, sprains, etc., **Agg.: Calc-c.** Grap. Lyc. **Rhus-t.** Sep.

LIGHT, **Agg.:** Aco. Arg-n. Ars. BELL. CALC-C. **Con.** Dros. EUPHR. **Glo. Grap.** Hep. **Lyc. Merc.** Merc-c. Nat-s. **Nux-v. Pho.** Pho-ac. Pul. RHUS-T. Sang. SEP. **Sil. Stram. Sul.**
Comp. **Twilight.**
Amel.; darkness, Agg.: Calc-c. Cann. Lyc. **Plb.** STRAM. **Stro.**
of sun, Amel.: Stro.

LOOKED AT, **when, Agg.: Ant-c.** Ars. **Cina.**

LOOKING **at bright objects, Agg.:** snow, water, etc.: **Bell.** Stram.

intently, fixedly, reading, **straining the vision,** etc., **Agg.**: Ap. **Arg-n.** CALC-C. **Cina.** Croc. Epiph. **Kali-c.** Lil-t. **Lyc.** NAT-M. **Nux-v.** Onos. Pho. **Rhod.** RUT. Seneg. **Sil.**

running water, at, Agg.; moving objects: **Bell.** Con. Fer.

up or down, Agg.: Calc-c.

MEASLES, **Agg.: Aco.** Kali-bi. PUL.

MENSES, **before, Agg.:** CALC-C. CUP. KALI-C. LACH. LYC. Nat-m. PUL. Sep. SUL. VER-A. Vib. Zin.

at start of, Agg.: Aco. Hyo. Lach.

during, Agg.: AM-C. Arg-n. **Cham.** Cimi. Cocel. GRAP. HYO. Ign. **Mag-c.** MAG-M. Nux-m. Nux-v. PUL. **Sep.** Stap. **Sul. Zin.**

after, Agg.: BOR. GRAP. Kre. Lach. Lyc. **Nux-v.** Sep.

MERCURY, **Agg.: Aur. Carb-v.** HEP. **Lach.** NIT-AC. **Stap. Sul.**

MESMERISM, magnetism, **gentle stroking** or rubbing, **Amel.: Cup. Pho.** Sep. Sil.

Comp. **Rubbing.**

MOON, **change of, Agg.:** Alu. Clem. Sil.

full, Agg.: Saba.

MOTION, **Agg.;** also while walking, etc.: Ant-t. **Arn.** BELL. BRY. Calad. **Cham. Chel.** Chin. **Coccl.** COLCH. Colo. Croc. Dig. Eupat. Flu-ac. Glo. Grap. Hell. Ip. Kali-n. Klam. LED. Lil-t. Merc. **Nat-m.** NUX-V. Petr. Pho. **Ran-b. Scil.** Sep. Sil. **Spig. Stan.** Stap. **Zin.**

Amel.; walking, Amel.; rest, Agg.: Ant-t. **Ars. Aur. Caps. Con. Cyc. Dulc. Euphor. Fer.** Flu-ac. **Kali-io.** Lyc. Mag-c. PUL. **Rhod.** RHUS-T. **Saba. Samb. Sep.** Sul. **Tarax. Val.** Zin.

Comp. **Restlessness.**

after, Agg.: Agar. ARS. **Cann. Pul.** RHUS-T. SEP. **Stan.** Sul-ac. **Val.**

arms, of, Agg.: Led. Ran-b. Rhus-t. **Spig.**

behind him, Agg.: Ign. Mar. Pul. **Sanic.** Sep.

raising the, see Position.

ascending, Agg.: Arn. ARS. BRY. **Calc-c.** Cup. **Nux-v.** Seneg. Sep. Spig. **Spo.** Thu.

beginning of, Agg.; change of position, starting to walk, etc.: CAPS. CON. EUPHOR. FER. Flu-ac. LYC. **Pho** PUL. RHUS-T. Saba. Samb. Sil.

downward, descending, **Agg.:** Bor. **Gel.**

gentle, Amel.: Amb. **Fer.** Gel. Kali-bi. Mag-m. **Pul.**

rapid, Agg.: Ars. Bry. Sil. **Sul.**

riding; on a boat, cars, carriage; swaying, etc., **Agg.;** seasickness, carsickness: Ars. COCCL. **Colch.** Lach. PETR. **SEP.** Sul. **Tab.** Ther.

Amel.: Ars. Grap. **Nit-ac.**
Comp. **Carried.**

shaking, concussion, **Agg.;** striking against anything; **jarring, stepping hard,** etc.: **Arn.** BELL. BRY. **Chin.** Cic. Colch. **Glo.** Led. Lyc. Nit-ac. **Nux-v.** Pho. RHUS-T. Sep. SIL.

violent, rapid, **Amel.;** running, dancing, etc. **Idleness, Agg.:** **Ars.** Brom. Flu-ac. **Sep.** Sul-ac. Taren. Comp. **Hurry.**

MOUTH, **opening, Agg.:** **Merc.**

MUSIC, **Agg.:** **Grap.** Lyc. **Nat-c.** Nux-v. **Pho-ac.** SEP. Thu.

Amel.: Taren.

NARCOTICS, **Agg.:** **Bell.** CHAM. **Coff.** **Lach.** NUX-V. **Pul.**

NOISE, **Agg.:** ACO. **Arn.** BELL. Bor. **Bry.** Caps. **Caus.** Cham. **Chin.** COFF. Con. **Ign.** Lyc. Nat-c. NUX-V. Plat. **Sep.** **Sil.** Spig. **Ther.** **Zin.**

penetrating, Agg.: Asar. Ther.

rattling, Agg.: Nit-ac.

sudden, Agg.; reports, etc.: Bor.

ODORS, **Agg.:** **Aur.** **Bell.** **Coff.** Grap. **Ign.** **Lyc.** NUX-V. **Pho.** Sang. Sul.

Comp. **Smell.**

of food, Agg.: Ars. COLCH. Eupat. **Sep.** **Stan.**

ONANISM, **Agg.:** **Chin.** **Con.** Merc. **Nat-m.** Nux-v. **Pho-ac.** Sep. **Stap.** **Sul.** **Ust.**

PAIN, **during the, Agg.:** Colo. Rhus-t. **Sep.**

POSITION, **changing, Agg.** See **Motion, beginning of.**

Amel.: Cham. **Ign.** Pho-ac. Rhus-t. Val. Zin.

crossing limbs, Agg.: Dig. Lyc. Pho. Rhus-t.

doubling up, Amel.: Canth. COLO. Pul.

drawing up the limb, Agg.: **Rhus-t.** **Sec-c.**

Amel.: **Calc-c.** **Sep.** **Sul.** **Thu.**

hanging down of part, Agg.: **Bell.** **Calc-c.** Carb-v. Pul. **Vip.**

Amel.: **Con.**

leaning against an object, supporting or resting the part, **Amel.:** Fer.

lying, Agg.: **Amb.** Ant-t. **Ap.** ARS. AUR. CAPS. CHAM. CON. DROS. **Dulc.** EUPHOR. FER. LYC. MEN. **Nat-s.** **Pho.** PLAT. PUL. RHUS-T. Rum. SAMB. **Sang.** Sep. Stro. Tarax. Verb.

Amel.: **Am-m.** **Arn.** **Asar.** **Bell.** BRY. **Calc-c.** **Nat-m.** NUX-V. **Scil.**

abdomen, on, Amel.: **Bell.** **Colo.** **Med.** Phyt. Pul.

back, on, Agg.: Ars. **Caus.** Cham. **Ign.** **Iod.** NUX-V. PHO. **Rhus-t.** Sep.

Amel.: BRY. CALC-C.

bed, in, Agg.: **Amb.** Calc-c. Chel. Dros. Hell. Hep. **Iod.** Kali-c. **Lyc.** **Merc.** Nit-ac. PUL.

Amel.: **Bry.** NUX-V. **Scil.**

hands and knees, on, Amel.: Par-b.

head low, Agg.: ARS. PUL.
Amel.: Psor.

side, on, Agg.: ACO. ANAC. BRY. CALC-C. CARB-A. **Kali-c.** LYC. **Pho. Pul.** STAN.
Amel.: Nux-v.
left, Agg.: Aco. Ap. **Bar-c.** Bry. Cact. Lil-t. Lyc. Naj. Nat-c. **Nat-m.** Nat-s. PHO. PUL. Sep.
right, Agg.: Bell. Caus. **Mag-m.** MERC. **Nux-v.** Spo.
pain goes to side lain on: Bry. Pul.
painful, Agg.: ACO. Am-c. Ant-t. **Ars. Bar-c. Calad. Cyc.** Dros. Grap. **Hep. Iod. Kali-c.** Kali-o. Lyc. Mag-c. Mag-m. Mos. Nit-ac. **Nux-m. Nux-v.** Par. **Pho.** Pho-ac. Rhe. **Rut.** Saba. Sele. **Sil.** Spo. Stap. Thu. Comp. **Pressure.**
Amel.: Amb. Arn. BRY. CHAM. COLO. Flu-ac. **Ign.** PUL. **Rhus-t.** Sec-c. Sep.

raising affected part, Agg.: Con.
Limb, Agg.: Calc-c.
arm, Agg.: Bar-c. **Con.** Cup. Fer. Sang. Spig.
Comp. **Motion of Arms.**

raising up, Agg.; erect posture: ACO. **Bell.** BRY. Cad-s. **Ign.** Merc-i-fl. **Nux-v.** Phyt. **Rhus-t. Sul. Ver-v.**
Amel.: Am-c. ARS. **Calc-c.** Glo. **Samb. Sep.**

seat, from a, Agg.: Berb. **Caps. Con.** Lyc. **Pho. Pul. Rhus-t. Spig.**

sitting, Agg.: Agar. Ars. Asaf. CAPS. **Cob.** CON. CYC. DULC. EUPHOR. LYC. Mag-m. Mur-ac. PLAT. PUL. RHUS-T. SEP. **Sul.** Tarax. **Val.** VERB. VIOL-T. **Zin.**
Amel.: BRY. COLCH. NUX-V.
bent, Agg.: ANT-T. DIG.
down, Amel.: CAPS. CON.
erect, Agg.: Kali-c.

standing, Agg.: Caus. CON. CYCL. Lil-t. **Plat. Pul. Sep.** SUL. VAL.
Amel.: Ars. BELL. Colch. Led. Pho. Ran-b. Scil.

stooping, Agg.: Am-c. BRY. **Calc-c. Mang. Sep. Spig. Val.**
Amel.: Colch. Hyo.

stretching, Agg.: Ran-b. Rhus-t.
limbs, Agg.: Calc-c. Colch. Iod. **Sep. Sul. Thu.**
Amel.: RHUS-T. **Sec-c.**

turning head, Agg.: Calc-c. Pul. Spig.
over in bed, Agg.: Lyc. **Nux-v. Pul.** Sul.
Comp. **Rolling over, as if.**

PREGNANCY, **Agg.: Caul. Cham.** Cimi. **Coccl. Croc.** Nux-m. PUL. **Sabi.** Sec-c. SEP. Sul. Ver-a.

PRESSURE, **Agg.; on affected part,** etc.; AGAR. Ap. BAR-C. CINA. HEP. IOD. **Lach.** LYC. Merc-c. **Ran-b.** Sep. SIL.
Amel.; bandaging, etc.: Am-c. **Arg-n.** BRY. **Chin. Cimi.** COLO. CON. Dros. **Lil-t.**

MAG-M. **Mag-p.** MEN. NAT-C. **Plb. Pul.**

clothes, of, Agg.: Bry. CALC-C. Hep. LACH. LYC. Nit-ac. NUX-V. Sep. Spo. Stan. Sul.

about neck, Agg.: Agar. Chel. Con. Glo. Kali-c. LACH. Sep.

hard edge, over a, amel.: Chin. Colo. Ign. Lach. Samb. Stan.

spine, on, Agg.: Bell. **Chin.** Sil.

PUBERTY AND YOUTH, at, **Agg.:** Bell. Calc-p. Hell. Kali-br. **Nat-m.** Pho-ac. PUL. **Senec.** Sul.

QUININE, **Agg.:** Arn. **Ars.** Carb-v. Fer. Ip. **Nat-m. Pul.**

RUBBING, **Agg.: Anac. Con. Pul. Stro.**

Amel.: Calc-c. Canth. Nat-c. Pho. Plb. Pod. **Rhus-t.**

Comp. **Mesmerism.**

RUNNING, **Agg.: Ars. Bry.** Sil. **Sul.**

Amel. see **Motion, violent, Amel.**

SCRATCHING, **Agg.:** ANAC. CAPS. **Lach.** Old. PUL. RHUS-T. Sul.

Amel.: Asaf. Calc-c. Cyc. Mur-ac. Pho. **Sul.**

SEA, **Agg.: Ars.** Mag-m. **Rhus-t. Sep.**

SEASONS, **Spring,** melting snow, etc.; **Agg.:** Amb. Bell. Calc-c. Cep. **Gel. Lach.** Lyc. Rhus-t. Sul.

Summer, Agg., hot weather, etc.: Aeth. Bry. Carb-v. Iod. Iris. Nat-c. Nit-ac. **Pod.** Pul.

Comp. **Cold, Amel.**

Autumn, Agg.: Colch. **Dulc. Merc.** RHUS-T. Ver-a.

Winter, Agg.: Aco. Ars. Aur. Bry. Cam. **Dulc.** Hep. Kali-c. **Nux-v.** Petr. Psor. RHUS-T. Ver-a.

SEDENTARY LIFE, **Agg.:** NUX-V. **Sul.**

SHAVING, **Agg.:** Carb-a. Pho. **Pul.**

SINGING, **Agg.: Carb-v.** PHO. Sele. Stan.

Sleep, **half asleep, if:** Cam. Mag-p-a. Val.

SLEEP, **just before, Agg.: Ars. Carb-v. Pho.** PUL. Sep.

at beginning of, Agg.: Aral-r. Ars. Bry. LACH. Lyc. Mur-ac. **Pul. Sep.** Sul. Tarax.

during, Agg.: Ars. Bell. Bry. Cina. Hep. Lach. Op. Pul. Sil. Stram. Sul.

after, Agg., awaking, on, opening eyes, etc.: **Amb.** Am-m. Arn. Ars. **Calc-c. Caus. Hep.** Kali-bi. LACH. **Lyc.** Naj. Nit-ac. Nux-v. Op. **Pho.** Pul. Rhus-t. Sele. SEP. **Stap. Stram. Sul.**

Amel.: loss of, Agg.: Ars. COCCL. Cup. Epiph. Nux-v. PHO. Sang. Sele. **Zin.**

SMOKE, **Agg.** Ars. Lyc. Sep. Spig.

SNEEZING, **Agg.: Ars. Bell. Lyc. Rhus-t.**

SNEEZING, **Agg.: Aco. Alc-Anac. Arg.** Arn. Aru-t. **Calc-c. Cann.** Carb-v. **Chin. Coccl.** Dros. Iod. Mang. **Nat-c. Nat-**

m. Pho. Pho-ac. Rhus-t. Sele. Stan. Sul.

STONECUTTERS, **Agg. in: Calc-c. Sil.**

STORMS, **Agg., on approach of:** Dulc. **Lach.** Nat-c. Nat-m. **Pho.** Psor. RHOD. **Rhus-t.** Sep. **Sil.** Sul.

snowstorms, Agg.: Con. Form. Sep. Urt-u.

thunderstorms, Agg.: Phos.

Comp. **Weather.**

SWALLOWING, **Agg.** also painful Swallowing; Ars. Bar-c. **Bell. Bry. Hep.** Hyo. **Ign.** Kali-c. **Lach. Merc. Merc-c. Nit-ac.** Nux-v. **Phyt.** Pul. Stram. **Sul.**

Amel.: Ign.

after, Agg.: Nux-v. Zin.

drinks, Agg.: liquids, **drinking,** etc.: Ars. **Bell. Canth. Crot-t. Lach.** Merc. Nux-v. **Pho.** Ver-a.

after, Agg. see **Food.**

empty, Agg.: Bar-c. **Coccl.** LACH. Merc. **Merc-i-r.** Rhus-t. Sul.

rapidly, Agg., hastily: **Nit-ac. Sil.**

SWEAT, **Agg. or sweats without relief:** Ars. **Caus.** Cham. **Chin. Form.** MERC. **Nux-v. Op. Pho-ac. Rhus-t. Sep. Stram. Sul. Tilia. Ver-a.**

Amel.: BRY. CHAM. **Gel.** Grap. Nat-m. Psor. RHUS-T.

Comp. **Discharges.**

TALK OF OTHERS, **Agg.:** Am-c. **Ars.** Chin. **Mang.** Mez. **Nat-c. Nux-v.** Rhus-t. **Sep.** Sil. Ver-a. Zin.

THINKING OF HIS SYMPTOMS, **Agg.:** Aur. Bar-c. **Nit-ac.** Ox-ac. Saba.

TONGUE, **protruding the, Agg.:** Kali-bi.

TOUCH, **Agg.:** ANG. **Ant-c. Ap.** Arn. BELL. Bry. Caps. CHAM. **Chin.** Cina. **Coccl.** COLCH. Cup. Grap. HEP. **Hyo.** Kali-c. Lac-c. LACH. LED. **Lyc.** Mag-p. Mez. **Nit-ac.** NUX-V. **Petr.** Pho-ac. Plat. Pul. RAN-B. **Rhod. Rhus-t.** SABI. SEP. SIL. SPIG. STAP. **Stram.** SUL.

Amel.: Asaf. Bism. Calc-c. Cyc. Mur-ac.

least, Agg.: Aco. **Ap. Bell. Chin.** LACH. **Nit-ac. Nux-v.**

TWILIGHT, **Agg.:** Calc-c. Plat. **Pul.**

Amel.: Pho. Sang. Tab.

Comp. **Light.**

UNDRESSING, **Agg.: Ars.** Coccl. **Dros. Nux-v.** Pul. **Rhus-t.**

Comp. **Cold, becoming.**

URINATING, **Amel.:** Chin-s. **Gel. Ign.** Lyc. Pho-ac. Sang. Sil.

Comp. **Discharges.**

at close of, Agg.: Equis. Sars.

VACCINATION, **Agg.:** Thu. Variol.

VAULTED PLACES, **Agg., damp cellars,** cold rooms, etc.: **Ars.** Dulc. Nat-s. **Pul.** Sep.

VERTIGO, **during, Agg.: Aco. Calc-c.** GEL. NUX-V. **Pho. Pul. Stram.**

VOMITING, **Agg.**: Aeth. **Ars. Cup.** IP. **Pul. Sul.**
Amel.: **Sang.**

WALKING, see **Motion.**

WASHING, **Agg.; bathing, getting wet, wet applications,** etc.: **Alu.** AM-C. ANT-C. **Bry.** CALC-C. CLEM. **Dulc. Lyc.** Psor. PUL. RHUS-T. **Sep.** Sil. SUL.
Amel.: Ap. Arg-n. ASAR. FLU-AC. Led. PUL.
feet, Agg.: Lyc. Nux-v. **Pul.** Rhus-t. Sep. **Sil.**
head, Agg.: Bar-c. **Bell.**
in cold water, Agg.: **Am-c.** Calc-c. Dulc. **Rhus-t.**
Amel.: Guai. Led. Pul. Sec-c.

WEATHER, **changing, Agg.** or **temperature, change of:** ARS. Calc-c. **Calc-p. Carb-v.** Colch. **Dulc.** Mang. NUX-M. PHO. Psor. **Pul. Ran-b.** RHOD. RHUS-T. Sep. SIL. Sul. **Verb.**
dry, clear, **Agg.**: ACO. Asar. **Bry.** CAUS. HEP. Kali-c. Med. NUX-V. SPO.
foggy, heavy, **Agg.**: Bap. Chin. Gel. Hyper. RHUS-T. **Sep.**
frost: Carb-v.
wet, Agg.: **Am-c.** Aran. Ars. Bar-c. CALC-C. Cimi. DULC. Merc. **Nat-s. Nux-m.** Pul. Rhod. RHUS-T. Rut. Tub.
Comp. **Washing.**
and warm, Agg.: Carb-v. Gel. Ip. **Ver-v.**
and cold, Agg.: Bar-c. CALC-C. Carb-v. DULC. **Lach. Merc.** Nat-s. **Nux-m.** RHUS-T.
windy, Agg.; stormy; wind, Agg.: **Aco. Bell.** CHAM. Chin. Cimi. Euphr. **Hep.** LYC. **Nux-m.** NUX-V. PHO. Pul. RHOD. **Rhus-t.** Sep. Spo.
Comp. **Air, drafts of.**

WEEPING, **Amel.**: Pul.

WIPING PART, **Agg.**: Alo. Grap. Mur-ac.
Amel., eyes, etc.: **Calc-c.** Cina. **Cyc.** Euphr. **Nat-c.**

WOOLENS, **Agg.**: Psor. Sul.

WRITING, **Agg.**: **Calc-c.** KALI-C. **Sil.**
Comp. **Motion of Arms.**

YAWNING, **Agg.**: **Cina.** IGN. **Kre.** NUX-V. **Rhus-t. Sars.**

GENERALITIES.

ACHING, general: Anac. **Arn. Bapt.** Bry. Chin. Cimi. Eupat-p. **Gel. Ign.** Lyc. **Nux-v.** Onos. Old. Phyt. **Rhus-t.** Stan.

ADHERENT SENSATION: Rhus-t.

AIR, see **Conditions.**

ALIVE FEELING: Cann. Cocc. **Croc.** Ign. Lyc. **Pul. Sil.** Sul. Ther. **Thu.**

ALTERNATIONS: Agar. **Alo.** Chin. Gel. **Lach. Lyc.** Pul. **Stan. Sul.**
of sides: Agar. Cocc. Lac-c. Lach. Lyc. Pho. Sep. Sul.
Comp. **Changing.**

ANAEMIA: Ars. **Chin.** **Fer.** Nux-v. **Pul.** Scil. Stap. Sul.
Comp. **Chlorosis.**

ANEURISM: Carb-v. Lach. **Lyc.** Pul. **Sul.**
Comp. **Bloodvessels.**

ANXIETY, physical: Ars. Cham. Nux-v. Pho-ac. Pul.

APOPLEXY: **Aco.** Arn. **Bell.** Cocc. Gel. Lach. Lyc. Nux-v. **Op.** Pul.

ARTHRITIC (gouty or rheumatic pains, etc.): **Aco.** Ag-c. Ant-c. Arg. **Arn.** Ars. **Bell.** **Bry.** **Calc-c.** Caul. Caus. **Cham.** **Chin.** **Colch.** Colo. Dulc. Fer. Hep. Kali-bi. Kali-c. Kali-io. Led. **Lyc.** **Merc.** Mez. Nat-m. **Nux-v.** Phyt. **Pul.** Rhod. **Rhus-t.** Rut. **Sabi.** Sep. Spo. Stap. Stro. **Sul.**
small joints: Caul. Rhod.

ASLEEP FEELING: Carb-a. Cocc. Croc. Grap. Kali-c. **Lach.** **Lyc.** Merc. Nux-v. Petr. Pul. Rhus-t. Sep. Sil.
Comp. **Numb.**

AWKWARDNESS: Ap. **Caps.** Ign.

BALL, globus, etc. (ascending), as of a: **Ign.** Sep. Zin.
Comp. **Knot.**

BAND: Anac. Cact. Con. Lyc. Nit-ac. Plat. Pul. Sul.
Comp. **Contraction.**

BEATEN, bruised, lame, **sore pain, as from a blow, hard bed,** etc.: Aco. **Ap.** **Arn.** **Bry.** **Carb-v.** Caus. **Chin.** Cimi. **Cocc.** Gel. Ham. **Hep.** **Ign.** Nat-m. **Nux-v.** Pho-ac. **Rhod.** **Rhus-t.** **Rut.** **Sil.** **Sul.** Ver-a.
glands, in: Con.
internally: Bels. **Cann.** Pul.
joints: Arg. Aur. Pul. **Sul.**
pains after the: Plat.
as if flesh were beaten from bones: Bry. **Rhus-t.**

BENUMBING PAIN: Cham. Nux-v. **Old.** **Plat.** Saba. Verb.

BILIOUS PERSONS, bilious attacks, stools, vomit, etc.: **Aco.** Ars. Bell. Bry. **Cham.** Colo. Eupat-p. Ign. Ip. **Iris.** **Merc.** Nat-s. **Nux-v.** Plat. **Pod.** Pul. Sep. Stap. Ver-a.

BITING, pungent sensation, etc.: Carb-v. Euphor. Lach. Led. Nux-v. Old. **Pul.** Ran-sc. Sul. Zin.

BONES: **Asaf.** Aur. **Calc-c.** **Calc-p.** Chin. **Eupat.** Flu-ac. Kali-io. Lyc. Mang. **Merc.** Merc-c. Nit-ac. Pho. **Pho-ac.** Pul. **Rut.** **Sil.** **Sul.** Symp. Syph.
cartilage: Calc-p. Sul. Symp.
curvature, softening, etc.: Calc-c. Sil. **Sul.**
marrow: Am-c. Naj. Stro.
pains in: Chin. **Eupat.** Merc. Stro. Sul.
periosteum: Kali-bi. Kali-io. **Mez.** Pho. **Phyt.**

BORING, grinding, piercing: Asaf. Bell. Bism. Dios. **Plb.** Pul. Ran-sc. Sep. Spig.
Comp. **Burrowing.**

BROKEN, AS IF: **Bapt.** Chel.

Coccl. **Eupat.** Ign. Pho. Rut. Ver-a.

Comp. **Torn.**

BURNING: **Aco. Ars. Bell.** Bry. Merc. Nat-m. Nit-ac. Nux-v. **Pho.** Pho-ac. Pul. Rhus-t. Sang. Sep. Sil. **Sul.**

Comp. **Heat.**

external: Asaf. **Carb-v. Caus.** Lach. **Lyc.** Merc. Op. Pho-ac. Pul. **Rhus-t.** Sec-c. Sil. Spo. Stan. Stap. Thu.

Comp. **Cold, Amel.**

internal: Canth. Iris. Saba. Sep.

painful, etc.: Aco. **Ars.** Canth. Carb-v. **Caus. Merc.** Pho. Sul.

BURNS: Canth.

BURNT, as if: Ap. **Ars.** Pul.

BURROWING, digging, etc.: Dulc. Rhod. Spig.

Comp. **Boring.**

BURSTING, splitting, distending pain, etc.: **Bell. Bry.** Calc-c. **Caus.** Chin. **Glo. Ign.** Merc. Nit-ac. **Nux-v.** Ran-b. Sep. Sil. **Spig.** Sul.

CANCER: **Ars. Con.** Grap. Kre. **Nit-ac.** Pho. **Sil. Sul.** Thu.

CARPHOLOGY, **picking at imaginary objects: Ars. Hyo. Lyc. Mur-ac. Op.** Pho-ac. Rhus-t. Stram.

lips; one spot; at real things; buttons, etc.: Ars. **Aru-t.** Kali-br. **Taren.**

CARRIED, desires to be: **Cham.**

Comp. **Riding.**

CHANGING PLACE, here and there, etc.: Am-m. Ant-t. Arn. Bell. Colch. Grap. Ign. Kali-bi. Kalm. **Lac-c.** Led. Mag-p. Nux-m. Plat. **Pul.** Rhus-t. Comp. **Alternations.**

CHEWING MOTIONS: Calc-c. Hell. **Lyc.**

CHILDREN, infants, nurslings: Aco. Ant-c. Ant-t. **Bell. Calc-c.** Caps. Cham. Chin. **Cina.** Coff. Ip. Merc. Phyt. Pod. Pul. Sep. Sil. **Sul.**

CHLOROSIS: Bell. **Calc-c.** Coccl. **Fer.** Lyc. Nit-ac. Plat. **Pul.** Sep. **Sul.**

Comp. **Anaemia.**

CHRONICITY, indolent processes: Ars. Calc-c. Caus. Con. Kali-bi. Lyc. Sul.

COATED OR FURRED FEELING: Dig. Pho. Pul.

COLD, TENDENCY TO TAKE: Aco. Bry. **Calc-c.** Calc-p. Carb-v. Cham. **Dulc.** Grap. Kali-c. **Nit-ac. Nux-v.** Ol-jec. Psor. **Sep.** Sil. **Sul.** Tub.

COLLAPSE, extreme debility, sudden weakness, shock, etc.: Aco. Aeth. **Arn.** Ars. Cam. **Carb-v.** Ip. Kali-c. Pho. **Ver-a.**

COLOR, **in general,** of discharges, skin, etc.; **black: Ars.** Chin. Crot-h. Cup. Kre. **Mag-c. Merc.** Rhus-t. **Sec-c.** Stap. Sul. **Ver-a.**

blue, purple, etc.: **Aco.** Aesc. Arn. Ars. Bell. **Cam. Carb-v. Cham.** Con. **Cup. Dig. Hyo.** Kre. **Lach. Laur.** Lyc. Mur-ac.

Nux-m. **Nux-v.** **Op.** Ran-b. Sec-c. Sul-ac. **Ver-a.** Ver-v.

brown: Ant-c. **Bry.** Carb-v. **Lyc.** Merc. Nat-c. Nit-ac. **Sep.** Sil. Sul. Ver-a.

coppery: Carb-a. Merc. Mez. Nit-ac. **Rhus-t.**

dark, dusky, livid: Ail. Am-c. **Bap.** Cham. Croc. **Crot-h.** Gel. Ham. Lach. Lept. Nux-v. Op. Psor. Pul. **Rhus-t. Sec-c.**

earthy, dirty, dingy: Calc-p. Iod. Nat-m. Psor. Sul.

glistening, glowing: Aco. Ap. Arn. Bell. Bry. Lach. **Mang.** Merc. Mur-ac. Rhus-t. Sul.

gray: Amb. Arg. **Ars.** Caus. Con. Dig. **Lyc.** Merc. Pho-ac.

greenish: **Ars. Cham. Con.** Ip. Mag-c. **Merc.** Pho. Pho-ac. **Pul.** Sep. **Sil. Ver-a.**

mottled, petechial, etc.: Ail. Ars. Carb-v. Caus. **Lach.** Lyc. Pho. **Plat.** Sep. Thu.

pale, white, watery, etc.: **Ant-c. Ant-t. Ars.** Bell. **Bry. Calc-c.** Carb-v. Chin. Cina. Coccl. **Dig.** Fer. Grap. Iod. **Lyc. Merc.** Nit-ac. Pho. Plat. **Pod. Pul.** Sep. Sil. **Sul. Ver-a.**

of red parts: Bor. Hell. Merc.

red: **Aco. Am-c. Ap.** Ars. **Bell.** Bry. **Cham.** Chin. Coccl. **Fer. Grap.** Hep. Hyo. Kre. **Melil. Merc. Nux-v.** Op. **Pho.** Pul. **Rhus-t.** Saba. Sep. Sil. Stram. **Sul.**

deep: Mur-ac.

orifices: **Sul.**

yellow, (also jaundice): **Aco.** Arn. Ars. Calc-c. Cham. **Chel. Chin.** Cic. Con. Fer. **Hyds.** Ip. Kali-bi. (bright) **Lach. Lyc. Merc. Nat-m. Nux-v.** Pho. Plb. Pod. **Pul. Sep.** Stan. **Sul.**

CONSUMPTION, **tuberculosis:** Ars. **Calc-c.** Iod. Kali-c. **Lach. Lyc. Pho. Pul.** Stan. Sul.

Comp. **Scrofula.**

CONTORTIONS: Bell. Plat. Stram.

CONTRACTION, **constriction, etc., sense of:** Alu. **Bell. Cact. Chin.** Dros. Grap. **Ign.** Nux-v. Plat. **Plb.** Pul. Rhus-t. Sep. Sul. Comp. **Band.**

glands, in: Ign. Iod.

joints: Anac. Aur. Grap. Nat-m. Nit-ac.

limbs, of, spasmodic: Calc-c. Caus. Colo. Grap. Lyc. Sec-c.

Comp. **Band, Squeezing.**

CONTRACTURES, **strictures, etc.:** Cic. **Clem.** Guai. **Merc.** Nux-v. Rhus-t.

Comp. **Distortions.**

orifices: Bell.

CONVULSIVE MOTIONS: **Bell.** Cam. Cham. **Cic.** Coccl. **Cup. Hyo. Ign. Ip. Nux-v. Op.** Sec-c. **Stram.** Ver-a. Zin.

bending backward, opisthotonos: Ang. Ign.

clonic, markedly, choreiform, etc.: **Agar. Ars. Bell.** Caus. **Cham.** Cic. Cimi. **Coccl.** Con. **Cup. Hyo.** Iod. Lach. **Lyc.**

Op. **Sep.** Sil. Stan. Stram. Taren. Ver-a.

epileptic: **Bell.** **Calc-c.** Caus. Cina. **Cup.** Hyo. Ign. **Lach.** Nux-v. Op. Sil. Stram. **Sul.**

consciousness, with: Cina. Ign. **Stram.**

unconsciousness, with: Calc-c. Canth. Cic. **Hyo.** Plb.

hysterical, of females, eclamptic, etc.: Coccl. Con. Hyo. **Ign.** Mag-m. Mos. Opi. **Plat.**

internal: Caus. **Coccl.** **Hyo.** **Ign.** Ip. Mag-m. Nux-v. Pul. Stan.

tonic: Ang. **Bell.** **Cham.** Cic. **Ign.** **Ip.** Mos. **Op.** **Petr.** **Plat.** Sec-c. Sep. **Ver-a.**

CRACKING IN JOINTS: Caps. Led. Nit-ac. Petr. Pho.

CRACKLING, like tinsel: Aco. Calc-c. Rhe.

CRAMP, colic, clutching, clamping, constriction, grasping, pinching, griping; **internal; tonic,** rigidity, with, etc.: **Ang.** **Bell.** **Calc-c.** Cam. Caus. **Cham.** **Coccl.** **Colo.** **Cup.** Dios. Dulc. Grap. **Ign.** **Mag-m.** **Nux-v.** Pho-ac. **Plat.** Plb. Pul. **Sil.** Stan. **Sul.** **Ver-a.**

joints, in: Ang. Calc-c. Pho-ac. Plat. Sul.

muscles, in: Anac. Ang. Bell. **Calc-c.** Cina. Con. **Lyc.** Merc. Nux-v. Plat. Sep.

Comp. **Pressure compressive.**

CREEPING OR RUNNING, as of a little animal: Lyc. Pho. Rhod. Sec-c. Stap.

Comp. **Formication.**

CUTTING: **Bell.** Calc-c. **Canth.** Colo. Dios. Hyo. Kali-c. Lyc. Merc. Nat-c. Nat-m. Nit-ac. Nux-v. Pul. Sil. Sul. Ver-a. Zin.

DEADNESS OF PARTS (sense of): **Calc-c.** Nux-v. Sec-c. Sul.

Comp. **Numbness.**

DEATH, apparent: Aco. Ant-t. Op.

DELICATE, tender, easily ennervated: Ars. **Caus.** Croc. **Ign.** Lyc. Nat-c. Stro. Sul. Ver-a.

Comp. **Nervous Affections.**

DIAGONAL EFFECTS: Agar. Calc-c. Mang. Pho.

DIRECTION of symptoms, **backword:** Bell. Bism. Bry. Kali-c.

downward: Caps. Carb-v. Cic. Coff. Fer. Ip. Lyc. Mos. Nux-v. Rhus-t. Stap. Val. Verb.

forward: Gel. Sang. Sil. Spig.

inward: Anac. Arn. Canth. **Ign.** Plat.

outward: Arg. **Asaf.** Bell. Calc-c. Chin. Con. Spig. Spo. Stan. Sul. Val.

upward, ascending: Aco. **Bell.** Chel. Glo. **Lach.** Led. Men. Pho. Saba. **Sang.** **Sil.** Sul.

DISLOCATED, as if separated, etc.: Rhus-t. Sep. Stram. Trill. Comp. **Sprained.**

DISTORTIONS: Ag-c. Calc-c. Lyc. Nat-c. Nat-m. Petr. Pho. **Rhus-t.**

DRAWING: Alo. Arn. Bry. Carb-v. Caus. Cham. Chin. Lyc. Merc. Nux-v. Pul. **Rhus-t.** Sul.
joints, in: Stap.
muscles, in: Ant-c. Ant-t. Bell. Cham. Coccl. Cyc. **Plat.** Pul. Rhod. Val.

DROPSY, oedema, etc., **in general:** **Ap.** Ars. Bell. Bry. Canth. **Chin.** Colch. Dig. **Hell.** Rhus-t. **Sul.**
external parts: Ant-c. Grap. Kali-c. **Lyc.** Old. Op. Pul. Scil. Zin.
joints: Sul.

DRY FEELING: Aco. Alu. **Bell.** Bry. Nux-m. Pul. **Rhus-t.**
joints: Nux-v. **Pul.**

DRYNESS (of moist parts): **Bell.** **Bry.** Calad. **Calc-c.** Cann. Lyc. Nat-m. Nux-m. Pho. Seneg. Sep. Sul.

DULL PAIN: Agar. Hyo. Ign.

DUST, featherdown, etc., as of: Am-c. Ars. Bell. **Calc-c.** Chel. Dros. Ign. Ip. Ver-a.

EBULLITIONS, surgings: **Aco.** Aur. **Calc-c.** Fer. Kre. **Lach.** **Lyc.** Sul.

ELONGATED, as if: Alu. Hyp. Pho.

EMACIATION, atrophy: **Ars.** **Chin.** Grap. **Iod.** Lach. **Lyc.** **Nat-m.** Nit-ac. Nux-v. **Pho-ac.** Stap. **Sul.**
affected parts, partial, etc.: Calc-c. Plb. Pul. Sul.
glandular: Con. Iod.
infantile, marasmus: Abro. Calc-c. Sul.
senile: Bar-c. Chin. Op.

EMPTY, hollow, sinking, etc.: Coccl. **Ign.** Lyc. **Pho.** Pod. Pul. **Sep.** Stan. Sul.
Comp. **Stomach.**

ENLARGED, swelled, as if: Arg-n. Par. **Pul.** Rhus-t. Spig.
internal: Bell. **Ign.** Old.

FAINTING: **Aco.** **Carb-v.** Caus. **Cham.** Chin. **Coff.** **Dig.** **Hep.** **Ign.** Lach. Mos. Nat-m. **Nux-v.** **Op.** Petr. **Sep.** **Stram.**

FALLING OUT FEELING: Bell. **Sep.**

FALLING DOWN: Con. Laur.
Comp. **Collapse.**
unconscious: Calc-c.

FIBROUS TISSUE: **Colch.** **Flu-ac.** **Guai.** Rhod. **Rhus-t.** Rut.

FISTULAE: **Calc-c.** Caus. Lyc. Pul. **Sil.** Sul.

FLOATING, levitation, flying, as if, etc.: Bell. Calc-c. **Cann.** Croc. **Lac-c.** **Sul.**

FLOWING, or dashed with water, as if: Aco. Arn. Ars. Chin. Glo. Merc. **Rhus-t.** Sep. Thu. Ver-a. Comp. **Wavelike.**

FORCING THROUGH, forward, etc., narrow as if: Bell. Pul. Comp. **Urging.**

FRACTURES: Calc-p. Sul. **Symp.**

FULNESS, internal: Aco. Alo. Bry. Chin. Glo. Kali-c. Lyc. Pho. Rhus-t. Sul.

GANGLION, bursae: Pho. Rut.

GATHERED TOGETHER SENSATION: Aco. **Arn.** Chin. Par. **Pul.** Zin.

GLANDULAR AFFECTIONS: Bar-c. **Bell.** **Calc-c.** **Calc-p.** Carb-a. Clem. **Con.** Dulc. Hep. **Iod.** **Lyc.** **Merc.** Merc-i-f. **Pho.** Rhus-t. **Sil.** **Sul.** Tub.

GNAWING, eating: **Ag-c.** Ars. Caus. Dros. Lyc. Mez. **Old.** Plat. **Ran-sc.** **Rut.** Spo. **Stap.** Sul.

Comp. **Ulcerative Pain.**

GONORRHŒA: **Cann.** Merc. Sep. Sul.

GREASY, oily, etc.: Chin. **Merc.** Thu.

GRIPPE: **Eupat-p.** **Gel.** Merc. Nux-v. Phyt. **Rhus-t.**

GURGLING: Alo. Berb. Crot-t. Gamb. Rhe. Scil. Sul.

HAIR, thread, etc., as of a: Kali-bi. **Sil.** Sul.

HANGING LOOSE, as of a skin, film, etc: Bar-c. Mang. Pho.

HARDNESS, induration: Aco. **Ant-c.** Ars. Asaf. Aur. **Bell.** **Bry.** Calc-c. Calc-fl. **Carb-a.** Carb-v. Chin. **Clem.** **Con.** **Grap.** Iod. **Lach.** Lyc. Mag-m. Merc. Pho. Phy. **Pul.** Rhod. **Rhus-t.** **Sep.** **Sil.** **Sul.** Taren-c.

glandular; nodes in: Bell. Carb-an. Clem. Con. Grap. Iod. Phy. Plb. Sil.

HEAVINESS (as of a load, etc.); Aco. **Alo.** Bell. Bism. Calc-c. Carb-v. Chin. Gel. Lyc. Merc. Nat-m. **Nux-v.** Pho. Pic-ac. **Pul.** **Rhus-t.** Saba. Sep. Sil. Spig. Stan. Stap. Sul. Vip.

Comp. **Knot.**

HEMORRHAGE and all bloody discharges: **Aco.** **Arn.** Ars. **Bell.** Calc-c. Canth. Carb-v. Cham. **Chin.** Coc-c. Croc. Crot-h. **Fer.** Ham. Ip. **Lach.** Led. Lyc. Merc. **Nit-ac.** Nux-v. **Pho.** **Pul.** Rhus-t. Sabi. Sec-c. Sep. Sil. **Sul.** Tereb. Trill.

altered blood of: Crot-h. Pul. Sec-c.

bright: **Aco.** **Bell.** **Dulc.** Fer. **Hyo.** Led. Mill. **Sabi.**

clotted, lumpy: **Cham.** Ip. Plat. **Rhus-t.**

passive: Chin. Crot-h. Ham.

streaked: Ars. Asaf. Bry. Chin. **Fer.** Hep. **Merc.** **Pho.** **Sul.** Zin.

HOLD THE PART, impulse to: Bry. Dros. Eup-p. Lil-t. Nat-s.

HOLDING HIMSELF UP or supporting himself, difficulty in: Cocl. Ver-a.

HUMMING, buzzing, whizzing, purring: Caus. Nux-m. **Old.** Pul. **Spig.** Sul.

Comp. **Vibration.**

HYDROPHOBIA: Bell. Canth. Hyo. Stram.

ILL OR SICK FEELING: Aco. Ars. Nux-v. **Pod.** Pul.

INCREASING AND DECREASING SLOWLY, **sun pains,** etc.: **Cact.** Kali-bi. **Nat-m.** Plat. Sang. Spig. **Stan.** Stro.

slowly but decreasing suddenly: Arg-n.

suddenly and leaving quickly, lightning like pains: Arg-n. **Bell.** Mag-p.

INFLAMMATION: **Aco.** Ap. Ars. **Bell. Bry.** Calc-c. Cann. Canth. Cham. **Gel.** Hep. Hyo. Iod. Kali-c. **Merc. Nux-v. Pho.** Pul. **Rhus-t.** Sep. **Sil. Stap.** Sul. **Ver-v.**

lymphatics, streaks: **Bell.** Buf. Merc. Pho. Sil.

INTERNAL AFFECTIONS: Calc-c. Canth. Nux-v. Pho.

IRREGULAR, incoordinate effects: **Agar. Ign.** Nux-v.

IRRITABILITY, SENSIBILITY, **decreased;** insensibility, absence of pain, etc.: **Carb-v.** Cocel. Con. Hyo. **Laur.** Lyc. Old. **Op. Pho-ac.** Plat. **Stram. Sul.**

increased, acute senses, sensitive to pain: Aco. Amb. Arn. Ars. **Asaf.** Aur. **Bell.** Canth. **Cham. Chin.** Cocel. **Coff.** Cup. **Hep. Ign. Lach.** Lyc. Merc. **Nux-v. Pho.** Pul. Sep. Sil. Spo. **Stap.** Zin.

glands, of: Con. Pho.

ITCHING, TICKLING, **glands: Con.** Sil.

internal: Amb. Coc-c. **Iod.** Nux-v. Pho. **Rum.**

JERKING PAIN, **external: Asaf.** Bell. Calc-c. **Caus.** Men. Nat-m. **Nux-v. Pul.** Rhus-t. Tarax.

internal: Chin. Ign. Kali-c. Pul. Sil.

JERKS, **internal:** Calc-c. Plat. Pul. Spig. Stan.

muscles: Cic. Colch. Sep. Sul. Sul-ac.

KNOT, lump, etc., sense of a: Amb. Arn. **Nux-v.** Pul. Spig. Sul.

Comp. **Ball, Heaviness.**

LABORLIKE PAINS: Aco. Bell. Cham. Fer. Nux-v. **Pul.** Sabi. Sec-c. Sep.

LETHARGY, lassitude: Chin. Gel. **Op.** Pho-ac.

LIE DOWN, inclination to: Aco. Alu. **Ars.** Calad. Cham. **Gel.** Lyc. **Nux-v.** Pic-ac. Stram.

LIGAMENTS: Guai. **Rhus-t.**

LIGHTNING LIKE PAINS, see **Increasing and Decreasing.**

LIMPING: Colo. Rhus-t.

LUMP, see **Knot.**

MEDICINE, oversensitive to: Nux-v. Pul.

Comp. **Reaction.**

MEMBRANES, **mucous:** Aco. Ant-t. Ap. **Arg-n. Ars. Bell.** Bor. **Bry.** Caps. Cep. **Cham. Dulc.** Euphr. Hep. Hydr. Ip. Kali-bi. Kali-c. **Merc. Nux-v.** Pho. **Pul.** Seneg. **Stan. Sul.**

Comp. **Secretions, mucous.**

serous: Ap. **Bry.** Canth. Hell. Kali-c. Sul.

sulci of: Kali-bi.

MOTION, **absent,** immobility (of affected part): Cocel. Hell. Rhus-t.

agile: Coff. Stram.

averse to: Aco. **Bry.** Calad. Caps. Guai. **Nux-v.**
difficult: Bell. **Bry.** Caus. Lyc. Petr. Rhus-t. Sep.
sense of, see **Floating.**
stepping backward: Stram.
high: Agar.

MUSCLES: **Agar.** Arn. Ars. **Bry.** Cimi. Colch. Cup. Gel. Hell. Kali-c. Mur-ac. Onos. Plb. Pul.
lax, flabby, limpness: **Aeth.** Ant-t. Calc-c. Caps. Carb-ac. **Chin.** Coccl. **Gel. Lyc.** Mur-ac. Pho-ac. Stram. Sul.
short: Am-m. Caus. Colo. Grap. Nat-m.
tense, tense tissues: Aco. Lach. Nit-ac. **Nux-v.** Pho. **Sep.**
tendons: Rhus-t.

NEEDLES see **Sticking.**

NERVOUS EFFECTS: **Aco.** Amb. Arn. Asaf. **Bell.** Bry. Calc-c. **Cham. Chin. Coff.** Con. Cup. Fer. **Ign.** Mag-p. Merc. **Nux-v. Pho. Pul. Sep. Sil. Val.**
Comp. **Excitement, Emotions.**

NET LIKE **capillaries:** Thu.

NEURALGIA: **Aco.** Arn. Ars. Bry. Cham. Coff. Ign. Merc. **Nux-v.** Spig. Ver-a.

NODES (calculous deposits), etc.: **Calc-c.** Caul. Caus. Dulc. Lach. **Lyc.** Mez. **Pul.** Rhod. Rhus-t. Sars. Sil. Stap. Sul.
Comp. **Urinary Deposits.**

NUMB FEELING (also painless complaints, etc.): **Aco.** Bry. Cham. Chin. Cimi. Con. Gnap. Kalm. Nux-v. **Old. Op. Pho. Pho-ac. Plat.** Plb. **Pul.** Rhus-t. Sul.
Comp. **Asleep.**

OFFENSIVENESS see **Secretions.**

OLD PEOPLE: Amb. **Aur. Bar-c.** Carb-a. Con. Lyc. Op. Sec-c. **Sul.**

OPPRESSIVE PAIN: Mos.

ORIFICES: Grap. **Nit-ac. Sul.**

PARALYSIS, **internal:** Ant-t. **Bell.** Dulc. Hyo.
limbs: Caus. Coccl. Nux-v. **Rhus-t.** Rut. Sec-c. **Sil.**
organs (single): Ant-t. Bar-c. Bell. **Caus.** Dulc. Gel. Hyo. Nux-v. Op. Pho. Pul. Sec-c. Sil. **Sul.**
painless: Coccl. Con. Lyc. Old. **Rhus-t.**
paraplegia: Ars. Nat-m. **Nux-v.** Rut. Sul.
sense of, internal organs: Lyc.
spasms, after: Cup. Sec-c.
unilateral: Caus. **Coccl. Lach.**

PARALYTIC OR LAMING PAIN, lameness, etc.: Bell. Carb-v. Cham. **Chin.** Coccl. Cyc. **Nux-v. Rhus-t.** Sabi. **Stap.**
joints, in: Aur. Caps. Euphor. Pul. Stap. Val.

PECKING, **hacking:** Chin.

PINCHING, **external:** Men. Rhod. Saba. Stan.
internal: Calc-c. Chel. Coccl. Ign. Lyc.

PLETHORA, obesity, etc.: **Aco. Bell. Calc-c. Caps.** Fer. Hyo. **Merc. Nux-v.** Pho. Pul. **Sul.**

PLUG, nail (clavus), as of a: **Anac.** Hep. **Ign.** Nux-v. Plat. Ran-s. Sul-ac. Val.

POISONED FEELING: Lach. Naj. **Vip.**

PRESSURE, **compressive,** crushing together, etc.: Alu. Asar. Cocel. Lyc. Plat.

Comp. **Squeezing.**

external parts, in: Caus. Old. Stan. Stap.

internal parts, in: Arn. Ars. Bell. Calc-c. Carb-v. **Chin.** Glo. Zin.

muscles, in: Cyc. Nux-m. Rut. Verb.

PRICKLING, **external:** Plat. Ran-sc.

PULSATION: Aco. Alu. Ant-t. Arn. Ars. **Bell.** Calc-c. Fer. Glo. Grap. Kali-c. Lach. **Mell.** Merc. **Old. Pul. Saba.** Sep. **Sil. Sul.**

bloodvessels, in: Bell. Glo.

QUIVERING, **external: Asaf. Kali-c.** Mez. Nat-c.

Comp. **Vibration.**

REACTION, poor: Am-c. **Carb-v. Op.** Sul. Tub.

REELING, tottering, staggering, etc.: Bell. Bry. Gel. Ign. Lach. Nux-v. Op. Rhus-t. Stram. Sul. Ver-a.

REMITTENT SYMPTOMS: **Gel.**

RENDING see **Torn to Pieces.**

RESTLESSNESS, uneasiness, etc., **physical, in limbs: Aco.** Anac. **Ars.** Bar-c. **Bell.** Bov. Bry. Calc-c. Chin. Cimi. Fer. **Hyo. Lyc.** Mag-c. **Merc.** Mur-ac. Nux-v. Pul. **Rhus-t.** Rut. **Sep.** Sil. **Stap. Stram.** Sul. Taren. Zin.

Comp. **Motion, desire for.**

RETRACTION, drawing backward or inward (of soft parts): Ang. Cup. Merc. **Plb.**

RICKETS: **Calc-c. Calc-p.** Pho. Sil.

ROLLING OR TURNING OVER, loose, etc., as if: Cact. Chin. Grap. **Lach.** Nux-v. Rhus-t. Sep. Sul.

Comp. **Position; Turning over.**

ROUGH, scratchy, raw feeling, **as of a rough body,** etc. **internal:** Aesc. **Alu.** Amb. Carb-v. **Nux-v.** Pho. Phyt. Sul.

Comp. **Smarting.**

RUNNING, like a mouse: Bell. **Calc-c.** Sul.

SCORBUTIC SYMPTOMS: Am-c. Carb-v. **Merc.** Mur-ac. **Nux-v.** Stap. Sul.

SCROFULA: Bar-c. **Calc-c. Calc-p.** Hep. Iod. Merc. **Sil.** Sul.

SECRETIONS, discharges, expectoration, etc., **bland:** Euphr. **Pul.**

bloody, streaked see **Hemorrhage.**

briny odor: Bell. Grap. Ol-an. Sele. Tell.

burning: Ars. Calc-c. Kre. Pul. Sul.

corrosive, acrid, biting: Alu. **Ars.** Aru-t. Carb-v. **Caus.** Fer. Flu-ac. Iris. Kali-c. Kali-io. Kre. Merc. **Nit-ac.** Pho. **Rhus-t.** Sep. **Sil. Sul.**

curdy: Bor. **Helo.** Merc.
foamy, frothy: Aco. **Arn. Ars.** Fer. Ip. **Mag-c.** Pho. Pul. Sul.
gelatinous: Alo. Arg. Colch. Colo. Hell. Kali-bi. **Rhus-t.** Sil.
glairy, albuminous, etc.: Am-m. Bor. **Coc-c.** Kali-m. Merc. Pul. Stan.
hardened, lumpy: **Kali-bi.** Psor.
hot: Bell. Pul. Sabi.
itching, causing: Calc-c. Led. Mang. Med. Par. Rhod. **Rhus-t.** Sul.
milky: Calc-c. **Pul.**
mucus, increased, catarrhal: **Ant-t. Calc-c.** Chin. Dulc. Euphr. Grap. Iris. **Kali-bi.** Merc. Nux-v. **Pho. Pul.** Stan. **Sul.** Thu.
Comp. **Mucous Membranes.**
musty, mouldy: Crot-h. Pho. **Rhus-t.** Stan.
offensive, bad smelling and putridity in general: Arn. **Ars. Bapt.** Bell. Bry. Calc-c. **Carb-v.** Cham. Chin. **Grap.** Guai. **Hep.** Kre. **Lach.** Lyc. Merc. Mur-ac. **Nat-c.** Nit-ac. Pho-ac. Pod. **Psor.** Pyro. **Rhus-t.** Sabi. Sang. **Sep. Sil.** Stan. **Stap.** Stram. **Sul.** Tell. Thu.
profuse: Am-m. Ars-iod. Calc-c. **Crot-t. Hep.** Plat. **Pod. Pul.** Rhus-t. Scil. Sep. Sul.
salty: Lyc. Pul.
Comp. **Briny.**
sanious: Sil.
scanty see **Discharges.**
slimy: Bor. Calc-c. Chin. **Kali-bi.** Lyc. Mag-c. Nat-m. Par. Phos. **Pul.**
sour: Ars. Asar. **Calc-c.** Cham. **Hep.** Iris. **Lyc.** Nit-ac. **Nux-v.** Pho. **Pul.** Rhe. Sep. Sil. **Sul.** Ver-a.
sticky, clammy, stringy, tenacious, tough, viscid: Bov. **Bry.** Calc-c. Caus. Cham. **Croc.** Cup. **Grap.** Hyds. **Kali-bi. Lach.** Lyc. Mag-c. Mang. Merc. **Pho.** Pho-ac. Stan. Sul-ac. **Ver-a.**
tarry: Lept. Mag-c. Nux-m. Plat.
thick: Croc. Hyds. **Kali-bi.** Pho. Pul. Stan. Sul.
urinous odor: Canth. **Colo.** Nit-ac. Urt-u.
watery, thin: Ars. **Asaf. Caus.** Cham. Crot-t. Cup. Gamb. **Grap.** Grat. Iris. **Merc.** Nat-s. Pho. **Pod.** Rhus-t. Sabi. Sec-c. Sil. **Sul.** Ver-a.

SENSITIVE **senses** see **Irritable.**

SENSORY ILLUSIONS: Rhus-t.

SHAKING, shocks, jerks, shuddering, shivering, shrugging: Anac. Ant-c. Ant-t. **Bell.** Brom. Bry. Cam. Cann. Chel. Chin. Cina. Coccl. Colch. Croc. Hell. **Ign.** Iod. Kre. Mar. **Nux-v.** Par. **Plat.** Rut. Spo. Stap. Stro. **Ver-a.**

SICKNESS, subject to attacks of; Calc-c. Con. Cup. Sil.

SIDE, **onesided effects**: Alu. Anac. Asaf. Bell. Bry. **Calc-c.** Cham. **Coccl. Colo.** Dig. **Grap.**

Kali-c. Lyc. Mos. **Nux-v.** Par. Pho-ac. Plat. **Pul.** **Rhus-t.** Sars. **Spig.** Sul-ac. Thu. Verb.

left: Arg-n. Asaf. Asar. Caps. Carb-v. Chin. Cimi. Cina. Clem. Croc. Euphor. Grap. **Lach.** Lil-t. Mez. Nit-ac. Old. **Pho.** **Rhus-t.** Scil. Sele. **Spig.** Stan. Sul. Thu.

upper and right lower: Anac. Arn. Carb-a. Flu-ac. Kali-c. Pul. Rhus-t. Scil. Stan. **Tarax.** Ver-a. Verb. Viol-o.

then right: **Lach.** Merc-i-r.

right: Agar. Alu. **Ap.** Arg. Aur. **Bell.** Bry. Calc-c. Canth. **Chel.** Colo. Con. **Gel.** Iris. **Lyc.** Nux-v. Pul. Ran-sc. Rhus-t. Sang. Sars. Sec-c. Stro. Sul-ac. Zin.

upper and left lower: **Amb.** Bor. Bov. Calc-c. Caus. Fer. Lyc. Merc-i-f. Nat-c. **Pho.** Plb. Sil. **Sul-ac.**

then left: **Lyc.** Merc-i-fl.

Comp. **Changing.** P. 15

SINKING, as if: Dulc. Lyc. Nat-m. Pho.

Comp. **Stomach.**

SIT, **inclines to**: Chin. Con. Grap. Nux-v. Pho. Scil.

SLIDES DOWN IN BED: Mur-ac.

SORENESS, smarting, as if raw, etc.: Ap. Aru-t. Grap. Ham. **Hep.** **Ign.** Kre. Lyc. Merc. Nit-ac. **Nux-v.** Pho. **Pul.** Rut. **Sep.** Sul. **Zin.**

Comp. **Beaten; Skin, excoriated. Bruised. Rough.**

SPOTS, sensations in, pain, as of drops of water, sparks, etc.: Alu. Arn. **Ars.** Bar-c. Caus. Clem. **Colch.** Con. Flu-ac. **Ign.** Kali-bi. **Ox-ac.** Petr. Pho. Plb. Sele. **Sep.** Sil. **Sul.** Sul-ac. Zin.

SPRAINED, TWISTING AND DISLOCATIVE PAIN, **external, and sprains, etc.**: Am-m. **Arn.** **Bry.** Calc-c. Carb-a. Ign. Lyc. **Nat-c.** Nat-m. Petr. Pho. Pul. **Rhus-t.** Rut. Sil. Sul.

Comp. **Lifting, Agg.**

SQUEEZING PAIN: Amb. Ang. Carb-v. **Colo.** Ign. Plat.

Comp. **Pressure.**

STARTS, jerks (of limbs): Aco. Agar. Ars. **Bell.** Bor. Bry. Kali-c. Lyc. **Nux-v.** **Stro.** **Sul.** Zin.

Comp. **Nervousness Twitching.**

STIFFNESS (joints): Caps. **Caus.** **Colo.** **Petr.** Pul. **Rhus-t.** **Sep.** **Sul.**

STIFFENING OUT OF BODY: Ang. Cam. **Cina.** Cup. **Ign.** **Ip.** Stram.

STITCHES, sticking, stinging, etc. **Aco.** **Ap.** **Arg-n.** Arn. Ars. **Asaf.** **Bell.** **Bry.** Calc-c. Canth. Carb-v. Chin. Fer. **Kali-c.** **Nit-ac.** **Pul.** Rhus-t. **Sep.** Sil. **Spig.** Spo. Stan. Sul. Val.

burning, in muscles: **Ap.** Asaf. Cocc. Mez. Nux-v. Rhus-t. Stap. Sul-ac. Thu.

crawling: Arn.

external: **Ap.** Bar-c. Bell. Caus. Clem. Cycl. Grap. **Merc.** Spo. Stap. Sul. Tarax. Thu. Viol-o.
glands, in: Ign. Merc. Pul.
internal: Arg-n. Chel. Ign. Pho. Verb.
jerky: Cina. Nux-v.
joints, in: **Ap.** Colch. **Hell. Kali-c.** Mang. **Merc. Rhus-t. Sil.** Tarax. **Thu.**
muscles: **Bry.** Merc. Rhus-t. Stap. Sul. Tarax. Thu.
needles, splinters, as from: Agar. (cold). Arg-n. Ars. (hot) **Hep.** Kali-c. **Nit-ac.** Pho. Sil.
pressive, in muscles: Sars.
tearing, joints, in: Stap.
muscles, in: Anac. Calc-c. Guai. Mang. Pul. Thu.
tensive: Spig.
STRANGLING, stifling pain: Sul.
Comp. **Oppressive Pain.**
STRETCHES, twists and turns: Alu. **Bell. Calc-c.** Chel. Cina. Ign. Nux-v. **Rhus-t.** Sul.
SUPPURATION, in **general,** abscess, boils, etc.: **Ant-t.** Arg-n. **Arn.** Ars. Asaf. **Bell. Calc-c.** Canth. Caus. Chin. Clem. Con. **Hep.** Kali-c. Kali-s. **Lach.** Lyc. **Merc.** Nit-ac. Pho. **Pul. Rhus-t. Sep. Sil. Sul.**
bones: Pul. Sil.
glands, of: Bell. Dulc. Hep. Lyc. Merc. Nit-ac. Sil. Sul.
SWELLING: Aco. Ap. **Bell.** Calc-c. **Merc.** Pul. **Rhus-t.** Sul.
puffy: Ant-c. Ap. Calc-c. Caps. Cup. Fer.
SYCOSIS: **Med. Nat-s.** Sabi. **Thu.**
TEARING, **shooting, drawing**: Bell. Bry. Caps. **Carb-v. Caus.** Kali-c. Lyc. **Rhod. Rhus-t.** Sil. Sul. Zin.
joints, in: Old.
muscles, in: Anac. Calc-c. Nat-c. **Plat.**
external: Aco. **Arn.** Cham. **Chin.**
glands, in: Chin.
internal: Bell. Cham. Con. **Merc.** Nux-v. **Pul.**
joints, in: **Arn. Chin. Fer.** Guai. **Hell. Hep. Merc. Pul. Rhus-t.** Stro.
muscles, in: Arn. Ars. **Calc-c.** Carb-v. Colch. **Lyc.** Merc. **Nit-ac.** Nux-v. Rhus-t. Sep. **Sil.** Stap. Stro.
paralytic, joints, in: Carb-v. **Stap.**
muscles, in: Chin. **Kali-c.**
pressive, joints, in: Carb-v.
muscles, in: Carb-v. Stan.
stitching, prickling, joints in: Led.
muscles, in: Colch. Merc. **Zin.**
twitching, jerking, **joints**: Chin.
muscles: Chin. **Pul.**
TEMPERATURE, **high,** hyperpyrexia: Bapt. Chin-ars. Iod. Pho.
low see **Collapse.**
TENSION, stretched feeling: Am-m. **Bry.** Caus.
external: Bar-c. **Caus. Colo.** Con. Pho. Plat. Pul. Rhus-t. Stro. Sul.
glands, in: Pho.

internal: Aco. Asaf. Bell. Lyc. **Nux-v.** Pul. Stro.
joints, in: **Bry. Caus.** Lyc. Nat-m. Pul. Seneg. Sep. **Sul.**

THROBBING, hard beating, pulsation, etc.: **Aco.** Am-m. Amy-n. Anac. Ant-t. Arn. Ars. **Bell. Bry. Calc-c.** Coccl. **Glo.** Hep. Ign. Iod. Kali-c. Kre. Merc. Pho. **Pul.** Saba. **Sep.** Stro. Sul. Thu.

external: Am-m. **Kali-c.** Saba. Sul.
glands, in: Con. Merc.
internal: **Aco.** Coccl. Pho.
painful: Aco. Am-m. **Bell. Fer. Ign.** Sep.
universal, general: **Carb-v. Pho.** Pul. **Sil.**

THRUSTS, stings, etc.: Ap. Arn. Cina. Plat. Rut. Sul-ac.

TINGLING, **formication,** crawling and tickling, **external: Aco. Arn.** Colch. Croc. Nux-v. **Plat.** Pul. Rhus-t. Saba. **Sec-c.** Sep. Sil. Spig. Sul.
internal: Colch. **Ign. Plat.** Rhus-t.

TORN, **loose, as if: Rhus-t.**
to pieces, shattered, rent: Coff. **Nux-v. Rhus-t.**

Comp. **Broken.**

out feeling: Calc-c.

TORPID: Asaf. Dros. Led.

TREMOR, **external: Agar. Ars.** Bell. **Cic.** Con. Gel. **Hyo. Ign.** Merc. Nat-m. **Op.** Plat. **Pul.** Rhus-t. **Sep. Stram. Sul.** Zin.
internal, sense of: Calc-c. Iod. Nux-v. Pho. **Rhus-t.** Spig. Stap. Sul-ac.

Comp. **Quivering.**

TRICKLING, as if: Cann.
TUBULAR TRACTS: Sil.
TUGGING, pulling, etc.: Pul.
TWINGES, nips, etc.: Am-m. Laur. Mos. Plb.
TWISTING, turning, as if, etc.: Sil.

TWITCHING: Agar. Amb. **Bell.** Caus. Hyo. Ign. Iod. Mez. Nat-m. Plb. Pul. Rhus-t. Sep. Sil. Zin.

Comp. **Muscles, Starts and Convulsive Motions.**

TYPHOID STATES: Ars. **Bapt. Bry.** Hyo. Lach. Mur-ac. Pho. Pho-ac. **Rhus-t.**

ULCERATION, erosion, necrosis, phagedena, etc.: Arg-n. **Ars. Asaf.** Bell. Calc-c. Carb-v. **Cham.** Grap. **Hep. Lach. Lyc. Merc.** Merc-c. Nat-c. Nit-ac. Petr. **Pho.** Pho-ac. **Pul.** Rhus-t. Sep. **Sil.** Stap. **Sul.**
areola, edge, etc.: Ars. Asaf. Hep. Lach. Lyc. Merc. **Pul. Sil.**
elevated: Ars. Merc. Sil.
deep, perforating, etc.: Calc-c. **Kali-bi.** Kali-c. Pul. Sil.
gangrenous: Lach.
ragged: Bor. Merc. Pho-ac.
shallow, flat: **Ars. Lach.** Lyc. Merc. Nit-ac.

ULCERATIVE, SORE PAIN, **in general:** Am-c. Am-m. Bry.

Grap. Ign. Kre. **Lach. Pho.** **Pul. Rhus-t. Sil.** Sul.

glands, in: Pho.

Comp. **Gnawing.**

URGING: Arn. Bell. Nux-v.

Comp. **Forcing Through.**

VAPOR **rising,** feeling of: **Ap.** Naj. **Pul.** Saba. **Ver-a. Zin.**

of sulfur, as of: Ars. Brom. Carb-v. **Chin.** Lyc.

VIBRATION, fluttering, etc., sense of: Bell. **Sep. Sul.**

Comp. **Humming, Quivering.**

VIGOR, strength, well being, etc. **sense of:** Op. Pho. **Psor.**

VIOLENT EFFECTS: Aco. Ars. Bell. Cham. Cup. Glo. Ign. Lach. Nux-v. Ver-a.

WALK, **impulse to:** Aco. Ars. Fer. Flu-ac. Lyc. Mag-c.

See **Motion, Amel.**

learns to, tardily: Calc-c. Sil. Sul.

WARMTH, sense of: Cann. Coff. Sul-ac.

WASHING, averse to: Am-c. Ant-c. Clem. Rhus-t. Sep. Spig. **Sul.**

WAVELIKE SENSATIONS, fluctuation, heats, flushes, overrunning chills, orgasms, rushes of blood, etc. in: **Amy-n.** Asar. Aur. Bar-c. Bry. Calc-c. Carb-v. Colch. Fer. **Glo.** Kali-bi. **Kali-c. Lach.** Lyc. Nat-m. Pho. **Pul.** Rut. Samb. **Sep.** Sil. Spig. **Sul.**

Comp. **Motion, Flowing, etc.**

WEAK, feeble, etc.: Arn. **Ars.** Bapt. Bar-m. Bry. Calc-c. **Carb-v. Chin.** Cup. Fer. Grap. **Gel.** Hep. Ign. Iod. **Ip.** Kali-bi. Kali-c. **Lyc.** Nat-c. Nat-m. Nit-ac. **Nux-v. Pho. Pho-ac. Rhus-t.** Sele. **Sep.** Sil. Stan. Stap. Sul. **Ver-a.**

in a. m.: Carb-v. Lach. Lyc. Sep. Stap.

joints: Aco. Arn. Calc-c. Kali-c. Lyc. Merc. Rhus-t. Sep. Sul.

muscles: Bapt. Bar-c. **Gel.** Nat-m. Nit-ac.

sickness, after; debility, etc.: **Chin.** Psor. Ver-a.

suddenly see **Collapse.**

WEARINESS: Cann. Croc. Pul.

WIND, draft, etc. sense of a: Cam. Chel. Corall. Laur. Mez. Pho-ac. Rhus-t.

MIND.

ACO. Alum. **Anac.** ANT-C. **Arg-n.** ARS. AUR. BELL. **Calc-c. Cann. Caus. Cham. Cimi. Coca. Coccl. Con.** Croc. **Grap. Hyo.** IGN. **Lach.** Lil-t. LYC. Med. **Merc.** NAT-C. **Nat-m.** Nux-m. **Nux-v. Op.** PHO. PLAT. PUL. **Sep. Sil. Stram. Sul.** Thu. Val. VER-A.

INTELLECT.

ACO. Anac. Aur. Bapt. BAR-C. BELL. **Cann. Coccl.** HELL. HYO. **Ign.** LACH. **Laur.** LYC. **Merc. Nat-c. Nux-v.** OP. PHO. PHO-AC. **Plat. Pul. Rhus-t.** SEP. STRAM. **Sul.** VER-A.

ABSENCE OF, abstraction, etc.: Aco. **Ap. Asar.** CAUS. CHAM.

Laur. Old. Plat. PUL. SEP. Sul.

ABUSIVE, scolding, quarrelsome: **Aur.** CHAM. Hyo. **Ign.** LYC. NUX-V. Ran-b.

ACTIVE, acute: COFF. OP.

ALTERNATIONS, great mobility, etc.: AUR. Croc. IGN. PLAT. STRAM. **Val. Ver-a.** Zin.

mental with physical: **Ign.** Lil-t. **Plat.**

nervous with physical: Saba.

AMATIVE, erotic, amorous, kissing, shameless, etc.: Ag-c. **Canth.** HYO. **Lach.** Lyc. **Pho. Plat. Ver-a.**

ANGER, irritability, bad humor, crossness, vexation, etc.: **Aco. Anac.** ANT-C. Ant-t. Ap. **Ars.** Asar. **Aur. Bell.** BRY. Calc-c. Carb-v. Caus. CHAM. **Cina.** Coccl. Coff. **Colo.** Con. Cup. **Hep. Ign. Kali-c.** Kali-io. Lil-t. LYC. **Nat-m.** Nit-ac. NUX-V. Op. Petr. **Pho. Plat. Sep.** Sil. **Stap. Sul.** Thu. Tub. Val. **Ver-a.** Ver-v. Zin.

fretful, peevish, petulant, touchy: ANT-C. Ars. **Aru-t.** Bell. CALC-C. Calc-p. Carb-v. CHAM. CINA. Kali-c. **Kre.** LYC. **Rhe. Stap.** SUL.

ANGUISH, agony: ACO. ARS. **Caus. Pul.** Ver-a.

ANIMATION, vivacity, cheerfulness, exaltation: Aur. Bell. CANN. COFF. **Croc.** Hyo. Nat-c. **Op. Plat.** Spo. **Stram.**

ANSWERS, **slow:** **Pho-ac.** Thu. Zin.

ANTHROPOPHOBIA, bashful, shy, cowardly, etc.: Amb. Anac. BAR-C. **Hyo. Lyc.** Nat-m. **Pul.** Sil.

Comp. **Alone.**

AVARICE, greed: Pul.

AVERSION **to his own family:** Crot-h. Flu-ac. Lyc. Pho. **Sep.**

BAD PART, **takes everything in:** **Nux-v.** Pul.

BESIDE HIMSELF, frantic, madness from pain, etc.: ACO. Ars. CHAM. **Coff.** Lyc. Nux-v.

Comp. **Sensations.**

BEWILDERED, dazed, things look strange, loss of sense of location, etc.: Bry. Coccl. Fluac. **Glo.** Hell. Nux-m. Petr. **Plat.** Sil. Stram. Tub.

Comp. **Confusion.**

BITE, impulse to: **Bell.** Phyt. Pod.

BOLDNESS, daring: **Ign. Op.**

CAUTION: **Ign.** Nux-v. PUL. Ver-a.

CHANGING MOODS, erratic, fitful, moody, capricious, variable: ALU. Amb. Croc. FER. Grap. IGN. LACH. PLAT. PUL. **Stram.** SUL-AC. Taren. **Val.** ZIN.

ideas, cannot hold one thought; dementia, etc.: Anac. Lach. Pho-ac.

CLAIRVOYANCE: **Aco.** Nux-m. Pho.

COMPLAINING, lamenting: Coff. **Ver-a.**

CONFUSION, incoherence, muddled, etc.: BELL. **Bry.** CALC-C. Caps. **Gel.** HYO. Lyc. **Nux-v.** PHO. PHO-AC. RHUS-T. Sep. **Stram. Ver-a.**
Comp. **Bewildered.**

CONTRADICTION or opposition, intolerant of: **Asar.** Fer. **Ign. Lyc.** Nux-v. **Sep.**

CRITICAL, **fault finding, exacting, overconscientious:** **Ars.** Lyc. Sil. Sul.

CRUELTY: Kali-io.

DECEIT, duplicity, lying, etc.: Buf. **Op.** Plb. Taren. Ver-a.

DELIRIUM: **Aco.** BELL. **Cup. Dulc.** HYO. Op. STRAM. VER-A.
- **anxious:** Aco. Op. **Stram.**
- **foolish:** Bell. Stram. Sul.
- **frightful visions, with:** **Bell. Stram.**
- **laborious,** see **Dreams.**
- **maniacal,** furibund, wild, raving: Aco. BELL. Bry. HYO. **Stram.** VER-A.
- **tremens:** Cimi. **Hyo.** Op. **Stram.**

DISCONTENT: **Bism.** PUL. **Sul.** Tub.

DISTRACTION; scattered thoughts, can't collect his ideas: **Aco.** Ang. Cocc. Grap. Hell. Old.

DUALITY, as if in pieces, separated, etc., sense of: Anac. BAPT. Petr. Pho. Stram.

DULL, dim, dazed, beclouded, stupefied, difficult comprehension: Ail. Arn. BAPT. BELL. BRY. CALC-C. GEL. **Hell.** HYO. LAUR. LYC. NAT-C. NUX-V. OP. Petr. PHO-AC. **Pul.** RHUS-T. SEP. SIL. **Stram.** Sul. **Ver-a.**
Comp. **Indifference.**

ESCAPING: Bell. Merc.

EXCITEMENT, agitation, nervousness, **nervous patients:** ACO. Amb. **Ap.** Arg-n. **Asaf. Asar.** BELL. Bor. Cann. CHAM. Cina. COFF. Colo. Con. Croc. Cup. Epiph. Fer. Hyo. **Ign.** LACH. Laur. Mag-m. **Mag-p.** Mar. **Mos.** Naj. Nat-m. **Nit-ac.** NUX-V. Pall. **Pho.** Plat. Sep. **Stan. Stap.** Stram. Sumb. TAREN. **Ther. Val.** Ver-a. Vib. **Zin.**
Comp. **Nervous Effects.**

FEAR, fright, terror, anxiety, mental shock, etc.: ACO. Amb. **Arn. Bell.** ARS. **Aur.** Bar-c. **Bry. Calc-c.** Caus. **Cham.** Con. Cup. Dig. **Gel. Grap.** Hell. Hyo. IGN. **Kali-c. Lyc.** Merc. Nat-c. **Nat-m. Nit-ac. Nux-v.** OP. **Pho.** Plat. **Psor.** PUL. Sep. **Sil. Spig.** Spo. **Stram.** Sul. **Ver-a.**
- **animals,** dogs, etc. of: Tub.
- **awaking in, night terrors:** Bell. Bor. **Lyc. Stram.** Sul. Thu.
- **crowds:** Aco. Arg-n. Aur. Gel. Nat-m. Pul.
- **dark, of:** Cam. **Cann.** STRAM.
- **falling, of:** Bor. Gel.
- **frightened or startled easily:** Aco. **Arn.** Cocc. IGN. Lyc. **Nat-m.** Petr. **Pho.**

future, death, misfortune, evil, forebodings, presentiments, etc., **dread of:** ACO. ARS. Bry. CALC-C. Caus. Cham. Cimi. Dig. Grap. Lil-t. Nat-m. **Nux-v.** Pho. Plat. Psor. PUL. Thu. Ver-a.

ghosts, of: Carb-v. Pho. **Stram.**

glistening objects: Stram.

insanity: Alu. **Calc-c.** Cann.

ordeals, dread of: Arg-n. Arn. **Gel.**

poison: Hyo.

robbers: Ars. Nat-m.

thunder: Pho.

FOOLISH, childish, silly, imbecile: ANAC. BAR-C. BELL. Buf. HYO. NAT-C. PHO-AC.

GENTLE, timid, amiable: Bar-c. Cocel. Petr. PUL.

GRIEF: **Caus.** IGN. Lach. Nat-m. **Pho-ac. Pul. Stap.**

HOMESICK: **Bry.** CAPS. Carb-a. Hyo. IGN. Pho-ac. Sil.

HOWLING: Aco. **Bell.** Cham. Cic.

HURRY, impatience: Alu. Ap. **Arg-n.** ARS. BELL. Cham. HEP. IGN. Ip. Lach. **Lil-t.** Med. Nat-m. NUX-V. **Stram.** Sul. Sul-ac. Taren.

Comp. **Motion, rapid, Amel.**

HYPOCHONDRIA: Ars. AUR. Con. Ign. **Nat-c.** Nat-m. **NUX-V.** Plat. PUL. Sep. Stan. Sul. Val.

HYSTERIA: **Asaf.** Aur. Con. IGN. Mos. **Nux-m. Nux-v.** Pul. **Val.**

IMAGINATIONS, illusions, fancies, etc.: Aco. BELL. Calc-c. **Cann.** COCCL. HYO. **Ign.** Lac-c. Op. PHO-AC. Plat. SABA. STRAM. SUL.

sensory: Rhus-t. Thu.

voices, of: Aco. Chlor-hydr. Stram.

IMPULSIVE, emotional, nervous mobility: Cup. IGN. PUL.

INDIFFERENCE, apathy: Ap. Arn. Ars. **Bapt.** CALC-C. **Chin. Con.** HELL. **Ign. Nat-c. Nat-m.** OP. PHO. PHO-AC. **Plat.** PUL. SEP. Sul.

Comp. **Dull.**

INDOLENT, lazy, sluggish, slovenly, dirty: Bor. **Caps.** Chel. **Grap.** Lach. **Merc.** Nux-v. **Pho.** Psor. Sep. SUL.

Comp. **Slowness and Motion.**

INSANITY: BELL. **Cup.** HYO. **Op.** STRAM. VER-A.

females, of: Aco. Bell. Plat. **Pul.** Stram. Ver-a.

INSENSIBLE, unconscious, etc.: Ars. **Bapt.** BELL. **Cup.** HYO. Nat-m. OP. PHO-AC. STRAM.

INTOXICATION: **Caps.** GEL. Mez. NUX-V. **Op.**

INTROSPECTIVE: Pul.

JEALOUSY: Ap. HYO. **Lach.**

JESTS, jokes: Caps. Hyo.

LAUGHTER: **Bell.** Croc. **Hyo. Stram.**

convulsive: Aur. **Ign.** Stram.

LOQUACITY: Cimi. **Hyo.** LACH. **Stram.**

MALICE, hatred, hatefulness: ANAC. **Cham.** Cup. Lyc.

Nat-m. Nit-ac. NUX-V. Taren.

MANIA, see **Delirium.**

MEMORY, **active:** BELL. HELL.

bad: **Aco. Ag-c.** ANAC. **Arg. Ars. Bar-c.** BELL. CALC-C. **Con. Guai.** Lach. Laur. LYC. **Petr. Sep. Staph.** VER-A.

lost: BELL. HYO. VER-A.

MISTAKES IN SPEECH: Alu. LYC. NAT-M. Sep.

MOANING, groaning: **Bry. Cham.**

MORAL PERVERSIONS: **Anac.** BELL. HYO. Nux-v. OP. Pho-ac. **Plat.** STRAM. VER-A.

MOROSE and sullen: NUX-V. **Pul. Sil.**

MUTTERING: **Hyo. Mur-ac.** STRAM.

NOISY: BELL.

PERSECUTED, as if: Chin. Dros.

PRAYING: Stram.

PRIDE, arrogance and disdain: Lil-t. **Lyc.** PLAT. Sul. **Ver-a.**

PROFANITY: ANAC. Lil-t. Lyc. Nit-ac. Stram. Ver-a.

RELIGIOUS IDEAS: Hyo. **Lach.** Pul. **Stram.** Sul. VER-A.

REMORSE, sense of guilt: Ars. **Dig.** VER-A.

REPROACHES: **Aco.** ARS. NUX-V.

RESTLESSNESS, fidgety, impulse to move: ACO. **Ap.** Arg-n. Arn. ARS. BELL. **Bor. Cham.** Chin. Cup. Fer. **Lyc.** Mag-c. NUX-V. Pho-ac. Pul. RHUS-T. **Sep.** Sil. Stan. **Ver-a.** Zin.

REVENGEFUL, **spiteful:** Calc-c. Lach. Nit-ac. **Nux-v.**

REVERIE, ecstasy, dreaminess: ACO. **Ant-c. Lach.** Nux-m. Old. OP. PHO. Sep. Ver-a.

SAD, depressed, hopeless despair, gloom, melancholy, etc.: ACO. **Arn.** ARS. AUR. **Calc-c.** Carb-a. **Cham.** Cimi. **Coccl.** Colo. Con. **Grap.** IGN. Kali-io. Lach. **Lil-t. Lyc.** Merc. NAT-M. **Nux-v.** Petr. **Plat.** PSOR. PUL. Rhus-t. Sep. **Stan. Sul.** Syph. **Ver-a.** Zin.

SENSITIVE, impressionable: ACO. **Amb. Arn. Asaf.** Asar. AUR. **Bell.** CHAM. Cic. COFF. Croc. IGN. Mar. NUX-V. **Stap. Sul.** Tub. **Val.**

to **offense:** Ars. Calc-c. Lyc. **Nux-v.** Plat. Pul. **Stap.**

SHRIEKS, cries: AP. BELL. **Cham. Cup.** Lyc. Mag-p. **Plat. Zin.**

SIGHS, groans, takes deep breaths, etc.: IGN.

SINGING: Hyo. **Spo.** STRAM.

SLOWNESS: BAR-C. Bry. **Con.** HELL. **Pho-ac.** Pul. SUL.

Comp. **Indolent.**

STUBBORN, obstinate: **Alu. Bell.** BRY. **Calc-c. Cham.** Chin. Kre. NUX-V. Sil.

SUICIDAL IMPULSES, weary of life, etc.: ARS. AUR. **Chin.** Dros. Merc. Nat-s. Psor. Thu. Tub.

SUSPICIOUS, distrustful: Aco. Anac. Ars. BAR-C. CAUS.

CIC. **Hyo. Lach.** LYC. Merc. PUL. Stram. Sul.
Comp. **Fear.**

TACITURN, silent, reticent: Ign. MUR-AC. PHO-AC. **Pul.** Stan. Thu. Ver-a. Zin.

THINKING, **difficult:** NUX-V. PHO-AC. **Sep.**
fixed ideas: Anac. Chin. **Ign.** Saba. Sul. Thu.
strange ideas: Arg-n.

TOUCHED or approached, averse to or fear of being: ANT-C. **Arn.** CHAM. Ign.

TRIFLES, occupied with; seem important, anger at, etc.: Ars. Calc-c. Caus. **Grap. Hep.** Ign. Nat-m. **Nux-v.** Sil. Thu.

VIOLENCE, desperation, ardor: **Ars.** BELL. Carb-v. CHAM. Hep. **Hyo.** Merc. NUX-V. **Stram.** Sul. VER-A.
impulse to do: Alu. Hyo. Iod. Lach. Merc. Nat-c. **Nux-v.** Taren.
Comp. **Delirium, maniacal.**

WEAK, exhausted, relaxed, brain fag: Anac. Bar-c. Lyc. **Pho.** PHO-AC. **Pic-ac.** Plb. Stap. Sul.

WEEPING: **Ap.** Aur. **Bell.** Calc-c. Caus. **Cham. Grap.** Ign. **Lyc. Nat-m. Plat.** PUL. Rhus-t. **Sep. Sul.** VER-A.

WHINING, whimpering: Ant-t. **Cham.** Cic. **Cina.**

WORD HUNTING: Pho-ac. **Thu.**

WORK, **dread or dislike for:** Arg-n. Carb-v. **Chin.** CON. GRAP. Lach. NAT-M. **Nux-v. Pho.** Pul. Rhus-t. SUL.
Comp. **Indolence.**

CONCOMITANTS.

ACO. CALC-C. NUX-V. PHO. PUL. STRAM.

VERTIGO.

Aco. Arg-n. Ars. **Bell.** BRY. **Calc-c.** Cam. **Chin. Cic.** Coca. COCCL. CON. **Dig.** GEL. Lyc. Nat-m. NUX-V. PETR. PHO. Pho-ac. PUL. Rhus-t. Sil. Stan. Sul. Tab.
intoxicated, as if: Gel. NUX-V. Pul.
reeling, feeling, etc.: Bell. Nux-v. **Rhus-t.**
whirling: Nux-v.

INTERNAL HEAD.

Aco. **Aeth.** Amyl-n. Ars. Aur. BELL. Calc-c. **Cic. Cina.** GLO. Hell. Hyo. Hyper. **Ign.** Melil. **Merc. Nat-m.** NUX-V. Op. **Petr.** PHO. **Pic-ac.** PUL. **Saba.** Sabi. **Sang.** SEP. SIL. Stram. SUL. **Verb.** Zin.

MENINGES: **Bell. Bry.** Canth. **Lyc.** Zin.

DEEP IN: Arg-n. Bov. Calc-c. Dulc. Lyc. **Nux-v.** Pho. Sul.

CEREBRO-SPINAL AXIS: **Agar.** Arg-n. Chin. Cimi. Cocel. **Gel.** Ign. **Nux-v.** Oenan. **Pho.**

FOREHEAD: ACO. **Am-c. Am-m.** ARS. BELL. **Bism.** BRY. **Caps.** Chin. **Con.** Dros. Hep.

Hyo. Ign. Laur. Merc. Mez. Nat-c. NAT-M. NUX-V. **Pho.** Phyt. Sang. Sil. Spig. Stan. Sul.

upper: Colo.

lower: Arn. Bar-c. Carb-v. Lach. Lyc. Naj. **Nat-m. Pho.** Pul. Sil.

TEMPLES: **Anac. Arg.** BELL. **Chin.** Cyc. Glo. Kali-c. Kre. Nux-m. Par. Plat. **Pul.** Sabi. Thu. Val.

SIDES: **Pho-ac. Zin.**

ONE SIDED SYMPTOMS: Alu. Anac. **Ars.** Asaf. IRIS. Kali-c. Pho-ac. Plat. **Pul. Sep.** Sars. Sul-ac. Verb.

right: BELL. **Calc-c.** Carb-v. Chel. Ign. **Iris.** Nat-c. Plb. Rhus-t. Saba. **Sang. Sil.**

left: Arn. Asaf. Brom. Colo. Ip. Kali-c. Merc. Naj. Nit-ac. Nux-m. Onos. Rhod. Sele. **Sep.** SPIG. Sul.

alternating: Agar. (O). Hell. Hyper. (T). Kali-c. (O). Lyc. (T). Pho. (F). Sep. (O). Sil. Sul. (T).

ears over: Merc. Pul.

VERTEX: **Cact.** Calc-c. **Calc-p. Lach.** Nit-ac. Pho. **Ran-sc.** SUL. **Ver-a.**

OCCIPUT: Agar. **Carb-v. Cimi. Coccl.** Fer. GEL. Ign. Nat-s. NUX-V. **Onos. Petr.** Pic-ac. Sep. Sil. **Zin.**

FONTANELLES OPEN: Calc-c. Calc-p.

PAINS EXTENDING **Backward:** Arn. BELL. BISM. BRY. Kali-bi. Lac-def. **Lach.** Lyc. Med. Mur-ac. Par. Rut. **Sep. Thu.** Verb.

Downward to nose, face, neck, etc.: **Agar.** Ant-t. Bism. **Bry.** Calc-c. Cham. **Chin.** Dulc. Ign. IP. **Lach. Led. Med.** Men. **Mez.** NUX-V. Pic-ac. Plat. **Pul.** Rhus-t. Sep. **Stap.** Stro. VERB. **Zin.**

Eyes, into: Carb-v. **Chin.** Cimi. Ign. LACH. Lith. Mang. Nat-c. NIT-AC. PHO. Pho-ac. Pul. **Sil.** SPIG. **Sul.** Val. **Zin.**

Forward: Aco. Alu. **Bell.** Canth. **Carb-v. Chin.** Cimi. **Con.** GEL. Laur. Mur-ac. Pho-ac. **Rhus-t.** SANG. **Sil.** SPIG. Verb.

Inward: Agar. **Anac.** Arn. Ars. Calc-c. Canth. Hep. Nit-ac. **Stan.**

Outward: Aco. Arn. Asaf. BELL. Bism. **Bry.** Canth. Cham. Chin. Con. Dulc. Lach. Lyc. **Mez.** Nat-c. Rhus-t. Sep. Sil. Spig. Sul. Val.

Comp. **Bursting.**

Upward, ascending: Aco. BELL. **Calc-c.** Canth. Chel. Cimi. **Gel.** Glo. MEN. Merc. Nat-m. Pho. **Sang. Sep.** SIL.

HEADACHE.

BORING: Arg-n. **Hep. Spig.**

BRUISED, crushed, etc.: Chin. **Ign.** Ip. **Nux-v.**
BURNING: **Aco. Merc.** Pho.
BURSTING: **Bell. Bry.** Chin. Glo. Merc. Nat-m. Nux-v.
CATARRHAL: Kali-bi. **Merc. Nux-v.**
COLDNESS in: Agar. **Bell. Calc-c.** Laur. Ver-a.
COMPRESSION, squeezing, etc.: **Ign. Lach.** (Cap-like) **Plat.**
vise-like: Nit-ac. Pul.
CONGESTION: **Bell.** Fer. Glo. Lach. Nux-v. Sul.
CONSTRICTION: Grap. **Merc.** Nit-ac. Sul.
CRAWLING, formication, etc. in: Arg. Colch. Hyo. Rhus-t.
CUTTING: Arn. **Bell.** Calc-c. Lach.
DRAWING: Carb-v. Cham. Chin.
DULL OR HEAVY ACHING: Ars. **Carb-v.** Chin. **Gel. Nat-m. Nux-v.** Pho-ac. **Pul. Sul.**
ENLARGED, as if: Arg-n. Bell. Glo. **Nux-v.**
FULNESS: **Aco.** Bry. Glo. Sul.
HAMMERING: Calc-c. **Fer.** Lach. Nat-m. Sul.
HEAT OF: **Aco. Bell.** Bor. Bry. Sul.
MOTIONS IN, shaking, **looseness,** splashing, fluctuation, etc.: Aco. Bell. Chin. Kali-c. **Rhus-t.**
NOISES in: Chin. Kali-c. Plat. Sul.
PLUG, nail, clavus: **Coff. Ign.** Thu.
PRESSURE: **Bry.** Chin. Ign. **Nux-v.** Saba. Stan. **Sul.**
STITCHES, stinging, etc.: Arn. **Bry.** Caus. **Kali-c.** Nat-m. **Pul.** Sul.
STUPEFYING PAIN: **Bell.** Calc-c. Gel. Hyo. **Nux-v.** Pho-ac.
TEARING, rending: **Chin. Lyc. Merc.** Nux-v. Pul. Sul.
THROBBING: **Aco. Bell.** Calc-c. **GLO.** Laur. Lyc. Sil. Sul.
TIGHTNESS: Nit-ac. **Nux-v.**
TWINGING, twitching, jerking: Bell. **Bry.** Chin. **Pul.** Sul.

EXTERNAL HEAD.

Ap. **Arn. Bar-c. Bell.** CALC-C. **Lyc. Nux-v. Rhus-t. Rut. Stap.** Sul.
right: **Calc-c.** Canth. Con. Mez. Sil.
left: Clem. Rut. Thu.
BONES OF: **Aco. Merc.** Nit-ac. **Pho.** Pho-ac.
SCALP: **Ars.** CALC-C. Clem. Merc. **Old. Rhus-t.** Sil. Stap. Viol-t.
FRONT OF: Hep. Led. Pho-ac. Sul.
bregma: Ars. Merc.
SIDES: Zin.
TEMPLES: Nat-m.
EARS, BEHIND: Bar-c. Caus. **Grap.** Petr. Sil. Stap.
OCCIPUT: Carb-a. **Carb-v. Petr. Sil.**
VERTEX: Carb-a. Grap.

BURNING **in vertex:** Grap. Lach. **Sul.**
DANDRUFF: Ars. Grap. **Pho.** Stap. Thu.
ENLARGED HEAD: **Calc-c.** Sul.
HAIR AFFECTED: Bell. Bor. Grap. Hep. Kali-c. Lyc. Nat-m. Sul.

blond: **Calc-c.** Caps. Cocc. Hyo. Sele. Seneg. Sil.
dark: Aco. Nit-ac. **Nux-v.** Pho. Pho-ac. Plat. Sep.
dry: Kali-c.
falling out: Calc-c. Grap. **Hep. Kali-c.** Nat-m. **Pho. Sul.** Thu.
bregma: Ars. Nat-m. Pho.
temples: Kali-c. **Nat-m.**
sides: Grap. Pho.
occiput: Carb-v. Pho.
vertex: **Bar-c.** Grap. Sep.
eyebrows: **Kali-c.**
headaches, after: Hep. Nit-ac.
margins of: Mez. Nat-m. Petr. Sep.
matted: Grap. Lyc. Vio-t.
painful: **Ars. Chin. Nux-v.**
tangled: Bor. **Lyc.** Mez. **Pho-ac.**
ITCHING: **Grap.** Lyc. **Nat-m.** Old. Pho. Sep. **Sul.**
MOTIONS OF: Alu. **Bell.** Cam. **Cic.** Cina. **Cup.** Hyo. Ign. Sep. Spo. Stram.
ROLLING OF: Ap. Bell. Cina. **Hell. Lyc.** Pod.
SENSITIVE, painful: Bell. **Chin.** Nux-v. Spig.
TENSION: Merc.

EYES.

Aco. Ap. **Bell.** Calc-c. Euph. Grap. Merc. Onos. Spig. **Sul.**
RIGHT: Am-c. **Bell.** Calc-c. Cann. **Colo.** Euphr. **Lyc.** Nat-m. Nit-ac. Petr. Pho. **Plat.** Rhus-t. Seneg. Sil.
LEFT: Ap. Ars. Asar. Bry. Chel. Chin. Hep. Laur. Mez. Nux-v. Plb. Scil. **Spo.** Stan. Sul. Tarx. Thu.
ALTERNATING BETWEEN: Aco. Agar. Ang. Bell. Cup. **Lyc.** Pul. **Ran-b.** Seneg.
BACKWARD FROM: Grind. **Par.** Rhus-t. Spi.
EYEBALL: **Aco.** Bell. Calc-c. Cimi. Euphr. Hep. Lyc. Phyt. Pru-s. **Spig. Sul.**
convulsions of: Cham.
oscillating: Cup.
sunken: Ant-c. Sul.
or drawn back, as if: Hep. Lach. **Par.** Pho. Sul.
CONJUNCTIVA: **Aco.** Ap. ARG-N. Ars. **Bell. Cepa.** EUPHR. Merc. PUL. Rhus-t. **Sul.**
SCLEROTIC: **Aco.** Rut. Sul.
CORNEA: CALC-C. **Cann.** Con. **Euphr.** Hep. Merc. **Pul.** Sul.
IRIS: Bell. Merc. **Merc-c.** Nit-ac. Sul.
LENS: Euphr. **Pul. Sil. Sul.**
PUPILS, **adherent:** Nit-ac.
contracted: Aco. **Chel.** Cocc. Sep. Sil. Sul. **Ver-a.**
dilated: BELL. CALC-C. Hep. **Hyo.** Op. Spig. **Stram.**
fixed: Bell. Cup. **Op.**
irregular: Merc. Sul.
BROWS: Bell. Caus. Kali-c. **Par.** Sele.
ORBITS: **Ap.** Spig. Rhus-t. Syph. Val.
CANTHI: Agar. Calc-c. Carb-v. Nat-m. Nux-v. Pho. **Pul. Sil.** SUL.
inner: **Agar. Bell. Stap.** Zin.

outer: Calc-c. Ran-b. Sul.

LIDS: Aco. Agar. Ap. Bell. Calc-c. **Caus.** Hep. Merc. Rhus-t. **Sep.** Spig. **Sul.**

upper: **Caus.** GEL. Kalm. **Sep.** **Spig.**

lower: **Calc-c.** **Pho-ac.** **Rut.** Seneg.

edges, tarsi: Bor. Merc. PUL. Stap. **Sul.** Val.

inner surface: **Arg-n.** Ars. **Rhus-t.**

agglutinated, suppuration: Caus. Euphr. Lyc. **Nux-v.** Pho. **Pul.** **Rhus-t.** Sep. Sul.

closed tightly, spasm: Bell. Cham. **Hyo.** Kali-c. Stram.

dry: Rhus-t. Ver-a.

heavy, falling, dropping, paralysis, opening difficult, etc.: Caus. Cham. Coccl. **Gel.** Nux-v. Sep. Spig. Ver-a.

inflamed: Aco. Ars. Bell. **Lyc.** **Pul.** **Stap.** Sul.

tarsi: Grap. Pul. **Sul.**

gonorrhoeal: Aco. **Pul.** Sul. Thu.

nodes: Grap. Stap.

open: Op.

one: Chin. Ign. Ver-a.

red: **Aco.** Lyc.

styes: Pul.

DULL: Op.

GLAUCOMA: Pho.

INJECTED: Glo. Merc.

ITCHING: Calc-c. Pul. Sul.

LACHRYMATION: Ars. Bell. Calc-c. **Cep.** **Euphr.** Kre. Merc. Nat-m. **Pul.** Rhus-t. **Rut.** Saba. Sil. **Stap.** Stram. **Sul.**

LIPPITUDE: Aco. Euphr. Merc. Pul. Rhus-t. Stram.

PROTRUDING: Aco. Bell. Chlor. Guai. **Hyo.** **Iod.**

RED: Asar. Bell. Merc. Rhus-t. Spig.

SPARKLING: Bell. **Stram.**

SQUINT: Alu. Con. **Hyo.**

STARING: Bell. Cic. Hell. **Hyo.** Op. Stram.

VISION.

IN GENERAL: Bell. Pho. Rut. Sil. Sul.

ACUTE: Hyo.

BLACK, suddenly, blind spells, etc.: BELL. Cic. **Con.** Glo. Hyo. Merc. **Nat-m.** Old. **Pho.** **Pul.** Sil. **Stram.**

BLINDNESS: Con. **Hyo.** Op. Pul. Sil. **Stram.**

DAZZLED: Kali-c. Sil.

DIM, blurred, etc.: Calc-c. **Cann.** **Caus.** Con. **Euphr.** Hep. **Pho.** **Pul.** Sil.

FARSIGHT: Calc-c. Nat-m. SEP. SIL.

FLICKERING, flames, red, etc.: BELL. **Cyc.** **Grap.** Hyo. Kali-c. **Pho.** Sep. **Spig.**

GLIMMERINGS: **Grap.** Iod. **Nux-v.**

ILLUSIONS OF: Bry. **Hyo.** Spig. **Stram.** Ver-a.

animals, bugs, etc.: Cimi. **Hyo.** STRAM.

bright objects: Hyo. Val.

colors: **Bell. Pho.**
black: Pho. Sil.
blue: Lyc.
dark, rich, etc.; Stram.
green: Pho.
rainbow: Pho-ac.
red: Sul.
Comp. **Fiery.**
striped: Sep.
yellow: Dig. Sep.
diplopia: **Aur.** Bell. Cic. GEL. **Hyo.** Nat-m. Pul. Sul. Ver-a.
fantastic, apparitions etc.: Bell. Stram. Ver-a.
fiery, bright, etc.: Bell. Hyo. **Kali-c. Pho. Spig.**
Comp. **Red.**
flies, musca volitantes, etc.: Agar. Sil. **Stram.**
halos: Lach. PHO. Pul. **Sul.**
hemiopia: **Lyc.** Nat-m.
large, as if too: Pho.
letters running together: Nat-m. Sil.
lightnings: Spig.
mist: Calc-c. Caus. Croc. **Pho.**
near, too: Bov.
small, as if too: Plat.
spotted: Am-m. Kali-c. **Pho.** Sil.
veil, as of a: Pho.
NEARSIGHT: Con. **Pho.** Pho-ac. **Pul.**
PALE: **Sil.**
PARALYSIS OF OPTIC NERVE: Bell. **Caus.** Con. **Gel.** Hyo. **Pho.** Pul. Sec-c. Sil. Stram. Sul.
PHOTOPHOBIA, see **Light, Agg.**
WEAK: **Anac. Bell.** Chin. Nat-m.

EARS.

RIGHT: **Bell.** Flu-ac. Iod. Kali-c. Kali-n. Nit-ac. Nux-v. Plat. Sil. Spo.
LEFT: Anac. Asaf. Bor. Grap. Guai. Ign. Old. **Viol-o.**
ALTERNATING BETWEEN: **Bry.** Caus. Chel. Cocc1. Fer-p. Glo. Kali-c. **Mag-m.** Mos. **Nit-ac.** Sul.
EXTERNAL: Alu. Kali-c. Kre. Merc. Pho-ac. **Sep. Spig.**
red: Pul. Sul.
INTERNAL: **Calc-c.** Caus. Grap. Kali-c. Lyc. Mang. Merc. **Nux-v. Psor. Pul. Sep. Spig.**
dry: Grap.
BEHIND; (also mastoids): Bar-c. Calc-c. Canth. **Caps.** Caus. **Grap.** Lyc. Old. Petr. **Pho.** Sil. Stap.
moisture: Grap. Lyc.
BELOW: Bell.
LOBULES: Bar-c. Caus. **Chin.** Kre.
GLANDS: Bell. Cham. Con. **Merc.** Rhus-t.

DISCHARGE FROM: Calc-c. Con. **Lyc. Merc. Psor. Pul.** Sil.
EARACHE: Cham. Fer-ph. Nux-v. **Pul.**
STITCHES in: **Bell.** Cham. Con. **Kali-c.** Merc. Nux-v. **Pul. Sul.**

HEARING.

BAD, dull, deafness, etc.: Aur. **Bell. Calc-c.** Caus. Chin-s. Hyo. Led. **Lyc. Nit-ac.** Op. Petr.

Pho. Pho-ac. **Pul.** Sec-c. Sep. **Sil. Sul.**

ILLUSORY SOUNDS: Bell. **Calc-c.** Caus. **Chin.** Chin-s. Grap. Pul. Spo. Sul.
echoing: Caus. Pho.
fluttering: Spig.
humming, buzzing, etc.: Calc-c. Caus. **Chin. Pul.** Sul.
pulsating: Bell. **Calc-c.** Cann. Nit-ac. **Pho.** Pul.
ringing: Calc-c. Caus. **Chin.** Nux-v. Pul.
roaring, rumbling, etc.: Bell. Caus. Grap. Nux-v. Pul. Spig. Sul.
rushing: Petr. Pho.

PARALYSIS, auditory: Bell. Hyo. Pul. Sil.

SENSITIVE, acute: Aco. Aur. Cham. **Coff.** Lyc. Sep. Spig.

STOPPED, as if: Con. Lyc. **Pul.** Sil.

NOSE.

Aco. Aur. Bell. Bry. Calc-c. Croc. Kali-bi. Kali-c. Kali-n. Mos. Nit-ac. Pul. Rhus-t. Sil. Sul.

ONE SIDE OF: Am-m. Ign. Phyt. **Saba.** Sinap. Sul.
right: Con. **Mar.** Spig.
left: Carb-v. Nat-m. Rhod. Sep.
alternating between: Lach. Mez. Nux-v. **Pho.** Rhod. Sinap.

EXTERNAL: **Aur.** Carb-v. Caus. Kali-c. **Merc.** Nat-c. Pho-ac. Pul. **Rhus-t.** Sep. Spig.

INTERNAL, nares: **Ars.** Ars-io. Aur. Bell. **Calc-c.** Cep. Euphr. Grap. **Kali-bi.** Kali-io. Mar. Saba. Sil. Spig. **Stict.**
posterior: Hydr. **Lyc. Merc.** Merc-i-r. **Nat-c. Nat-m.** Sep. **Spig.** Stap. Sul.

ROOT **and above:** Aco. Ars. Calc-c. **Hyo. Ign.** Merc. Pho. **Pul.** Sang. Zin.

BONES: **Aur. Merc.**

BRIDGE: Pho-ac. **Sep.**

TIP: Carb-a. Carb-v. Caus. **Sep.**

WINGS: Lyc. Thu.

BORING **into,** with fingers, picking at, **itching:** Aru-t. **Cina.** Lyc. Pho. Sil.

CORYZA (fluent discharges): **Aco. Ars. Cham. Cep. Gel.** Kali-io. Lach. **Merc. Nux-v. Pul.** Rhus-t. Sele. Sul.
chronic: Hep. Kali-bi. Sil. Sul.

CRUSTY: Merc. (inside). Sul. (outside).

MOTION OF ALAE:: Ant-t. **Lyc.** Pho.

ODOR FROM, ozoena: **Aur.** Kali-bi. Merc. **Pul.** Sul.

PAINFUL: Hep. Merc.

RAW, excoriated: Ars-io. Nit-ac. **Nux-v.** Pho.

RED: Aur. Sul.

SMELL, **acute:** Ars. Aur. Bell. Chin. Coff. **Colch.** Grap. Lyc. **Nux-v. Pho.** Sep. **Sul.**
Comp. **Odors, Agg.**
illusory: Bell. Calc-c. Par. Sul.
catarrh, as of: Pul. Sul.

earth, as of: Ver-a.
foul: Bell. Par. Pho.
sulphur, as of: Nux-v.
weak, dulled: Bell. Calc-c. Hyo. Nat-m. Plb. **Pul.** Sep. Sil.
SNEEZING: Ars-io. Carb-v. Cepa. Cina. **Gel.** Kali-io. **Nux-v.** Pul. Rhus-t. **Saba.** Sil. Sul.
abortive: Carb-v. Sil.
violent: Nux-v. Saba.
STOPPED, obstructed, suppressed coryza, etc., see **Discharges, Suppressed.**
SWELLED: Bell. Caus. Kali-c. Merc. Nat-c. Pho-ac. Pul. Rhus-t. Sep.
ULCERATED: Merc. Pul.
YELLOW: Sep. (across).

FACE.

Aco. Ant-c. **Ap.** Ars. **Bell.** Bry. Caus. Cham. Chin. Fer. Hyo. Lyc. **Merc. Nux-v.** Op. **Rhus-t.** Stram. **Sul.** Ver-a.
RIGHT: Ap. Bell. Calc-c. Canth. Lyc. Nat-c.
LEFT: Colo. Con. Rhus-t. **Spig.**
ALTERNATING SIDES: Chin. Lyc. Pho.
FOREHEAD: Hep. Led. Pho-ac. Rhus-t. Sep.
TEMPLES: Ang. **Bell.** Lyc.
NOSE, ON: **Rhus-t. Sep.** Sul.
ZYGOMAE AND MALAR BONES: **Kali-bi.** Old. Stan. Stap. Verb.
CHEEKS: Bell. Caus. **Rhus-t.** Stap.
EYEBROWS: Nat-m.
EYES, AROUND: Hep. Merc.
JAW BONES: Pho. Sil.
UPPER JAW: Am-c. Carb-v. Chin. Kre. Zin.
MAXILLARY JOINT: Bell. Ign. Merc. **Rhus-t.**
LOWER JAW: **Bell.** Caus. Cham. Laur. Nat-c. Plb. Stap. **Zin.**
ABOUT MOUTH: Ars. Bry. **Kre.** Nat-m. Rhus-t. Sep. Stap. **Sul.**
LIPS: Ars. Aru-t. **Bell.** Bry. **Nat-m. Rhus-t.** Sep. Sil. **Sul.**
cracked: Bry. Nat-m. Pul.
upper: Bar-c. Kali-c. Sul.
cracked: Hep. Nat-m.
lower: Bry. Ign. Pul. Sep.
cracked: Cham. Nat-m. Pho. **Pul.** Sep.
corners: Ant-c. Bell. Merc. Pho.
cracked: Arn-t. Grap. Nit-ac.
CHIN: Caus. Plat. Sil.

BLUISH, **about eyes:** Ars. **Chin.** Ip. Old. Rhus-t. Sec-c. Stap. Ver-a.
lips: Cup. Lyc. Nux-v.
about mouth: Cina. Cup. Ver-a.
See **Color in General.**
CHANGING COLOR: Aco. Bell. Ign. Pho. Plat.
COLD: Cina. Lyc. **Ver-a.**
CONGESTED: Aco. **Bell.** Hyo. Nux-v. Op. **Stram.**
DEATHLY, pinched, collapsed, etc.: Ars. **Ver-a.**
Comp. **Collapse.**
DISTORTED: Ars. **Bell.** Cocc. Hyo. Ip. Lyc. Op. **Stram.**
Comp. **Convulsions.**

DRY LIPS: **Bell.** Bry. **Chin.** Merc. **Nux-v.** Rhus-t. Sul. Ver-v.
DUSKY, dark, sooty: Ant-t. **Bap.** Hell. Op. **Pho.**
EARTHY: **Ars. Chin. Fer.** Lyc. **Merc.** Nux-v.
EMACIATED: Calc-c. Sele.
ERUPTION: Ant-c. Kre. Led. Rhus-t. Sep.
about lips: Ars. **Nat-m.** Rhus-t.
eczematous: **Bor. Rhus-t.** Sars.
pimples: Carb-v.
EXPRESSION, altered: Stram. Ver-a.
HECTIC: **Ars.** Calc-c. Chin. Iod. Kali-c. Lyc. Pho. Pul. Sang. **Sul.**
HOT: **Bell. Calc-c.** Cham. Fer. Nux-v.
ITCHING: Calc-c.
LOCKJAW, mouth closed spasmodically, etc.: Ang. **Bell. Cam.** Cann. Cic. Hyper. Ign. Merc. **Nux-v.** Op. Sec-c. Ver-a.
NUMB: Gel. Plat.
PAIN, neuralgia, migraine, prosopalgia, etc.: Bry. Caus. Chin. **Colo.** Kalm. **Mag-p.** Mez. **Nux-v.** Pho. Pru-sp. Sep. **Spig.** Verb.
PALE, **about nose and mouth:** **Aeth.** Ant-t. **Cina. Pho.**
PEELING **lips:** Nux-v.
RED **cheeks:** Aco. Arn. Chin. **Fer.** Lyc. Pho.
one side: Aco. Ars. (r). **Bar-c. Cham.** Ign. Lyc. (l). Merc. (r). Mos. **Nat-m.** (l). **Pho.** Ran-b. Rhus-t. (l).
alternating: Nat-p.
SICKLY: **Chin.** Nux-v.
SPOTTED: Carb-a. **Rhus-t.** Sil. Sul.
SUNKEN: **Ars.** Cam. **Chin.** Op. Rhus-t. Sec-c. **Ver-a.**
hollow eyed: Chin. Ver-a.
SWEAT ON: Lyc.
SWOLLEN, puffed, turgid: Am-m. **Ap. Ars. Bell.** Bry. Cham. Kali-c. **Lyc.** Nux-v.
cheeks: Arn. Cham. Merc.
eyes, under: Ap. Pho.
between and brows: **Kali-c.**
lips: **Ars.** Bell. Calc-c. (up.) Merc-c. Nat-m. (up.) **Sep.** (low.) Sul. (up.).
TENSION: Pul. Verb. Viol-o.
TWITCHING, trembling, etc. **lips:** Cham.
VESICLES, hydroae: **Nat-m.**
WRINKLED: Alu. Calc-c. **Lyc.**
YELLOW **across nose:** SEP.

TEETH AND TOOTHACHE.

Aco. Bell. Bry. **Calc-c. Cham.** Chin. Kre. **Merc.** Nat-c. Nux-v. Plant. Pul. Rhod. **Rhus-t. Sep.** Spig. **Stap.** Zin.
RIGHT: Bell. Flu-ac. Stap.
LEFT: Caus. Cham. Clem. Euphor. Mez. Sep. Sul. **Thu.**
ALTERNATING SIDES: Iod. Psor. Sul. Zin.
between upper and lower: Pul.
CHANGING ABOUT: Grap. Pul.
ROW, **in a whole:** Ars. Aur. Lach. Mag-c. Mag-p. **Merc.** Nat-m. Nux-v. Psor. Sep. Spig. **Stap.** Zin.

UPPER: Am-c. Bell. **Carb-v.** Chin. Kre.
LOWER: Bell. Canth. **Cham.** Nat-c. Plb. Stap.
CANINE: Calc-c. Nux-v. Sep. Sul-ac.
INCISORS: **Colch.** Sul.
MOLARS: Bry. **Kre.** Stap. Zin.

BRITTLE, crumbling: Euphor. **Stap.**
EXTENDING TO EARS, **head or face, pain:** Ant-c. Cham. Lach. **Merc.** Mez. Pul. Rhod.
GRINDING, clenching: Bell. **Cina.** Phyt. Pod.
HOLLOW, early decay: Bell. Bor. Cham. **Kre.** Merc. Mez. Nat-c. Plb. Sep. **Stap.**
LOOSE: Bry. (as if). **Hyo. Merc.**
SORDES, slimy: Rhus-t.

GUMS.

Bor. Carb-v. Kre. **Merc.** Nux-v. Stap.
UPPER: Calc-c. Rut.
LOWER: Sars.
INNER: Pho. **Stap.**

BLEEDING: Pho-ac. Stap.
EXCORIATED: Carb-v. Sep.
RECEDING: Carb-v. Merc.
SORE: Carb-v. Merc.
SUPPURATING, pyorrhœa: Cist. **Merc.** Stap.
SWELLED: Merc. Nux-v. Sep. Stap. Sul.

MOUTH AND THROAT. (INNER).

Ap. Arg-n. Aru-t. Bell. Carb-v. Coc-c. **Kali-bi. Lach. Merc. Nux-v. Pho.** Phyt. Pul.
RIGHT: Am-c. Ap. **Bell. Lyc.** Merc-i-fl.
LEFT: Kali-c. **Lach.** Merc-i-r. Pho-ac. Rhus-t. Sep.
ALTERNATING SIDES: **Lac-c.** Colo.
BACK OF: Aco. Cocc. Kali-c. **Merc.** Nit-ac. Rhus-t.
PALATE: Aur. Bell. **Merc. Nux-v.** Pho.
  hard: Bell. **Nit-ac.** Nux-v.
  soft: **Ap.** (uvula). **Merc.** Merc-i-fl. (rim).
TONGUE: **Bell.** Hyo. **Merc.** Nux-v. **Pho. Plb. Pul.** Rhus-t. **Sul.**
  down center (stripe): **Arn. Bap.** Pho. Rhus-t. **Ver-v.**
  edges: Nat-m.
  tip: **Rhus-t.** Sul.
TONSILS: Bar-c. **Bell.** Guai. **Lach.** Merc. **Merc-i-fl.** Phyt.
  enlarged: **Bar-c.** Lyc. Merc. Merc-i-r. Nit-ac. Stap.
ADENOIDS: Agrap. Calc-c. **Merc.** Tub.
EUSTACHIAN TUBE: Merc-dulc.

ANGINA, simple, sore throat: Aco. Bell. Merc. Merc-i-fl. Sep.
APHTHAE: Ars. Bor. **Merc.** Nit-ac. Nux-v. Sul-ac.
BLUISH **tongue:** Ars. Dig. Gym.
BURNING: Bell. Petr.

BURNT, scalded, as if: Ars. Hyds. Iris. Pul.

CHOKINGS, **constriction, spasm, narrow, as if:** Bell. Hyo. **Ign. Lach.** Merc-c. Merc-i-r. Stram. **Ver-a.**

COATED TONGUE: Bell. **Bry.** Chin. Merc. **Nux-v.** Pho. Pul.

white: Ant-c. Ars. Bell. Chin. Kali-m. Pul. Sul.

yellow: Bry. Chin. Merc-i-fl. (at base).

CRACKS, fissures: Aru-t. **Bell.**

CUTTING: Nit-ac.

DIPHTHERIA AND TONSILITIS: Ap. Ars. Kali-bi. Lac-c. **Lach.** Lyc. Merc-cy. **Merc-i-fl.** Mur-ac. Phyt. Rhus-t. Sul-ac.

laryngeal: Brom. Iod. Lach.

nasal: Kali-bi.

DRY, **in general:** Aco. **Bell.** Lyc. Merc. Pho. Pho-ac. Sep. Stram. Sul. Ver-a.

palate: Pho-ac.

tongue: Ars. Bry. Calc-c. Pho. **Rhus-t.**

EAR, extending to: Hep. Kali-bi. Lach.

FOAM **at mouth:** Bell. Hyo. Ign. Stram.

beads of, near edge of tongue: Am-c. Ap. **Nat-m.** Pho.

HAWKING (mucus): Caus. **Kali-bi.** Lach. Lyc. Pho. Pul.

from posterior nares: Hydr. Kali-bi. Nat-m. Nux-v. Spig. Sul.

HEAVINESS: Bell. (tongue).

INDENTED TONGUE: **Merc** Rhus-t.

INFLAMED: Nux-v.

ODOR FROM, bad breath: **Arn.** Bapt. Cham. **Carb-v.** Lach. **Merc. Nux-v.** Pul. Sul.

OPEN: **Bell.** Lyc. Mur-ac. Op.

PARALYSIS: Caus. Gel. (palate). Op. (tongue).

PATCHY, mapped tongue: Ars. Kali-bi. **Nat-m.** Nit-ac. Rhus-t. **Tarx.**

RANULA: Thu.

SORE, palate: Bell. Lach. Merc. Phyt.

STICKY, clammy, pasty: Bapt. Kali-bi. Lach. Pho-ac. Sul-ac.

SWALLOWING, **impeded** see **Swallowing, Agg.**

urging to: Bell. Caus. Lach. Merc.

SWELLED: Ap. (uvula), Arg. (palate). Lach. (palate). **Merc.** Nux-v. Pul. (as if)

VESICLES on tongue: Ap. (tip). **Nat-m.** (edge). Pho. (edge).

SALIVA.

IN GENERAL: Merc. Sul.

DIMINISHED: **Bell.** Kali-bi. Nux-v. Pho. Stram. Sul. **Ver-a.**

INCREASED: Dig. **Merc.** Nit-ac. Nux-v. Pho. Pul. **Rhus-t.** Stram. **Ver-a.**

THIRST.

Aco. Arn. **Ars.** Bell. **Bry. Calc-c.** Caps. **Cham. Chin.** Cina. Croc. **Dig.** Lyc. **Merc. Nat-m.** Pho. **Rhus-t.** Sep. Sil. **Stram. Sul. Ver-a.**

with aversion to drinks: Hell. Stram.

with the chill: Bry. Caps. **Ign. Nat-m.**

ABSENT: Ant-c. Ant-t. **Ap.** Ars. Chin. Cyc. **Gel.** Hell. **Ign.** Men. **Mur-ac.** Nux-m. Pho. Pho-ac. **Pul. Saba. Samb.** Sep. Spig.

during the heat: Ap. Carb-v. **Gel.** Hell. **Ign.** Ip. Nux-m. **Pul.** Saba. Sep.

COLD DRINKS, FOR: Aco. **Ars.** Pho. Rhus-t. **Ver-a.**

LITTLE AND OFTEN, for: **Ars.** Bell. Chin. **Lyc.** Rhus-t.

MUCH AT A TIME: **Bry.**

VIOLENT burning: **Aco.** Arn. **Ars.** Bry. Colo. Cup. Merc. Nux-v. Saba. **Ver-a.**

TASTE.

ALTERED, in general: Chin. **Pul.** Rhus-t.

ACUTE: Chin. Coff.

AFTERTASTE, of food eaten: **Ant-c.** Caus. Dio. Nat-m. **Pho. Pho-ac. Pul.** Sil.

ASTRINGENT: Alu. Arg-n. Arn. Ars. Euphor. **Pho.**

BAD, foul, nauseous, repulsive, etc.: Arn. Merc. **Nux-v. Pul.** Rhus-t. Stap.

in the morning: Bry. Nat-s. **Nux-v. Pul.**

BITTER: Aco. Ant-c. Ars. **Bry.** Cham. **Chin.** Lyc. Merc. **Nux-v. Pul.** Sep. Sul. Ver-a.

to food: Chin. Pul.

BLOODY: Ip.

DULLED, flat, watery, etc.: **Bry.** Chin. Ign. **Pul.** Stap.

EARTHY: Pul.

GREASY, fatty: Asaf. Caus. Iris. **Pul.** Val.

HERBY: Nux-v.

LOST: **Nat-m.** Pul. Sil.

to food: Pul.

METALLIC: Cocc. Cup. **Merc.** Nux-v. Rhus-t.

SALTY: **Ars.** Kali-io. Lyc. Merc. Pho. Pul. Sep.

SLIMY: Kali-bi. Pul.

SOUR: Bell. **Calc-c.** Chin. **Lyc. Nux-v.** Pho. Pul. Sul.

SWEET: Pho. Plb. Pul. Saba. Scil. Stan.

APPETITE.

AFFECTED, IN GENERAL: Chin. Lyc. **Nux-v. Pul.** Sul.

HUNGER: Calc-c. Chin. **Cina.** Grap. Pho. **Pul.** Sep. Stan.

eating, after: Cina. Lyc.

gluttony, with: Chin.

ravenous: Calc-c. **Chin. Cina. Iod.** Lyc. Nux-v. Saba. Sil. **Sul.** Ver-a.

relish, without: Nat-m. Op. Rhus-t.

VARIABLE, capricious: Calc-c. Cina. **Coc-c. Iod.** Lach. Nat-m. Petr. Syp.

AVERSIONS.

TO FOOD, etc.: **Ars. Nux-v.** Pul.

loathing, disgust, repugnance, etc. with: **Ant-c.** Arn. **Ars.** Cham. Colch. Ip. **Kali-c. Nux-v.** Op. Pul. Sep.

after a little food; quick satiety: Cyc. Ign. **Lyc.** Rhod. Rhus-t. Thu.

acids: Sul.
beer: Chin.
bread: Kali-c. **Nat-m.** Pul. Sul.
coffee: Nux-v.
fats: Nat-m. **Petr. Pul.**
fluids, drinks: **Bell.** Hyo. **Pul.** Stram.
meat: Grap. Mur-ac. **Petr. Pul.** Sep. Sil. **Sul.**
milk: Ign. Sep. **Sil.**
sweets: Caus. Sul.
tobacco: Calc-c. **Ign.** Nux-v.
water: Bell. Chin. **Stram.**
wine: Lach. Merc.

CRAVINGS AND DESIRES.

BEER: Stro. **Sul.**

BITTERS: Dig. Nat-m.

CABBAGE: Cic.

CHALK: Nit-ac. Nux-v.

COFFEE: Bry. Nux-v.

COLD THINGS: **Ars.** Bism. Pho. Rhus-t. **Ver-a.**

FAT FOODS, bacon, etc.: Calc-p. Nit-ac. Nux-v.

JUICY THINGS, fruit: Pho-ac. Stap. **Ver-a.**

LIQUIDS: Stap. Sul.

MILK: Rhus-t. Saba.

PREGNANCY. during: Sep.

REFRESHING THINGS: Pul.

SALTY THINGS: Caus. **Nat-m.** Ver-a.

SOUR THINGS: **Aco. Arn.** Ars. Sul. **Ver-a.**

SPIRITS, alcoholic: Arn. **Ars. Calc-c. Lach.** Nux-v. **Op.** Stap. Sul.

SWEETS AND DAINTIES: Arg-n. **Chin. Kali-c. Lyc.** Saba. Sul.

WINE: Calc-c.

WATERBRASH.

(Also raising mucus):

Ars. **Bry.** Calc-c. Carb-v. Mez. Nat-m. **Nux-v.** Par. **Pho.** Saba. Sep. **Sil.** Stap. Sul.

HEARTBURN.

Calc-c. Carb-v. Con. Croc. **Nux-v.**

QUALMISHNESS.

Ars. Caus. Nat-c. Sul.

HICCOUGH.

Am-m. Cic. Cyc. Hyo. Ign. Mar. NUX-V. Pul. Ran-b.

NAUSEA.

Aeth. Ant-c. **Ant-t. Ars.** Bry. Carb-v. Cham. Colch. Cup. Dig. Hep. Ign. **Ip.** Lyc. Nit-ac. **Nux-v.** Pho. Pul. Rhus-t. Sep. Sil. Sul. **Ver-a.**

CONTINUOUS: **Ip.**
DEATHLY, anxious: Ant-t.
MORNING: Cimi. Nux-v. Pul. Sep.
STOMACH, felt in: **Ver-a.**
THROAT, in: Cyc. Pho-ac. Stan. Val.

GAGGING.

Cham. Pul. Rhus-t. Ver-a.

REGURGITATION.

Aeth. Ant-t. Arn. **Bry.** Nux-v. **Pho.** Pul. Sars. Sul. Sul-ac.
ingesta of: Bry. **Pho.**

RETCHING.

Bell. **Ip. Nux-v.** Ver-a.

VOMITING.

Ant-t. Arn. **Ars.** Bry. Cham. Cina. Cup. Fer. **Ip.** Kre. **Nux-v.** Pul. Sil. Sul. **Ver-a.**

BLACK: **Ars. Nux-v.**
CURDS: **Aeth.**
FECAL: **Op.** Rhus-t.
FLUIDS ONLY: **Ars.**
after they become warm: **Pho.**
FROTHY: Aeth. Arg-n.
INGESTA: Ars. Bry. Cina. **Fer.** Ign. **Nux-v.** Pul. Sil. Sul.
MUCUS: Dros. Ip. **Pul.**
OFFENSIVE: Ars. Nux-v. **Sep.**
PURGING with: Ant-t. Ars. **Cam.** Colch. Cup. Ip. Iris. Sec-c. Sul. **Ver-a.**
VIOLENT: Ant-t. Ars. Cup. Kali-bi. **Nux-v.** Phyt. **Ver-a.**
WATERY: **Bry.** Caus.
WORMS: Cina.

ERUCTATIONS.

Arg-n. Asar. Bell. **Bry. Carb-v.** Cocel. Con. **Lyc.** Merc. Nat-m. **Nux-v.** Saba. Sep. Sul. Ver-a.
ABORTIVE: Con.
ACRID: Merc.
EGGS, like bad: Arn.
EMPTY: Bry. Calc-c. Carb-v. Con. Grap. Pho. Sep. Sul.
FROTHY: Kre.
INGESTA, tasting of: **Ant-c.** Bry. Pul.
LOUD, noisy: Arg-n. Asaf. Kali-bi. Petr. Pho.
NAUSEOUS, foul: Asaf. (rancid). Carb-v. Pul. Sul.
SOUR: **Lyc.** Nat-m. **Nux-v.** Pul. Sul.

FLATULENCE.

Arg-n. Asaf. **Carb-v.** Cham. **Chin.** Grap. Ign. **Lyc. Nux-m. Nux-v.** Pho. Plb. Pul. Stap. Ver-a.

DISCHARGE OF: **Carb-v.** Chin. Grap. Kali-c. Old.
FERMENTING, as if: Rhus-t.
FOUL, putrid: Ars. Asaf. **Carb-v.** Cocel. Pul. Scil. Sul.

GENERATION OF: Carb-v. Kali-c. **Mar.**

NOISY, rumbling, growling, etc.: Ant-c. **Carb-v.** Caus. Chin. Hell. **Lyc.** Nat-m. **Nat-s. Nux-v.** Pho. Pho-ac. Pul. Sep. Sil. Sul. Ver-a.

OBSTRUCTED, crowding, etc.: Ant-t. Aur. (1). Carb-v. (upward). Cham. Chin. **Coccl.** Grap. **Ign. Lyc.** Nat-c. Nit-ac. Nux-v. Plb. Pul. Stap.

PAINFUL, wind colic: Carb-v. Cham. Chin. Lyc. **Nux-v.** Pul. Rhod. Stap. Ver-a.

SOUR: Nat-c.

EPIGASTRIUM.

Bry. Kali-c. Lyc. Nat-m. **Nux-v. Sil.**

ACHING: Sil.

ANXIETY AT: **Ars.** Lyc. Nux-v. Pul.

BURNING: Ars. Nux-v. Sep. Sil.

CRAMP, pinching, etc.: Sil. Ver-a.

PAIN IN: Ars. Nux-v. Ver-a.

PRESSURE: Cup. Nux-v. **Pho. Pul.** Ver-a.

SENSITIVE: Calc-c. Kali-c. **Lach. Ver-a.**

STICKING: Arn. Bry. **Nit-ac.** Rhus-t. **Sep.** Sul.

SWELLED: **Calc-c.** Nux-v.

THROBBING: Asaf. Kali-c.

STOMACH.

Aeth. **Ant-c.** Arg-n. **Ars.** Bry. Calc-c. **Carb-v. Cham.** Coccl. Ign. Ip. Kali-bi. **Nux-v.** Pho. (cardiac end). **Pul.** Rhus-t. Sep. Sul. Ver-a.

ACIDITY: Calc-c. Chin. Lyc. **Mag-c.** Nat-p. Nux-v.

BACKWARD, pain goes: Bell. **Chel.** Nux-v.

BORING: Stan.

BURNING: **Ars.** Carb-v. Cic. **Pho. Sul.**

CANCER: Lyc. Pho.

DISORDERED DIGESTION: **Ant-c.** Arg-n. **Ip.** Nat-c. **Nux-v. Pul.**

DISTENDED, swelled, full, etc.: Ant-c. **Calc-c. Carb-v.** Chin. **Kali-c. Lyc. Pho.** Sul.

EMPTY, hollow, gone, sinking, weak, hanging down, etc., also epigastrium; **Ign.** Ip. Petr. **Pho. Sep.** Stap. **Sul.**

not ameliorated by eating: Cina. Lach. Lyc. Mur-ac. **Pho. Sep.** Ver-a.

FULNESS: Chin. **Kali-c. Lyc.** Pho. Sul.

GNAWING, eating, ulcerative pain, etc.: **Carb-v. Pho. Sep.**

PAIN, aching, indefinite distress, etc.: Ars. Cup. **Nux-v.** Pul. **Sep.**

PRESSURE, **heaviness, as of a load,** etc.: Ars. **Bry.** Calc-c. Cham. Hyo. Lyc. **Nux-v. Pul.** Sil.

SPASMODIC PAIN: Caus.

TENDER, painful: Ars. Chin. Lach. **Nux-v.**

THROBBING: Nux-v. **Pul.** Sep.

HYPOCHONDRIÆ.

Aco. Chin. Ran-b.

RIGHT, liver and gall ducts: and bladder: Aco. Alo. **Am-c.** Am-m. Ars. **Aur.** Bar-c. **Bell.** Berb. Bry. **Chel. Chin. Coccl.** Colch. Dios. Gel. Hydr. Iris. **Kali-c. Lach. Lyc.** Mag-m. Merc. Nat-s. **Nux-v.** Pod. Rhe. **Sep.**

posterior: Calc-c. Kali-bi.

LEFT, spleen and pancreas: Arn. Asaf. **Carb-v. Chin.** Con. Flu-ac. Ign. Iris. **Nat-m.** Nit-ac. Ran-b. **Sul.**

ABSCESS: Lach.

GALL STONES: Calc-c. Chel. **Chin.** Lyc. Nux-v.

INDURATION: Grap. (liver).

INFLAMMATION: Mag-m. (liver)

PAIN, liver: Bry.

PRESSURE, L.: Mag-m.

STICKING: Ign. (S). Sil.

TENSION: Aco. Lyc.

ABDOMEN.

Alo. Ars. Bell. Bry. Cham. **Chin.** Cina. Colo. **Nux-v.** Plb. **Psor. Pul. Rhus-t. Sep. Sul.**

UPPER: Caus. **Cham.** Chin. **Coccl.** Nux-v. Pul.

ABOUT NAVEL: Bry. **Colo.** Dios. Kre. Nux-v. Pho-ac. **Rhus-t. Ver-a.** Verb.

SIDES: Asaf. Carb-v. Chin. Ign.

Right: Ars. **Lyc. Rhus-t.**

Left: Alu. Arg. Asaf. Brom. Dulc. Flu-ac. Hep. Plb. **Rhe. Sul.** Tarax.

alternating: Arn. Pul.

LOINS (flanks): Canth. Rhe. Thu. Zin.

LOWER: **Bell.** Bry. Carb-v. Lyc. **Merc.** Ran-b. Scil. **Sep.**

ANXIETY, emotions, etc., in: **Ars.** Carb-v. Pho. Ver-a.

BORING IN: Plb. Stan.

BURNING in: **Ars.** Canth. **Pho.** Ran-b. **Sec-c.** Sep. **Ver-a.**

CUTTING: Bell. **Bry.** Chin. **Colo.** Ip. Merc. Nit-ac. Nux-v. **Pul.** Rhe. **Sul.** Ver-a.

DIARRHŒA, sense of: Dulc. **Nux-v.** Pul.

DISTENDED, tympanitic, inflated, etc.: Aco. **Arg-n.** Ars. Bell. **Carb-v. Chin.** Colch. Grap. Kali-c. **Lyc.** Merc. Nat-c. Nat-m. (Side). **Nux-v.** Pho. Rhus-t. Stram. Sul. **Tereb.** Ver-a.

DRAWING: Pul.

FERMENTATION IN: Chin.

FULNESS: Chin. Carb-v. Kali-c. **Lyc. Nux-v. Sul.**

GURGLING IN: **Alo.** Crot-t. Gamb. Pod. **Sul.**

HARD: Grap. Merc. Sil.

HEAVY: Alo. **Grap.** Kali-c. Nux-v. Sep.

ILEUS: Nux-v. **Op.** Plb. Thu.

INACTIVE PERISTALSIS: Con. Grap. **Nux-v.** Op.

INFLAMED: Aco.

LUMP, ball, stone, etc.: Pul. Sul.

PAIN, dull, aching, etc.: Colo. Cup. Plb. **Pul. Ver-a.**

PRESSURE: Arn. Calc-c. Nux-v. Pho-ac. (lower). Sep. Sul.
RAWNESS: **Ars.** Bell. Canth. Nux-v. **Ran-b.**
TEARING, shooting: Cham.
TENSION: Arn. Caps. **Carb-v.** Chin. **Colo.** Sil.
THROBBING: Sele.
TWISTING: Colo. Dios.
ULCERATIVE FEELING: **Ran-b.**
WEAK, sinking, hanging, etc.: Ign. Pho.

EXTERNAL ABDOMEN.

Ap. Bry. Merc. Nux-v. Plb. **Pul.** Sele.
BRUISED SORE, tender, etc.: Aco. **Ap.** Bell. **Nux-v.** Stan. Sul. Tereb.
PENDULOUS, enlarged, pot-bellied: **Calc-c.** Caus. **Sep.** Sul.

GROINS.

RIGHT: Calc-c. Kali-c. Lach. **Lyc.** Nux-v. Pul. Rhod. Rhus-t. Sul-ac. **Thu.**
LEFT: Euphor. Mag-c. **Zin.**
INTERNAL RING: Am-m. Aur. Lyc. **Nux-v.** Sul-ac.
EXTERNAL RING: Ars. Merc.
GLANDS: Calc-c. **Hep.** **Merc.** Nit-ac. **Thu.**
HERNIA: Am-m. Aur. Lyc. **Nux-v.** Sul. Sul-ac. Ver-a.
  incarcerated or protruding: Nux-v. Ver-a.
MONS VENERIS: **Rhus-t.**

ANUS AND RECTUM.

ANUS: Aesc. Carb-v. Grap. **Kali-c.** Mur-ac. Nit-ac. **Nux-v.** **Pho.** Sep. **Sul.**
RECTUM: Aesc. **Alo.** Calc-c. **Ign.** Lyc. **Merc-c.** Nat-m. **Nux-v.** Pho. **Pod.** Rat. Sep. **Sul.**

DRAWING: **Lach.**
EXCORIATION: Sul.
FISSURE: **Grap.** **Ign.** Nat-m. **Nit-ac.** Paeo. Rat. Syp. Thu.
HEMORRHOIDS: Aesc. Alo. Grap. Kali-c. Mur-ac. **Nux-v.** **Pul.** **Sul.**
  blind: Nux-v.
  painful: Mur-ac. Nit-ac. Paeon. Stap.
  protruding: Alo. Calc-c. Mur-ac. Sul.
INACTIVE, powerless, open, etc.: **Alo.** Alu. Ap. Ign. Kali-c. **Pho.** Sec-c.
ITCHING: Caus. Lyc. Nit-ac. **Sul.**
MOISTURE AT: Caps. Carb-a. Caus. **Pho.** Sil. Sul.
PRESSURE, fulness, etc.: **Aesc.** **Nit-ac.** Sul.
PROLAPSE: **Ign.** Lyc. Merc. **Pod.** Sep.
SHOOTING: **Ign.**
SORE, sensitive, smarting, painful: Carb-v. Grap. **Mur-ac.** Pul. Sul.
TENESMUS: **Caps.** Merc. **Merc-c.** **Sul.**
UPWARD, pain goes: **Ign.** Lach. Sep. Sul.

PERINEUM.

Ag-c. Alu. **Carb-a.** Carb-v. Cyc. Sul.

PROSTRATE GLAND: Dig. **Pul.** Sul. Thu.

STOOL.

ACRID: **Ars.** Chin. Colch. Gamb. Ign. Iris. **Merc.** Pul. **Sul.**

BAD ODOR: **Ars.** Asaf. Bapt. **Carb-v.** Nux-v. **Pod. Psor.** Pul. Sul.

BLACK: **Ars.** Lept. Stram. **Ver-a.**

BLOODY: Canth. Ham. **Ip.** Merc. **Merc-c. Nux-v.** Pul. Rhus-t. (water). Sep. **Sul.** (streaked).

CHANGEABLE: Pul.

CONSTIPATED: **Bry.** Calc-c. Cocel. Lyc. **Nux-v.** Op. Plb. Sil. Stap. Sul.

alternate days, on: Calc-c. Cocel. Kali-c. Nat-m.

chronic: Bry. **Nux-v.**

hard faeces, from: Bry. Mag-m. Nux-v. Op. Plb. Verb.

inactivity, from: Alu. Hep. Kali-c. Nat-m. **Nux-v.**

CRUMBLING: Mag-m. Nat-m.

DARK, brown, etc.: Ars. **Bry.** Grap. Nux-v. **Psor.**

DIARRHŒA: Alo. Ars. Cham. Chin. Cina. Colo. Con. Crot-t. Gamb. Iris. Merc. **Nat-s. Pho.** Pho-ac. **Pod.** Psor. Pul. Rhe. Rhus-t. Sul. **Ver-a.**

chronic: Ars. Calc-c. Pho. **Sul.**

constipation, alternating with: Ant-c. Calc-c. Lyc. Pho.

morning: Bry. Nat-s. **Sul.**

painful: Colo. Merc-c. Rhe. Rhus-t.

painless: Ars. Chin. Fer. Hyo. Lyc. **Pho.** Pho-ac. **Pod.** Stram.

DIFFICULT: **Bry.** Chin. Mag-m. Nat-m. **Nux-v.**

DRY: Bry. Nat-m.

DYSENTERIC: Canth. Caps. **Merc-c. Nux-v.** Sul.

EGGS, LIKE BAD: Cham.

FREQUENT: **Aco.** Calc-c. Caps. **Cham. Merc-c. Nux-v. Pod. Ver-a.**

GELATINOUS: Alo.

GUSHING, pouring: Alo. **Crot-t.** Gamb. Jat. **Pod.** Sec-c. Ver-a.

HACKED, chopped: **Cham.**

HARD: Alu. **Bry. Grap.** Mag-m. Nat-m. Nit-ac. Plb. Sil. Sul.

INSUFFICIENT: Arn. Caps. Cham. Mag-m. **Merc-c.** Nat-c. **Nux-v.** Sul.

INVOLUNTARY, hurried, etc.: **Alo.** Ap. **Arn.** Gel. Hyo. **Pho.** Pho-ac. Pod. **Sul.** Ver-a.

KNOTTY, lumpy, like sheep dung, of little balls, etc.: Alu. Grap. **Mag-m.** Merc. **Op. Plb.** Sep. Sil. Sul. Verb.

LARGE CALIBER: **Bry.** Kali-c. Ver-a.

MUCUS: **Ars.** Asar. Bor. Caps. **Cham.** Colch. **Merc.** Merc-c. Nux-v. Pho. **Pul.** Sul.

bloody: Merc. Merc-c.

coated: Am-m. Cham. **Grap.** Hyds. **Pul.**

NOISY: Arg-n. **Nat-s.**

RETAINED: Coccl. Sil. **Stram.**
SHREDDY: Arg-n. Canth. **Merc-c.**
SLENDER: Caus. Pho.
SOFT, mushy, etc.: Chin. Nit-ac. Pho. Pul. **Sul.**
UNDIGESTED: Ars. **Calc-c. Chin.** Fer. Old. Pho-ac.
URGING: Caus. **Merc.** Sul.
ineffectual (also tenesmus): Caps. Merc. **Merc-c.** Nux-v. Rhe. Rhus-t. **Sul.**
WHITE: Ars. Dig. **Merc.** Pho-ac. **Pod.**
WORMS: **Aco. Calc-c.** Chin. **Cina.** Nat-p. **Saba. Sil.** Spig. **Sul.**
pinworms: Calc-c. Chin. Cina. Fer. Ign. **Mar.** Sul.
tapeworm: Calc-c. Grap. Plat. Pul. Saba. Sil. Sul.
YELLOW: Ars. Crot-t. Merc. **Pod.**

CONCOMITANTS.

BEFORE STOOL: Calc-c. Merc. **Nux-v. Ver-a.**
DURING STOOL: Ars. Cham. **Merc.** Pul. **Sul.** Ver-a.
AFTER STOOL: **Caus. Merc-c.** Nux-v. **Pho.** Pod. Sele.

MICTURITION.

DESIRE, urging, etc.: Ant-t. Bry. **Canth.** Caus. **Merc-c. Nux-v.** Pho-ac. Pul. Sabi. Sars. Scil. Stap. **Sul.**
fruitless: Ars. **Canth. Dig. Nux-v.** Sars.
DIFFICULT, painful, drop by drop, strangury, etc.: Cann. **Canth.** Cham. **Merc-c. Nux-v.** Pul. Stap. Sul.
DRIBBLING: Canth. Pul. **Sul.**
FEEBLE, slow, etc.: Alu. Arn. Hep. Mur-ac. Sars. Sep.
FREQUENT: Arg. Bar-c. Caus. Guai. Kali-n. Lyc. Mang. **Merc. Merc-c. Nux-v.** Rhus-t. Scil. Stap. Sul.
HURRIED, irresistible: Bry. Kre. Pho. Pul. Sul.
INFREQUENT: Canth.
INTERRUPTED, intermittent, etc.: Agar. Ant-c. Carb-a. Caus. **Clem. Con.** Gel. Kali-c. Led. Lyc. Op. Sars. Sul. Thu.
INVOLUNTARY: **Caus.** Fer. Pul. Rhus-t.
in bed, bed wetting: **Bell.** Caus. Cina. **Pul.** Rhus-t. Sil. **Sul.**
during first sleep: Sep.
coughing, on: **Caus.** Pho.
NIGHTLY: Rhus-t. Lyc.
PROFUSE: Arg. Lyc. Mur-ac. Pho. **Pho-ac.** Rhus-t. Scil. Spig. Verb.
RETENTION, suppression, tardy, etc.: Aco. Arn. Cam. **Canth.** Hep. **Lyc.** Op. Pul. **Stram.** Comp. **Discharges and Feeble.**
SCANTY: **Ap. Canth.** Colch. Dig. Grap. **Hell. Op.** Rut. Stap.

URINE.

ALTERED IN GENERAL: **Pul.** Sep. Sul.
ACRID, biting: Hep. **Merc.**
ALBUMINOUS: Ars. Canth. **Merc-c.** Rhus-t.

CLOUDY: **Cina.** Con. **Merc.** Pho. Saba.
turning: **Bry.** Cham. **Pho-ac.**
DARK: **Aco.** Ant-t. Bell. **Bry.** Colch. **Merc.** Sep. **Ver-a.**
DIABETIC: Pho-ac.
FLOCCULENT: **Canth.** Mez.
FROTHY: Lach. Spo.
GREENISH: Cam. Ver-a.
HOT: Ars. **Bell.** Hep. Merc.
MILKY: **Pho-ac.**

ODOR, **ammoniacal,** strong: Asaf. Nit-ac. Pho.
foul, repulsive: **Benz-ac.** **Dulc.** Pul. **Sep.**

PALE: Con. Kali-n. **Pho-ac.**

PELLICLE ON: **Par.** Pho. Psor. Pul.

VISCID: Colo.

WATERY: **Scil.**

SEDIMENT.

Canth. Colo. **Lyc.** Pho-ac. Pul. **Sep.** Val. Zin.
Comp. **Calculous Deposits.**

ADHERENT: Colo. Pho. Pul. **Sep.**
BLOODY: Canth. Pho-ac. Pul. Sep.
CLAYEY, earthy: Zin.
CLOUDY: **Pho-ac.**
FLAKY: Canth. **Mez.** Zin.
MUCOUS, OF: Pul.
RED, brickdust, etc.: Canth. Chin. **Lyc.** Nat-m. **Pul.** **Sep.**
SANDY: **Lyc.** Sars.
WHITE: Pho. **Rhus-t.**
YELLOW: Zin.

CONCOMITANTS.

Cann. Merc. Pul.
BEFORE URINATION: Bor. Colo. **Nux-v.** **Pul.**
AT START OF URINATION: Merc.
DURING URINATION: Cann. Canth. Hep. Lyc. **Merc.** Pho-ac. **Pul.** Sep. Thu.
AFTER URINATION: **Canth.** Colo. Hep. **Merc-c.** Nat-m. **Thu.**

URINARY ORGANS.

Bell. **Cann.** **Canth.** **Lyc.** **Merc.** **Nux-v.** **Pul.** Thu. Zin.
KIDNEYS: Ap. Ars. Berb. **Canth.** Merc-c. Rhus-t. Stro. Tereb.
Right: Cocc-c. **Lyc.** **Nux-v.** Sars.
Left: Chin. Merc. **Par-b.**
URETERS: Berb. Canth. Ocim-c. Polyg.
BLADDER: **Canth:** Caus. **Dulc.** Hyo. Lyc. Merc-c. Nux-v. **Pul.** Rut.
paralysis of: **Ars.** Hyo.
URETHRA: Arg-n. **Cann.** **Canth.** Caps. Clem. Lyc. Merc. Pho. Pul. Sul. Thu.
stricture: Clem. Petr.

GENITALS.

Ag-c. Arn. Calad. Merc. Nit-ac. **Pul.** Rhus-t. **Sep.** Sul.
RIGHT: Ap. Calc-c. Caus. Hep. **Lyc.** Merc. Nux-v. Spo. Sul-ac. Ver-a.
LEFT: **Lach.** Naj. Pul. Thu.
MALE: Arn. Cann. Merc. Nit-ac. Nux-v. Pul. Sul. **Thu.**

PENIS: Arn. **Cann.** Canth. Clem. **Merc.** Dulc. Thu.
GLANS: Merc. Nit-ac. Rhus-t. Thu.
PREPUCE: Calad. **Merc.** Rhus-t.
SPERMATIC CORD: **Pul.** Spo.
TESTES: Arn. **Aur.** Clem. Merc. Nux-v. **Pul.** Rhus-t. Sep. Spo.
SCROTUM: Arn. Crot-t. **Petr. Sul.**
FEMALE ORGANS: Caul. Cimi. Cyc. Grap. Kre. Lil-t. Mrx. Nux-v. Plat. **Pul.** Sec-c. Sep. **Sul.** Thu. **Vib.**
external: Sep. Thu.
VAGINA: Calc-c. Kali-c. Lyc. Merc. Pul. **Sep.** Sul.
UTERUS: **Bell.** Cham. Kali-c. Plat. **Pul.** Sabi. **Sec-c.** Sep.
painful: Ign.
prolapsus: Grap. Lil-t. **Sep.**
OVARIES: Ap. Bell. Canth. **Lach.** Lyc. Stap. **Thu.**

ABORTUS: Bell. Cham. Croc. Ip. **Sabi. Sec-c. Sep. Vib.**
ADHERENT PLACENTA: Pul. Sec-c.
AFTER PAINS: Arn. Cham. **Cimi. Pul.** Rhus-t. Sabi.
LABOR PAINS, **ceasing,** weak, etc.: Bell. **Kali-c.** Op. **Pul. Sec-c.**
false: **Pul.**
inefficient: Coff. Nux-v.
too painful, laborious or violent, etc.: Cham. Pul. Sec-c. Sep.
spasms, with: Cham. **Hyo.** Ign. Pul.

SENSITIVENESS: **Plat.**

SEXUAL IMPULSE.

EMISSION, **seminal**: Chin. Con. Fer. **Pho. Pho-ac.** Sele.
ERECTIONS: **Canth.** Grap. Merc. Nat-c. Nat-m. **Nux-v. Pho.** Pul. Thu.
deficient: Bar-c. **Con.** Lyc. Sul.
painful: Canth. Merc. Nux-v.
IMPOTENCY, sexual weakness: Ag-c. Calad. Con. **Lyc.** Sele.
NYMPHOMANIA: Ag-c. Hyo.
PROSTATIC LOSSES: Ag-c. Con. Hep. Nat-c. **Nit-ac. Pho-ac.** Sele. Sep. Stap. Sul.
SEXUAL DESIRE, **too strong: Canth.** Carb-v. Chin. Nux-v. **Pho. Plat.** Pul. Sil. Ver-a.
too weak: Caus. Lyc. Sul.
STERILITY: Merc.

MENSTRUATION.

IN GENERAL, affected: Aco. Bell. Plat. **Pul.** Sep. Sul.
MENSES, **early**: Amb. **Bell.** Bor. Bov. **Calc-c.** Carb-v. **Caul. Cham.** Cocc. Ip. Mang. **Nux-v.** Pho. **Plat.** Rhus-t. Sabi.
interrupted, reappearing, etc.: **Kre. Lach.** Nux-v. Pul.
irregular: Cimi. Cocc. Ign. Iod. Senec.
late: Caus. Con. Cup. Dulc. Grap. Kali-c. **Lach.** Lyc. Mag-c. Nat-m. **Pul.** Sep. Sil. **Sul.** Vib.
too long: Cup. Lyc. Nat-m. **Nux-v.** Plat. Sec-c.

profuse, excessive: Ars. Bell. Calc-c. **Chin.** Croc. Fer. Ip. Nat-m. Nux-m. **Nux-v. Pho.** Plat. **Sabi.** Sec-c. Stram.
scanty: Am-c. Con. Dulc. Grap. Kali-c. Lach. Mag-c. **Pul.** Sul.
Comp. **Discharges.**
short: Am-c. **Pul.** Sul.
suppressed: Hell. Lyc. Pho. Sil. Sul.
Comp. **Discharges.**
tardy at puberty: Pul.
vicarious: Bry. Grap. Lach. Pho. Pul. Senec. Sul.
MENSTRUAL BLOOD see **Hemorrhage.**

LEUCORRHŒA.

Alu. Calc-c. Kre. **Merc.** Nat-m. Pul. **Sep.**

FLOWING (down thighs): Senec.
MENSES, **before and after:** Grap.
URINATING, **when:** Sil.

CONCOMITANTS.

Kre. Merc. Nat-m. Sep.

RESPIRATION.

Aco. Ant-t. **Ars.** Bell. Bry. Cham. **Ip.** Kali-c. Lach. **Naj.** Pho. **Pul.** Rhus-t. Sep. **Sul.** Zin.

ANXIOUS: **Aco.** Ip. Pho. Pul. Scil. **Stan.**
COLD BREATH: Carb-v. **Ver-a.**
DEEP: Bry. Caps. **Ign.** Ip. **Op.** Sele. Sil. Comp. **Sighing.**
DIFFICULT: Ant-t. Ars. **Bry. Ip.** Kali-c. Lach. Pho. **Sul.**
HOT: **Bell. Cham. Coff. Zin.**
IRREGULAR: Ang. **Bell.** Cup. **Op.**
LIGHT, shallow: **Bell.** **Pho.**
LOUD, noisy: **Cham.** Chin. Samb. **Spo.**
OPPRESSED: **Aco. Ars.** Bell. Bry. **Carb-v.** Cup. Ign. **Ip.** Nux-v. **Op. Pho. Pul.** Sep. **Sul. Ver-a.**
PANTING: Bry. Calad. **Ip.** Stram.
PARALYSIS: Ant-t. Grind. **Lach.**
QUICK: **Aco.** Bell. **Carb-v.** Cup. Ip. Lyc. Pho. Sep. **Sul.**
RATTLING: Am-c. **Ant-t.** Cup. **Hep. Ip.** Lyc.
SHORT: **Aco. Ars. Bry.** Carb-v. Con. Cup. **Ip.** Kali-bi. Merc. Nat-m. Rhus-t. **Sep. Sil. Sul.**
SIGHING, takes deep breaths: **Ign.** Lach. Sil.
SLOW: **Bell. Op.**
SNORING: Hyo. Op.
SUFFOCATING ATTACKS, choking, asthma, etc.: Aco. Ant-t. **Ars.** Brom. Chlor. Cup. Hep. Ign. Iod. **Ip.** Kali-bi. Kali-io. **Lach.** Op. **Pul.** Samb. **Spo.** Sul.
TIGHT, wheezing: Ars. Brom. **Caus.** Con. **Ip.** Kali-bi. Kali-c. Lach. Lyc. Nat-m. **Nux-v. Pul.** Sabi. Sil. Stan. Sul. **Thu.**
WHISTLING, hissing, etc.: Chin. Hep. **Samb.** Spo.

CONCOMITANTS.

Ars. Bell. Cup. Ip. Pho. Pul. Sep.

COUGH.

Ars. Bry. Calc-c. Pho. Pul. Rhus-t. Sep. Stan. Sul.

See **Also Voice.**

INCESSANT: **Dros.**
SHORT: Aco. Caus. Merc. Rhus-t.
SPASMODIC, VIOLENT WHOOPING, etc.: **Bell. Carb-v.** Cina. Coc-c. Cor-r. Dros. **Ip. Nux-v. Pul.**
catarrhal phase: Aco. Dulc. Ip. Nux-v. Pul.
spasmodic phase, also concussive **cough:** Carb-v. Cina. Coc-c. Dros. Kali-c. **Nux-v.** Pul.
defervescent stage: Ant-t. Pho. Pul.
SUFFOCATING, choking: Ant-t. Brom. Cup. Ip. Op.
WITH EXPECTORATION: Ars. **Calc-c.** Led. Lyc. Pho. **Pul. Sep.** Stan.
in morning: Carb-v. Hep. Par. Pho. Pul. Scil. Sep. Sul-ac.
by day: Ars. Cham. Hep. Merc. Pul. Sil.
bloody: Aco. Am-c. Arn. Ars. Bell. Bry. **Chin.** Fer. Hyo. **Ip.** Nit-ac. **Pho.** Pul. Rhus-t. Sabi. Sec-c. Sul. Sul-ac.
Comp. **Hemorrhage.**
difficult: Ant-t. Caus. Kali-bi.
easy: Arg. Stan.
swallowed, must be: Caus.
taste of see **Taste in General.**
WITHOUT EXPECTORATION, **dry:** Aco. Ip. Nux-v. Pho. Spo. Sul.
VOMITING, with: Alu. **Ant-t.** Bry. Coc-c. Cor-r. Dros. Ip. Pul.

TIME, **morning:** Lyc.
evening: Bry. Calc-c. Nux-v. Rhus-t. Sep.
night: Bar-c. Bell. Calc-c. Hyo. Nux-v. Pho. Pul.

LARYNX.

Aco. Bell. Brom. Carb-v. Caus. Dros. Hep. Iod. Nux-v. Pho. Pul. **Spo.**

TUBERCULOSIS OF: Carb-v. Dros. Spo.

TRACHEA (Throat pit).

Brom. Nux-v. Pho. Pul. Rum. Spo. Stan.

MUCUS IN: Lyc. Pho. Seneg.
RATTLING IN: Ant-t. Hep. Ip.
TICKLING: Caps. Laur. Nux-v. Psor. Rhus-t. **Rum. Sang.** Sep.

VOICE AND SPEECH.

Bell. Caus. Dros. Gel. Hyo. Pho. **Stram.**

BARKING: **Bell. Canth.** Lyc. Spo. Stram.
BROKEN, cracked: Grap. Spo.
CROAKING: Aco.
DEEP: Dros.
DIFFICULT: Stram.
HASTY: Bell. Lach.

HOARSE, croupy: **Aco.** **Brom.** Calc-c. Carb-v. **Hep.** **Iod.** Kali-bi. Lach. Mang. Nit-ac. **Pho.** **Spo.**
HOLLOW: Bell. Spo. Ver-a.
HUSKY: Merc.
INDISTINCT: **Caus.** Lyc.
LOST: Ant-c. **Carb-v.** Caus. Pho.
LOW: Ang. Canth. Hep. Ver-a.
NASAL; Bell. Lyc. Pho-ac. **Stap.**
ROUGH: Pho.
SHRILL: Aco. Spo. Stram.
SLOW: Ars. Thu.
STAMMERING: **Bell.** Stram.
TONELESS, loss of timbre: Dros.
TREMULOUS: Merc.
WEAK: Ver-a.

EXTERNAL THROAT.

Bell. Lyc.

RIGHT: Caus. Flu-ac. Merc. Nat-c. Nat-m. Nit-ac.
LEFT: Asaf. Calc-c. Con. Sul.
ALTERNATING SIDES: Am-m.

GLANDS OF (Goitre): Am-m. **Bar-c.** Bell. **Calc-c.** Cham. Grap. Iod. Kali-c. Lach. Lyc. **Merc.** Nat-m. Rhus-t. **Spo.** Stap. Sul.
Parotitis: Rhus-t.

NECK (Nape).

Aco. Bar-c. **Calc-c.** Cimi. Gel. **Nux-v.** Phyt. Pul. Rhus-t. Sep. Sil. Stap.
CONSTRICTION, as of a band: Glo. **Lach.** Sep.
EMACIATION: Nat-m.
STIFF: Bell. Calc-c. Kali-c. Lyc. Mag-c. Nit-ac. Pho. Stict.

INNER CHEST.

Aco. Am-c. Ant-t. Ars. Aur. Bell. **Bry.** Cam. Chin. Cocel. Fer-ph. Kali-bi. Kali-c. Nux-v. **Pho.** **Pul.** Seng. Spig. Stan. **Sul.** **Ver-v.**
RIGHT: Arn. Ars. **Bell.** Bry. Carb-a. Chel. Colch. Colo. Iod. **Kali-c.** Lach. **Lyc.** Mur-ac. Psor. Pul. Sil.
LEFT: Am-m. Calc-c. Con. Euphor. Flu-ac. Kali-c. Kali-n. Laur. Lyc. Nit-ac. **Nux-v.** **Pho.** Rhus-t. Seneg. Stan. Sul.
CHANGING ABOUT in: Alu. Arg-n. Bell. Colch. Lyc. Mag-m. Merc. Nat-c. Pho. **Pul.**
ALTERNATING SIDES: **Agar.** Ars. Calc-c. Cimi. Dulc. Hyp. Lyc. Plb. Ran-b. Rum. Thu.
UPPER: Calc-c. Iod. Mang. Stan.
MIDDLE: Calc-c. Dulc. Kali-bi. Phel. Sep.
LOWER: Carb-v. Chel. Chin. **Kali-c.** **Pho.** Pho-ac. Sabi. Scil.
BACKWARD, EXTENDING: Kali-bi. Kali-c. Lil-t.
ANXIETY IN: Bry.
CONSTRICTION, cramp in: Cact. Fer. Mos. Nux-v. Sul.
LUMP WITHIN, as of: Amb. Sul.
PLEURISY: Aco. Bry. Sul.
PNEUMONIA AND BRONCHITIS: **Aco.** Ant-t. Bry. Kali-bi. Lyc. Merc. **Pho.** Rhus-t. Sul. Ver-v.

PRESSURE (as of a load): Ant-t. Aur. Fer. **Nux-v.** Pho.
SORENESS: Pho. Stan.
TIGHTNESS: Pho.
WEAKNESS: Calc-c. Carb-v. Kali-c. **Stan.** Sul.

EXTERNAL CHEST.

Arn. Bry. Pho. Ran-b. Ran-sc. Spig. Sul.

AXILLAE.

Carb-a. Carb-v. **Hep.** Pho. **Sep.** Sil. Sul.

ERUPTION **in:** Sep.
EXCORIATION: Carb-v. Mez.
GLANDS, **engorged:** Sul.
ITCHING: Pho.

MAMMAE.

Bell. Bry. Carb-a. Cham. **Con.** Hyds. Lac-c. **Pho. Phyt.** Sil.

MILK **in breasts:** Pul.
altered: Bell. Merc.
escaping: Calc-c.
increased: Bell. Bry. Phyt. **Pul.**
scant, absent, etc.: **Ag-c.** Bry. Calc-c. **Dulc. Pul.** Rhus-t. Urt-u.
spoiled: Aeth. Cham. Sil.
SWELLED MAMMÆ: Bell. **Bry.** Con. Pho. **Phy. Pul. Sil.**

NIPPLES.

Arn. Cham. Grap. Lyc. Pul. **Sul.**

HEART.

Aco. Ars. Aur. Buf. **Cact. Calc-c.** Carb-v. Dig. Glo. Kali-c. Kalm. **Lach.** Lil-t. Naj. **Nat-m. Pho.** Pul. (r). **Spig.** Sul.
VALVES: Bar-c. Calc-c. **Kali-c. Lach.** Pho. **Pul.**

CUTTING: Colch.
INFLAMED: Aco. **Lach.** Pul. **Spig.**
PALPITATION see **Heart beat.**
STICKING: Caus. Kali-c.

BACK.

RIGHT: Calc-c. Cic. Flu-ac. Zin.
LEFT: Dros. Glo. Sil.
ALTERNATING SIDES: Agar.
CHANGING HERE AND THERE: Berb. Cimi. Kali-bi.

SCAPULAR REGION.

Chin. Dulc. Kali-c. Kre. Merc. Rhus-t. **Sep.**
BETWEEN SCAPULÆ: Am-m.

DORSAL REGION.

Arn. Ars. **Bell.** Calc-c. Caus. Chin. **Coccl.** Gel. Ign. Lyc. **Nat-m. Nux-v.** Pho. Pic-ac. **Pul. Rhus-t.** Rut. Sep. Sil. **Sul.**

CURVATURE: Aur. Calc-c. Merc. **Pul. Sul.**

EMACIATED **in; Nux-v.**
SENSITIVE: Agar. Hyper.
STIFF: Caus. Rhus-t.
WEAK: Pic-ac.

LUMBAR REGION.

Aesc. Alu. **Ant-t.** Ars. Berb. **Calc-c.** Caus. Cimi. Kali-c. **Nux-v.** **Pul.** Rhus-t. **Sep.** Sul. Variol.

SACRUM.

Grap. Hep. Hyper. **Rhus-t.**

UPPER LIMBS.

Arn. Ars. Bell. **Calc-c.** Chin. Lach. Lyc. **Nux-v.** Pho. **Pul.** Rhod. **Rhus-t.** Sep. Sul.

RIGHT: Bell. Bism. Bry. Calc-c. Caus. Colo. Grap. Nat-c. Ran-sc. Sars. Sec-c. Sil. Stro.

LEFT: Anac. Arn. Asaf. Cact. Kali-c. Nit-ac. Rhus-t. Sabi. Scil. Stan. Stram. Sul.

ALTERNATING BETWEEN: Caus. Chin. **Coccl.** Colch. **Lyc.** Mag-m. Plat. Sep. Zin.

SHOULDER: Aco. Bry. Fer. Kali-c. Mag-c. Pul. Rhus-t. Sang.

heaviness, load, etc.: **Anac.**

UPPER ARM: Coccl. Fer. Nat-m.

FOREARM: Calc-c. Caus. Merc. Rhus-t. Stap.

HANDS: **Calc-c.** Caul. Lyc. Nux-v. Pho. **Sul.**

backs of: Nat-c. Rhus-t. Sep.

palms: Anac. Ran-b. Sele. Spig.

FINGERS: Am-m. Lyc. Rhus-t. Sil. Sul. Thu.

between: Grap. Sele.

clenched thumbs: Hyo. Merc.

felon: Ap. Hep. Flu-ac. Nat-s. **Sil.** Sul.

nails: Grap. **Sil.** Sul.

brittle: Sil.

deformed, thickened: Grap.

discolored: Grap. Nit-ac.

hangnails: Nat-m. Nat-s. Rhus-t. Sul.

ingrown: Sul.

painful: Grap.

ulcerative pain: Grap. Pul.

tips: Am-m. Lach. Mar. Pho. Thu.

JOINTS: Calc-c. Caus. Kali-c. Led. Lyc. Merc. Rhus-t. Sep. Sul.

shoulder: Calc-c. **Fer.** **Fer-p.** Ign. Kali-c. Nat-m. Pul. Rhus-t. **Sang.** Sep. Stap. Sul.

elbow: Caus. Kali-c. Rhus-t. Sep. Sul.

bend of: Kali-c.

tip of: Hep.

wrist: Bov. Calc-c. Caus. Kali-c. Rhus-t. Rut. Sabi. Sep. Sul. Viol-o. (r).

finger: Calc-c. **Caul.** Sep. Spig. Sul.

BONES: Asaf. Chin. Coccl. Rhus-t. Sil. Stap.

RESTLESS: Caus. Mur-ac.

WEAKNESS: Anac. Bell. Calc-c. Cic. **Kali-c.** Sul.

LOWER LIMBS.

Arn. **Ars.** Aur. Bry. Calc-c. Caps. Carb-v. Chin. Led. Lyc. Nat-m. **Nux-v.** Pul. **Rhus-t.** Rut. **Sep.** Sil. Stram. **Sul.**

RIGHT: Ars. Bell. **Bry. Colo. Grap.** **Lach. Nux-v. Pho. Pul. Rhod.** Sars. Sec-c. Sep.

LEFT: **Amb. Asaf. Calc-c. Cina.** Con. **Fer. Hep. Lyc. Nit-ac.** Rhus-t. Sil. Stram. Sul.

ALTERNATING BETWEEN: Aco. Calc-p. Cham. Dios. Grap. Kali-bi. Kali-c. Lach. **Nat-m.** Nat-s. Rhus-t. Sul.

HIPS AND LOINS: Arn. Caus. Euphor. Lyc. Phyt. Rhus-t. Rut. Sep. Sul.

BUTTOCKS: Grap. Pho-ac. Stap. Sul.

red: Carb-v. Cham. Sul.

THIGHS: Ars. Chin. Clem. Guai. **Merc. Nat-m.** Phyt. Sep.

anterior: Anac. Spo.

posterior and sciatic nerve: Colo. Gnap. **Rhus-t.** Sul. Zin.

outer side: Caus. Helon. **Pho-ac.** Phyt.

inner side: Petr. Rhod. Stann. Sul.

LEGS: Am-c. Calc-c. Lyc. Pul. Sep. Sil. Stap.

restless: Ars. Kali-c. Nit-ac. Rhus-t. Sul. **Zin.**

TIBIA, shin: Agar. **Asaf.** Calc-c. Carb-v. Merc. Mez. **Pho.** Pul.

CALF: Alu. Arg-n. Ars. Calc-c. Grap. Nit-ac. Pul. Sep. Stan. Stap. Sul. Val.

cramp in: Cham. **Cup.** Ign. **Nux-v.** Sec-c. Sul.

TENDO ACHILLES: Anac. Mur-ac. Sep. Zin.

FOOT: Arn. Ars. Bell. **Bry. Caus.** Kali-c. Lyc. **Pul.** Sep. Sil.

coldness of one: Bar-c. (r). **Carb-v.** (l). **Chel. Con. Lyc.** Psor. (l). Pul. Rhus-t (l). **Sabi.** (r). Sul. (l).

numb: **Ars.** Cocl. Nux-v. **Plat.**

sweating of: Bar-c. Calc-c. Carb-v. Iod. Lyc. Pul. **Sep. Sil.** **Sul. Thu.**

foul odor: Bar-c. Kali-c. Nit-ac. Pul. **Sil.** Thu.

heels: Calc-c. Caus. Grap. **Ign.** Led. Nat-c. Pul. Sabi. Sep.

dorsum: Cam. **Caus.** Hep. **Pul.** Spig. Tarax.

soles: Cup. Pho-ac. Pul. Sul. Tarax.

painful: **Kali-c. Lyc.** Med. Pul.

swelled: Fer. Lyc. Pul.

toes: **Arn. Caus. Grap.** Plat. Pul. Ran-sc. Sabi. **Sul.** Thu.

great: Arn. Asaf. Caus. Kali-c. Nat-s. Plat. Sabi. (Podagra). Sil. Zin.

tips: Kali-c.

balls of: Led. Petr. Pul. Spig.

nails: Grap. Saba.

corns: **Ant-c.** Bry. **Calc-c.** Ign. **Lyc.** Rhus-t. **Sep. Sil.** (soft). Sul.

inflamed: Sil.

JOINTS: Bry. Calc-c. **Caus.** Kali-c. Led. Lyc. Nat-m. **Rhus-t.** Sep. Sil. Stro. Sul.

hip: Bry. **Caus.** Led. Merc. Pho-ac. Rhus-t. Stram.

knee: Caus. Chin. **Gel.** Led. Nat-m. Nux-v. Petr. Pul. **Rhus-t.** **Sep.** Sul.
 weak: Coccl. **Gel.** Sep.
popliteal space: Bell. Nat-m. Pho.
patella: Bell. Con.
ankles: Caus. Lyc. Nat-m. Rhus-t. Sep. Sul.
toe joints: Aur. Caus. Kali-c. Led. Mar. Sabi. Sep. Sul. **Zin.**

BONES: Merc. Pho. Pul. Rut. Sil. Stap.

SKIN.

Ant-c. **Ap.** **Ars.** Asaf. **Bell.** Bov. **Calc-c.** Clem. Coff. **Grap.** **Hep.** Kali-s. **Lach.** Lyc. Merc. **Mez.** **Petr.** Psor. Pul. **Rhus-t.** Sep. Sil. **Sul.** Thu.

folds, angles, etc.: **Grap.** Petr. Psor. Pul.

CRACKS, fissures, etc.: Alu. **Calc-c.** **Grap.** Hep. Petr. **Pul.** Rhus-t. **Sep.** **Sul.**

CORNS see **Feet and Hardness.**

CYSTS AND WENS: Bar-c. Calc-c. Pho. Sil.

DESQUAMATION: Am-c. **Bell.** **Canth.** Dulc. **Mez.** Sep.

DRY, sweat and moisture, scanty or absent: Alu. Ars. Bell. Bry. Colch. Grap. **Kali-c.** Lyc. Nux-m. **Sil.** **Sul.**
Comp. **Discharges.**

ECCHYMOSES, petechiae, purpura, etc.: Arn. Ars. Bry. **Lach.** **Pho.** Rhus-t. Sul-ac.

ERUPTIONS (tendency to): **Aco.** **Am-c.** Ars. **Calc-c.** **Caus.** Dulc. Grap. Lyc. Merc. **Rhus-t.** Sep. Sil. Sul.
acne: Hep. Kali-bro.
acuminate: Ant-c. Pul.
circular (ringworm): Sep. Tell.
clustered, grouped, etc.: **Calc-c.** Nat-m. Rhus-t.
dry: Bar-c. Calc-c. **Sep.** Sul. Ver-a.
erysipelatous: Aco. **Ap.** **Bell.** **Grap.** Hep. Merc. **Rhus-t.**
favus: Ars. Sul.
fine: Carb-v. Nat-m. Rhus-t.
flat: Lach. Pho-ac. Sep.
granular: Ars. Carb-v. **Hep.**
impetigo: Sul.
indented: Thu. Variol.
lichen: Aco. Lyc. Sul.
measly: Aco. Kali-bi. Pul.
mentagra: Calc-c. Grap.
miliary: Aco. Bry. Coff. **Ip.** Merc. Sul.
painful: Arn. **Bell.** Pho-ac.
painless: Lyc.
pedunculated: Thu.
pimples: Ant-c. Caus. Nit-ac. Sep. Zin.
prurigo: Sep.
psoriasis: Ars-io. Sep.
pustular see **Suppuration.**
scabby, crusty: **Calc-c.** **Con.** Grap. **Lyc.** **Rhus-t.** Sars. Sil. **Sul.**
 bloody: Merc. **Sul.**
scaly: Calc-c. **Clem.** Pho. Sul.
scarlatinous: Am-c. **Ap.** **Bell.** Cham. Merc. **Mur-ac.** Sul.

serpiginous: Ars. Sul.
tettery (eczema and herpes): **Ars.** Bov. Calc-c. **Cham.** Con. **Dulc. Grap.** Lyc. **Merc. Nat-m.** Petr. Pho. **Rhus-t.** Sep. Sil. **Sul.**
urticarious, hives, etc.: **Ap. Calc-c.** Caus. Dulc. Hep. Rhus-t. Sep.
variola: Ant-t. Rhus-t. Thu. Variol.
vesicular, blisters, etc.: **Ars. Aru-t. Canth.** Caus. **Dulc.** Grap. Lach. Pho. **Ran-b. Rhus-t.** Sep.
zoster: Ars. Lach. Merc. Ran-b. **Rhus-t.**

EXCORIATED, denuded, raw: Arn. Aru-t. Aur. Carb-v. Cham. Chin. **Grap.** Hep. **Ign. Lyc.** Merc. Petr. Psor. **Pul.** Sep. **Sul.**

Comp. **Soreness.**

FLABBY, relaxed: **Calc-c.** Ver-a.
FRECKLES: **Lyc.** Pho. Sep. **Sul.**
FUNGUS GROWTH, excrescences, figwarts, condylomata, polypi, proud flesh, spongy, fungus haematodes, etc.: Ars. **Calc-c. Carb-a.** Cina. Con. Dulc. **Lach. Lyc.** Merc. Nat-s. **Nit-ac. Pho. Pho-ac.** Psor. **Sabi.** Sep. **Sil. Stap.** Sul. **Thu.**
GANGRENE: **Ars.** Bell. **Carb-v.** Chin. **Lach.** Plb. Sec-c. Sil.
GOOSESKIN: Hell. **Nux-v.** Par. Ver-a.
HEALS WITH DIFFICULTY, vulnerable: **Ars.** Cham. Con. **Hep.** Kali-bi. **Lach. Lyc.** Petr. Sil. **Sul.**
INACTIVE: Anac. **Con.** Kali-c. **Lyc. Pho-ac.**
INSENSIBLE, numb: Anac. **Sec-c.**
ITCH: Carb-v. Caus. Merc. Sele. Sep. Sil. **Sul.** Ver-a.
ITCHING: Am-c. Ap. Caus. Clem. Hep. **Lyc.** Mang. **Merc.** Petr. **Pul. Rhus-t.** Sep. **Sil.** Spo. **Stap. Sul.**
burning: Agar. Ap. Caus. **Lach.** Petr. Rhus-t. Sil. **Sul.**
painful: Bar-c.
pleasurable: Sul.

LUPUS: Ars. Grap. Sil. Stap. Sul.
MOIST: Carb-v. **Grap.** Lach. **Lyc. Rhus-t.**
NAEVI: Flu-ac. **Sul.**
OILY, greasy: Merc. Nat-m.
PARCHMENT LIKE: **Ars.** Sil.
PUFFED, bloated: Ant-c. **Ap.** Calc-c. Caps. Cup. Fer.
ROUGH: **Calc-c. Sep.** Sul.
SCURFY, mealy: **Ars. Calc-c.** Lyc. Rhus-t. **Sil. Sul.**
SHRIVELLED, withered, wilted, wrinkled: Ars. **Chin. Sec-c.** Ver-a.

Comp. **Face.**

SOFT, boggy: Ars. Lach. Sil.
STICKY: Pho.
STIFF: **Rhus-t.** Ver-a.
TENSE: Caus. Nit-ac. **Pho.** Stro.
THICKENED AND HARD: Ant-c. **Grap. Rhus-t.** Sep.
ULCER see **Generalities.**

WARTS: Ars. Bell. **Calc-c. Caus.** Dulc. Nat-c. Nit-ac. Sul. **Thu.**

WENS see **Cysts.**

SLEEP.

YAWNING: Caus. Cina. Croc. Hep. **Ign.** Nux-v. Op. Plat. Rhus-t.

and stretching: Cham. Nux-v. Rhus-t.

SLEEPINESS (by day): **Aeth.** Am-c. Ant-c. **Ant-t.** Calad. Croc. **Gel.** Hep. Ign. **Nux-m. Nux-v. Op. Pho. Pho-ac.** Plb. Pul. Saba. Sul.

morning: Calc-c. Con. Grap. Nux-v. Sep.

forenoon: Ant-c. Saba.

afternoon: Chin. Nux-v. Rhus-t. **Sul.**

evening: Ars. Calc-c. Kali-c. Nux-v.

---

accompanied by: Ant-t. Nux-m. Pul.

caused by other complaints: **Ant-t.** Nux-m. Rhus-t.

eating: Chin. Nux-v. Rhus-t. **Sul.**

SLEEP, **anxious:** Aco. Ars.

coma vigil: Aco. Op.

comatose: Croc. Nux-v. Op. Pul. Ver-a.

restless, tossing about, etc.: **Aco.** Ars. Bar-c. **Bell.** Chin. Pul. **Rhus-t. Sil.** Sul.

stupid, deep, etc.: **Aeth. Ant-t.** Bapt. Bell. Con. **Led. Nux-m. Op.**

unrefreshing, awakes tired, etc.: Bry. Chin. Con. Hep. Op. **Sul.**

---

lying on back: Bry. Pul. Rhus-t. Stram.

with hands over head: Pul.

---

during, nightmare: Aco. **Nux-v.** Op. Sul.

saliva, flow of: **Merc.** Pho. Rhus-t.

shrieks, screams, etc.: Ap.

snoring: Op.

somnambulism: Pho.

starting up, jerks, etc.: Aco. Ars. **Bell.** Cham. **Lyc. Pul.** Sep. **Stram.**

talking: Lach. Pul.

WAKING, **frequently,** catnaps: Calc-c. Hep. Pho. Pul. Sep. Sul.

too **early:** Kali-c. Nat-c. Nux-v. Ran-b.

late: Calc-c. Grap. Nux-v. Sep.

anger, in: Cham. **Lyc.**

confusion, in: Chin.

jerks, with a: Bell.

SLEEPLESSNESS: Aco. **Anac.** Ap. Ars. Bry. Calc-c. **Cham. Chin. Coff.** Hep. **Kali-c.** Merc. Nit-ac. Op. **Pul.** Rhod. **Rhus-t.** Sep. Sil. Thu.

early (late falling asleep): **Ars.** Bry. Calc-c. **Carb-v. Merc.** Pho. **Pul. Rhus-t.** Sep.

late (after midnight): **Caps. Coff.** Kali-c. **Nux-v.** Sil.
altho sleepy: Bell. Cham. Hep. Pho. Pul. Sep.
caused by: Ars. Bry. Calc-c. **Cham.** Chin. Coff. Merc. Pho. Pul. Rhus-t. Sep.
once awaking: Nat-m.
restlessness: Aco. Ars. Cham.
rush of ideas: Calc-c. **Coff.** Hyo. Ign. Nux-v. Op. Pul.
twitchings: Ars. Bell. Ign. Sul.

DREAMS: Bry. **Chin.** Mag-c. **Nux-v.** Pho. Pul. **Rhus-t.** Sil. Sul.
Comp. **Mind, Fear.**
agreeable: Calc-c. Nat-c. Nux-v. **Op.** Pul. Sep. Stap. Viol-o.
days work, difficulties, etc.: Am-m. Ars. Bry. Nux-v. Pul. **Rhus-t.**
dead, of the: Ars. Mag-c. Pho. Thu.
falling: Thu.
vivid, fire, etc.: Cann. Hyo. **Pho.** Pul. Rhus-t. Sil. Sul.

BLOOD AFFECTED: Ail. Am-c. Ap. Arn. **Ars. Bapt.** Bry. Carb-v. **Chin.** Crot-h. Cup. Elap. **Fer.** Grap. Kali-c. **Kre. Lach.** Merc. **Mur-ac.** Nat-m. Nit-ac. **Pho.** Pul. Pyro. **Rhus-t.** Sec-c. **Sul.** Sul-ac.

BLOODVESSELS.

Aco. **Amy-n. Arn. Ars. Bell.** Carb-v. Chin. Fer. **Flu-ac.** Glo. **Ham. Lach.** Lyc. Pho-ac. **Pul.** Sil. Sul. **Thu. Vip.** Ver-v.

CIRCULATION.

Aco. Ars. Bell. Calc-c. Carb-v. **Fer. Glo.** Hyo. **Lach. Pho. Pul. Rhus-t.** Sep. Spig. **Sul. Thu.** Ver-a.
As if stagnated: Lyc. Saba. Zin.

CONGESTION.

Aco. Arn. Aur. Bell. Bry. Calc-c. Carb-v. **Chin.** Croc. **Fer. Gel. Glo.** Hep. Iod. Kali-c. **Lach.** Melil. **Merc. Nux-v.** Op. **Pho. Pul. Rhus-t. Sep.** Sil. **Sul.** Thu. Ver-v.

HEART BEAT AND PULSE.

AUDIBLE: Ang. Bism. Saba. **Spig. Pul.** Sul.
CEASING, **as if: Aur.** Cic. Dig. Gel.
FULL: **Ant-t. Bell. Bry.** Calc-c. Canth. Colo. Fer. **Fer-ph. Gel. Glo.** Grap. Hep. **Hyo.** Merc. Mez. **Nux-v.** Pho. **Ran-sc. Spo. Stram. Sul. Ver-v.**
HARD: **Aco.** Am-c. **Bell. Bry.** Canth. Chin. Colch. Colo. Fer. Grap. Hep. **Hyo.** Ign. Iod. Mez. **Nit-ac. Nux-v. Pho.** Sil. **Stram.** Sul.
INTERMITTENT: Ars. **Carb-v.** Mur-ac. **Nat-m.** Ver-a.
IRREGULAR: Dig. Op. Ver-a.
LARGE: **Aco.** Pho.
PALPITATION: **Aco.** Ars. Aur. Cact. **Calc-c.** Cham. **Chin.** Dig. **Iod.** Kali-bi. **Lyc. Merc. Nat-m.** Nit-ac. **Nux-v. Pho.**

Pul. Rhus-t. **Sep. Spig. Sul.** Thu. **Ver-a.**

QUICK: **Aco. Ant-t. Ars. Bell.** Glo. **Lach. Nux-v. Pho. Rhus-t.** Spo. **Sul.**

SHAKING THE BODY: Nat-m. Rhus-t.

SLOW: Cic. **Dig.** Gel. Kalm. Stram.

SMALL: **Aco. Ars.** Cam. Carb-v. **Cup.** Hell. **Rhus-t. Ver-a.**

TREMULOUS: Ant-t. Calc-c. **Spig.**

UNEQUAL: Agar.

VISIBLE: Lach. Spi. Sul.

WEAK: **Ant-t. Ars. Carb-v. Mur-ac. Pho-ac.** Rhus-t. **Ver-a.**

CHILL, COLDNESS, ETC.

IN GENERAL: Ant-c. Arn. Aur. **Cam.** Caus. Chin. Chin-s. Eupat. Ip. Lyc. Men. **Mos. Nat-m. Pul.** Saba. Stap. **Ver-a.**

partial: Amb. Ars. **Bell. Bry.** Calc-c. Carb-v. Caus. Cham. Chel. Cist. Coccl. **Ign.** Lyc. Men. **Nux-v. Pul.** Rhus-t. Saba. Sep. **Spig.** Stro. Sul. Thu. **Ver-a.**

onesided: Bar-c. (r). **Bry.** Carb-v. (1). **Caus.** Con. **Dros.** Lyc. **Mos.** Nux-v. **Par. Pul.** Rhus-t. (1). Sabi. (r). Sul. (1). Thu.

external: Ign. Nux-v. **Ver-a.** Zin.

internal: Ars. Calc-c. Laur. Sul.

abdomen: Amb. Ars. Pho. Sep. **Ver-a.**

back: Bell. Caul. **Caus. Coccl.** Eupat. **Gel. Pul. Rhus-t.** Sec-c. Sep.

extremities: Bell. Caus. **Pul.** Sec-c. **Sep.**

affected part: Ang. Bry. **Led. Rhus-t.**

HEAT.

IN GENERAL: Aco. Ant-t. Ap. Ars. Bell. Fer. Nat-m. **Op.** Scil. Sec-c. Sil. Spo. Stram. Comp. **Cold Ameliorates.**

external: Aco. Bell. Canth. **Ign.**

internal: Aco. Ars. Bell. Nux-v. Ver-a.

flushes, in: Calc-c. **Lach.** Pho. Sep. Sul. Sul-ac. Comp. **Wavelike Sensations.**

partial: Am-m. Ars. Bell. **Bry.** Pho. Pho-ac. Sul.

external: Ars. **Bell. Merc.** Pho. Pho-ac. Sul.

internal: Aco. Bell. **Bry. Canth. Laur.** Pho. Sul.

SWEAT.

IN GENERAL, **easy tendency to, etc.:** Agar. Ant-t. **Calc-c. Chin.** Fer. Grap. Hep. **Lach.** Lyc. Merc. Nat-c. **Nat-m.** Nux-v. Op. Pho. **Pho-ac.** Samb. Sep. Stap. Sul. Ver-a.

cold: Ant-t. **Ars.** Cam. **Carb-v.** Chin. Merc-c. Sec-c. **Ver-a.**

on forehead: Ant-t. **Carb-v. Cina. Merc-c.** Op. **Ver-a.**

hot: Bell. **Cham.** Ign. Ip. **Op. Saba.** Sep. Stan. **Stram.** Viol-t.

MATERIA MEDICA

PART II

THE SYNOPSIS

ABROTANUM.

REGION.
NERVES.
Nutrition.

WORSE.
Cold Air. Night.
Checked Secretions.
BETTER.
Motion. Loose Stool (Nat-s. Zinc.)

Numb and weak. Paretic effects. **True metastases.** Receding gout. Alternations; piles alternating with rheumatism (Sabi.) or dysentery, etc. Ascending emaciation. Marasmus.——Cross, irritable children. Pale, hollow-eyed, old face. Nosebleed (youths). Bulimy. Stomach seems to swim in water. **Bloated abdomen.** Weak joints; can't hold up head. Cold, prickling, numb fingers and toes. Emaciated legs. Flabby skin.

Related: Led.

ACONITE.

REGION.
MIND. **Brain.**
NERVES.
HEART.
ARTERIAL CIRCULATION.
VISCERA { CHEST. **Abdomen.** }
Joints.

WORSE.
Violent Emotions { FRIGHT. SHOCK. }
NOISE. LIGHT.
CHILLED BY { **COLD DRY WINDS. When Sweating.** }
Dentition. Lying on side. **Night.**
Toward midnight.
BETTER.
Open Air. Repose. Warm Sweat.

Robust habit. **Sudden, intensely acute effects.** Beside himself from violence of the PAIN, FEAR OR NERVOUS RESTLESSNESS; screams, moans, gnaws the fists, wants to die, etc. **Sticking, tearing pains. Acute congestion;** often apoplectic. **Bright red hemorrhage** (Bell.). **Inflammation.** Convulsions. Parts feel changed, too big, full, **burn, tingle,** prickle or crawl; painful or **numb,** < after the pains (Caus. Cham. Colo. Gnap. Kalm. Mez. Sec-c. Verb.). Neuralgia. Crepitation (Rhe.).——FEAR; **agonizing; of death; of crowds;** obsessed by. Delirium. **Forebodings;** predicts death. Music saddens (Amb.). **Head,** crackling in (Calc-c. Coff.); heavy, outpressing in forehead or eyes; throbs in l. forehead (r. Ant-t. Bell. Ign.); aches, with more urine; burning in. Shooting in eyeballs.

Numb nose; with epistaxis (Bell. Med.). Coryza. ANXIOUS LOOK (Spo.). **Hot, irregularly red face;** pales on rising. **Faintness.** Toothache. Everything tastes bitter. Chokes on swallowing. BURNING THIRST; craves acids, beer; < after ices. Violent, bilious or bloody vomitus. **Stools of pure blood; slimy, grass green or white;** < hot days and cold nights. Dysentery. Itching sticking at anus. Retained, scanty, red or bloody urine. Cystitis. Dysuria. Orchitis. Short, hard, anxious breath; **sits** erect. **Dry, hoarse, painful cough;** must grasp larynx (Aru-t. Cep. Iod. Naj. Pho.); < night; drinking. Laryngitis. Raises blood. Pneumonia. Croup. Stitches in chest. . Pleurisy. Powerless legs. DRY, HOT SKIN or as of ice water on it. **Restless and sleepless.** Palpitation; with cutting in l. arm. Rapid or tumultuous pulse; **hard and forcible or thready. Arterial** tension (Ver-v.). Carditis. Chilliness; alternating with heat. HIGH FEVER. **Burning heat;** in eyelids; lungs (Tub.); **on palms.**

Complementary: Sul. Related: Bell. Cham. Coff.

AESCULUS.

REGION.

Veins { RECTUM. LIVER.

Mucous Membranes. Occiput.

LUMBAR REGION.

Right Side.

WORSE.

Morning on Awaking. After Stool.

Motion. Walking.

BETTER.

COOL OPEN AIR. Cool Bathing.

Continued Exertion.

INTERNAL DRYNESS, BURNING OR ROUGHNESS. Sticking pains. **Full, congested or paralyzed feeling.** Parts purple, puffy. Venous stasis. Varicose veins.——**Irritable.** Crushing in occiput. Follicular pharyngitis. Leucorrhœa. **Hard, dry stool. Full, sore rectum; as if filled with sticks** (Nit-ac. Sanic.); after stool (Agar.). As of a bug crawling from anus. **Painful, purple, external piles; with** BACKACHE. Laming pain in **small of back; it gives out; repeated efforts at rising** (Agar. Petr. Sul.); < walking.

Related: Bry. Collin. Pul.

AETHUSA.

REGION.

BRAIN. STOMACH.

Liver. Nerves.

WORSE.

MILK. Hot Weather.

Too Frequent Eating.

Sudden, violent weakness. Complaints that cause speechlessness. **Convulsive effects.** Parts feel screwed together. Cutting pains.——Headache,

> passing flatus. Eyes turn down. **Deathly countenance.** WHITE LINEA NASALIS (Ip.). Tongue feels too long. DEATHLY NAUSEA. **VOMITS MILK IN LARGE, HARD CURDS** (Calc-c. Sanic. Val.), **THEN LIMPNESS AND DEEP SLEEP** (Ant-t.). Digestion ceases from brain exhaustion. Cholera infantum. Stomach seems turned upside down. Bubbling at navel. Eruptions that itch from heat. Ecchymoses. Cool, clammy skin. Heat without thirst. Sweat with aversion to uncovering.
Complementary: Calc-c. Related: Ant-c.

AGARICUS.

REGION.

SPINAL AXIS { OCCIPUT. / **NERVES.** / Lumbar Region.

Heart.
Chest.

WORSE.

AIR { COLD. FREEZING. / OPEN. Stormy.

Exhaustion { **Mental.** / Debauchery. / **Coition.**

Alcohol. Pressure. Touch.
Morning. During Menses.

BETTER.

Gentle Motion.

Gradual onset. **Many symptoms** (Tub.). IRREGULAR, UNCERTAIN AND EXAGGERATED MOTIONS (Ign.); he reaches too far, steps too high, drops things, etc. **TREMBLING, TWITCHING, JERKING or fibrillar spasm; < EYELIDS.** Restlessness. Chorea. Pains with coldness or crawling; as of cold needles, a cold drop or a weight on parts.——Hilarious or dull and dizzy, as if drunk. **Turns head to and fro.** Headache > after stool or urine. Oscillating eyeballs. Musca volitantes. Angle of mouth droops. **As of a lump in epigastrium.** Rumbling and fermenting in bowels. Hot flatus or semen; cold urine. Isolated coughing attacks, then sneezing; seemingly from spine (Tel.); easy expectoration of flocculi or balls of mucus. Indistinct, jerky speech. Pressure or burning sticking from heart to left scapula. Angina pectoris, has excessive pain only. Metastases from suppressed milk. Shooting burning along spine; stiff; seems short on stooping. **Sensitive spine** (Chin. Cimi. Hyp. Ign. Zin.) > pressure. **BURNING-ITCHING** (Ap.), **< IN SKIN; AS IF FROZEN**; changing place on scratching. Chilblains (Abrot. Hep. Petr.). **Yawning**; before pains or spasms. Chills or sweats easily. Sweats on alternate sides. Night sweats.
Complementary: Calc-c. Related: **Phys. Tub.**

AGNUS CASTUS.

REGION.
SEXUAL ORGANS. MIND.
Nerves. Eyes.

WORSE.
VENERY. **Sprains.**

IMPOTENCY AND PREMATURE OLD AGE. **Jaded rakes.**——BAD MEMORY. Sad and despairing; repeats that he will soon die. Cold, relaxed genitals. Gnawing-itching. Agalactia.

Related: Pho-ac.

AILANTHUS.

REGION.
BLOOD. THROAT. **Skin. Mind.**

WORSE.
Sight of Food. Raising Up.

Rapidly prostrated. LIVIDITY, STUPOR AND MALIGNANCY.——Faintness on rising. **Foul, acrid discharges;** from nose. Sordes on teeth. Throat livid and swelled. Deep ulcers stud the tonsils. Lacunar tonsilitis. Diphtheria. **Eruptions in dark, spare patches.** Mottled skin. Scarlatina. Crawling over body.

Related: Bapt.

ALETRIS.

REGION.
Female Organs (r). **Blood.**

WORSE.
Loss of fluids.

BETTER.
Passing Flatus. Bending Backward.

Debility. Always tired. **Heaviness in many parts.** Uterine reflexes. Hemorrhages. Anæmia.——Frothy saliva. The least food **distresses.** Abdominal colic. Constipation. Early, profuse menses.

Related: Chin. Trill.

ALOE.

REGION.
ABDOMINAL VEINS { **RECTUM. LIVER. Intestines.**
Female Organs. **Lumbar Region.**

WORSE.
HEAT. **Summer.**
Early Morning (in Bed).
Stepping Hard.

BETTER.
Cool Open Air.

Relaxation; parts seem full and heavy (Lil-tig.). DRAGGING, AS OF A HEAVY LOAD. **Drawing.**——Heavy pressure on vertex. Headache alternating with abdominal symptoms (Calc-ph.). Pain from navel to rectum (Crot-t. Dios.). Heavy lower abdomen (Am-m. Grap. Nux-v. Sep.). A plug seems wedged into pelvis. **GURGLING IN BOWELS; SUDDEN URGING; THE RECTUM FEELS INSECURE, THEN THE PATIENT HURRIEDLY PASSES A GUSHING, WATERY STOOL. Diarrhœa.** Stool escapes with the flatus (Old.) or when urinating (Mur-ac.). Passes a solid stool unnoticed (Caus.). Urging to stool; passes flatus only (Carb-a. Carb-v. Mag-m. Nat-c. Pho. Sep.). **Gelatinous** (Colch. Kali-bi. Sep.) **or lumpy stools. Prolapsing piles,** like a bunch of grapes, > cold bathing. **Internal heat.** Hot stool or flatus. Burning in anus, rectum, piles, etc. Heat in skin.

Related: Sul.

ALUMINA.

REGION.

CORD { LUMBAR. RECTUM. **Lower Limbs.** }

MIND.

Mucous Membranes.

Skin.

WORSE.

WARM { ROOM. **Bed.** }

Foods { **Potatoes.** Artificial. }

Using Voice. Early on awaking. After Menses. **Dry Weather.** **Sitting.**

BETTER.

Evening.

Moderate { Exertion. Temperature. }

Open Air.

Scratching until it **bleeds.**

Dry, thin, wrinkled, inactive and inclined to lie down. PARALYTIC LOSS OF POWER. **Dry mucous membranes.** Scanty, thick, acrid discharges (Hyds.). Sensory illusions; of being larger, numb, heavy, etc. **Chronicity.** ——**Hasty,** but slow of execution, hence makes mistakes in speaking, writing, etc. **Timorous;** fears his own impulses; the sight of knives; the loss of reason, etc. Bad memory. Dry, falling hair. Weak eyelids. **Double** squint; <dentition. Inflamed, burning eyes. Old look. As of white of egg or a cobweb on face (Bar-c. Bor. Brom. Grap. Ran-sc. Sul-ac.). Toothache, pain extends to other parts (Kali-bi.). Twitching of lower jaw (Gels.). Uvula hangs down. Throat feels full of sticks or constricted. Craves coarse food. **Inactive rectum and bladder;** must strain to pass a soft stool;

hard ones cause severe cutting. **Must strain at stool to urinate** (Alo. Lil-t. Tub.); **slow flow** (Hep. Zin.). Increased sexual desire. Dry, hacking cough, with sneezing. Sudden loss of voice. As of a hot iron thrust through spine. Heavy lower limbs staggering (Calc-c. Nat-c. Pic-ac. Pul. Sul.). Locomotor ataxia (Gel.). Gnawing under nails (Lach. Lappa.). Bones feel squeezed. Dry, rough skin. Induration. Intolerable itching from heat of bed. Chilliness, > open air. Heat, with itching.

Related: Bry. Plumb.

AMBRA.

REGION.	WORSE.
NERVES { Pneumogastric. Spinal.	SLIGHT CAUSES { AGITATION. PRESENCE OF OTHERS. Embarrassment. Thinking of it. Music.
Mind.	Warmth. **Old Age.** Warm Milk.
Female Organs.	
One Side.	

WORN OUT, YET OVERIMPRESSIONABLE NERVES. Early senility. **Slight things affect the breathing and heart, start the menses, etc.** Symptoms suddenly change place; asleep, numb feeling (in spots), twitchings, itchings, trembling, ebullitions, etc. General pulsation.——Dreamy, flitting ideas. Fixed, disagreeable fancies. Slow grasp. Sadness. Vertigo. Coldness in abdomen. **Flatulency. Can't tolerate the presence of others when urinating** (Hep. Nat-m.) **or during stool;** < during pregnancy. Spasmodic cough; then eructation (Ver-a.). Bluish white expectoration. **Sense of a lump in left chest** (Am-m. Tarax.). **Palpitation. Sleeplessness.**

Complementary: Mos. Related: Ign.

AMMONIUM CARB.

REGION.	WORSE.
HEART. CIRCULATION.	**COLD** { WET. WASHING. RAW OR OPEN AIR.
Blood. Lungs.	Falling Asleep. 3-4 A. M.
RESPIRATION.	DURING MENSES. Motion.
Right Side.	BETTER.
	PRESSURE. Lying on Abdomen.

LOW VITALITY. LIVID, WEAK, DROWSY AND WANTING IN RE-

ACTION (Ant-t.). Old people. **Averse to cold. Internal burning-rawness. Acrid, hot secretions. Dark, thin hemorrhage.** Scorbutic states. Malignancy.——Sad. Peevish. **Brain feels loose. Shocks thro head on biting** teeth together. Pulsation. Bursting fulness in forehead. **Nose stops up at night** (Ant-c. Lyc.) **or bleeds if face and hands are washed** (Kali-c.). Loose teeth. Sensitive, bleeding gums. Menses with choleraic symptoms (Sil.); dark, lumpy, flow, < night; ending with dyspnœa. **Shortness of breath,** > cool air (Carb-v.). Rattling in chest, but gets up little. **WEAK HEART,** causing stasis, dyspnœa, emphysema, etc. **Palpitation;** with cold sweat and lachrymation. Bones ache as weather changes (Calc-ph.). Red or mottled skin. Scarlatina. Coldness.

Related: Carb-v. Glo. Lach. Mur-ac.

AMMONIUM MUR.

REGION.
MUCOUS MEMBRANES { CHEST. **Gall Ducts.**
Blood.
Female Organs.

WORSE.
Morning (Head, Chest).
Afternoon (Abdomen).
Evening (Skin, Fever, Limbs).
Sprains (Chronic).
BETTER.
Open Air. Rapid Motion.

Fat and puffy, with thin limbs (Ant-c.). **Irregular circulation; ebullitions, burnings or localized throbbings.** Many symptoms are accompanied by cough or PROFUSE SECRETIONS. GLAIRY CATARRHS. **Tightness, as if too short; tendons,** hamstrings, lumbar region, etc. Tired and sore. Festering pain.——A rough body obstructs upper nares (Rut.). Acrid, watery coryza; closing one nostril. Anosmia. Pulsation in tonsils. Tense, sprained feeling in groins; must walk bent. Prolapsus uteri. Scanty, hard, crumbling stools; changing color. Blood from anus or diarrhœa during menses. Polyuria. Cough, with salivation (Am-c.) or liver symptoms. Can't breathe for coughing. **Noisy, rattling, tenacious mucus in chest.** Cough with salivation. Bronchial catarrh. Hoarseness, with burning in larynx. Pulsating, burning spots in chest. **Swelled cervical glands. Soreness or coldness between scapulæ** (Caps. Lachn. Petr.). Lumbago. Desquamation between fingers. **Sciatica < sitting > lying.** Ulcer on heel. Chilly as often as he wakes. Sense of heat; > open air; alternating with chill.

Related: **Caus.**

AMYL NIT.

REGION.
VASO MOTOR NERVES { **CIRCULATION. HEAD. Heart.**
Respiration.

WORSE.
CLIMACTERIC. Emotions.
Heat. Close Room.

FLUSHINGS; then drenching (unilateral) sweat.——Surging of blood to head. Easy blushing. **Throbbings.** Migraine with pallor (Ars.). Constriction at heart. Tumultuous palpitation. Stretching and yawning with hiccough.

Related: Glo. **Lach.**

ANACARDIUM.

REGION.
MIND.
NERVES { Stomach. **Skin.** Palms.
Muscles.
Joints.

WORSE.
MENTAL EXERTION.
Emotions { **Anger,** etc. Fright.
Motion. **Stepping Hard.** Drafts.
Open Air. Cold. 4 P. M.
BETTER.
While Eating. Hot bathing.

Tremulous weakness, on slight exertion, < knees (Staph.) or arms. DULL PRESSURE, **as of a plug or a band. Blunting of one of the senses, sight,** hearing, touch, etc. Paralysis.——FAILING MEMORY; **suddenly forgets,** names, etc. Brain fag. As if in a dream (Nux-m. Ver-a.). **Illusions or fixed ideas;** imagines others present, behind her (Brom. Med. Sanic.), etc. **Ill natured** and cowardly. Vascillating; at odds with himself (Bar-c.). **Pressure in temples.** Illusory smells. **Bad breath and taste. Stiff, swelled tongue. The rectum seems plugged. Breath stops on coughing or drinking. Cough with pain in occiput** (Fer.), **then yawns and sleeps.** Occasional double stitch at heart; pain goes into lumbar region. **Heaviness, as of a load, on shoulders** (Lach. Pho. Pul. Stap. Sul.). **Insensible skin** (Arg-n.). Yellow itching vesicles. Eczema. **Easily chilled, > sunshine** (Stro.). Clammy sweat on palms.

Related: **Ign. Rhus-t.**

ANTHRACIN.

REGION.
Cellular Tissue.

Terrible burning pains, with much prostration. **Malignancy. Sepsis. Carbuncle.** Quinsy. Succession of boils. Black or blue blisters. Gangrene.

Related: Ars. Taren-cu.

ANTIMONIUM CRUDUM.

REGION.
STOMACH.
DIGESTIVE TRACT.
MIND.
SKIN.
Changing Sides.

WORSE.
COLD { BATHING. WATER (on Head). Dampness. }
OVEREATING.
HEAT { SUMMER. Of Sun. **Being Overheated.** Radiated. }
IF LOOKED AT OR TOUCHED.
Motion. Sour Foods.

Gross feeders, with gastric and skin symptoms. LUMPY EFFECTS; stool, leucorrhœa, skin, nails. Unexpected absence of pain. Gouty metastases (Abrot.).——FRETFUL, PEEVISH (Sul.); **children cry if looked at, touched** (Cham.) or washed. **Loathing;** of life, food, etc. **Ecstatic, dreamy state.** Red, moist canthi (ext.) (Grap.). Sore, scabby nostrils. Pimples about mouth (Ast-r.). TONGUE THICKLY COATED LIKE WHITEWASH (Bism. Cob.). No thirst. **DISORDERED STOMACH;** food leaves an after taste or causes belching. VOMITING; after eating or drinking; without nausea or relief. Stomach is painful to pressure. Gout of stomach. **Fulness in abdomen. Watery stool,** mixed with lumps. Gastro-intestinal catarrh. Aphonia from overheating. Violent cough, each bout grows a little weaker. Horny or split nails; growths beneath. Gouty pain in fingers. Footsweat, wilting the skin. **Callosities on soles (Bar-c.** Grap. Sep. Sil.). Eruptive tendency. Honey colored crusts (Viol-t.). Warts. **Sleepy and weary.**

Related: Sul.

ANTIMONIUM TART.

REGION.

PNEUMO- | **GASTRIC** | **NERVE** — BRONCHI. **LUNGS.** HEART. **RESPIRATION.**

STOMACH. BOWELS.

CIRCULATION. SLEEP.

Lumbar Region.

Skin.

WORSE.

WARM — ROOM. WRAPS. WEATHER.

ANGER. LYING DOWN.

Morning. Overeating.

Cold. Dampness.

BETTER.

Motion. Expectoration.

Depression. WEAK, DROWSY, RELAXED AND LACKING IN REACTION. MUCH SECRETION OF MUCUS. Complaints arising in digestive sphere. Old people and children.——**Apathetic** or easily annoyed; wants to be let alone. Whining and moaning. Waning consciousness on closing eyes. Sooty looking nostrils (Hell.). Sickly, sunken, pale, bluish or twitching face; covered with cool sweat. Papillæ show thro white coat on tongue. Craves acids, which disagree. Eructations like bad eggs. NAUSEA; waves of; **with weakness and cold sweat** (Lach.), **loathing** or anxiety. **Forcible vomiting** (Nux-v.); then exhaustion and sleep (Aeth.). Retching. Sinking at stomach (Lob.). Gastroses. Mucous or grass green stools. **Diarrhœa;** of eruptive diseases. **Unequal breathing. SUFFOCATIVE SHORTNESS OF BREATH;** a leaflet seems over trachea. **LOOSE, COARSE, RATTLING COUGH, THE CHEST SEEMS FULL, YET LITTLE IS RAISED** (Tub. Ver-a.); then vomiting or sleep; $<$ anger. Coughs and yawns alternately. Thick expectoration. Capillary bronchitis. Paralytic depression of heart and lungs (Bar-c.). **Violent (lumbar) backache;** motion excites retching and cold sweat. Restless arms. Dropsy of legs. SOMNOLENCY; from warmth. **Torpid, cool,** SWEATY SKIN. **Delayed,** blue or pustular eruptions. Weak, quick pulse.

Complementary: Bar-c. Related: Ascl. Ip.

APIS.

<table>
<tr>
<td>
REGION.
CELLULAR TISSUES { EYES. FACE. FAUCES. Ovaries.
SKIN. SEROUS CAVITIES.
Kidneys. Nerves.
Respiration.
RIGHT SIDE.
</td>
<td>
WORSE.
HEAT { ROOM. Weather. Fire. Bed. Drinks.
Touch. After Sleep. 4 P. M.
BETTER.
COOL { AIR. Bathing. Uncovering.
Motion. Slight Expectoration.
</td>
</tr>
</table>

Violent onset. SHARP STINGING, **itching-burning** (Agar. Bell. Ign. Merc.) **or bruised, sore pain.** Stiffness. Saccular (Ars.) or **puffy swelling** (Pho.). Rapid effusion. Oedema (Rhus-t.). Infections. Inflammation.——Irritable, fidgety or apathetic. Absent-minded. SUDDEN PIERCING SHRIEKS. ROLLS THE HEAD (Zin.). Stabbing head pains. **Numb,** tired headache. Painful hair. **Red eyes.** Puffy conjunctiva. Profuse, hot tears. Photophobia; yet can't bear coverings. Blindness, > stool. **Puffy face, < about eyes,** or waxy pallor. Tongue raw; as if burnt; sore or vesicles on edge; swelled; red. Mouth and anus feel raw. Glazed or **trans**lucent pharynx; >cold things. **Oedema of uvula** (Kali-bi. Rhus-t.). **Angina.** Diphtheria (Pho.). ABSENCE OF THIRST. **Bruised, sore, painful abdomen.** Anasarca (Ars. Lyc.). Yellow or tomato sauce stools, < motion. Anus swelled. oozing blood or stands open (Pho.). Burning urination. Dysuria. Scant urine; coffee grounds sediment. Nephritis. Bruised numbness in ovaries. Feels as if he could not breathe again (Bell. Helo.). Stitches backward from apex of heart. Pale, **rosy redness or rough eruption on skin.** Erysipelas. Scarlet fever. Skin alternately dry and hot or sweating. Sleepy, but too nervous. CRYING OUT (Hyo. Lyc. Zin.); **with sopor.** Kicks off bed covers. Weak, quick pulse. Very sensitive skin. Irregular temperature of skin. Chill with smothering, urticaria or desire to uncover. BURNING HEAT; **without thirst.** Gushes of sweat.
Complementary: Arn. Merc-cy. **Nat-m.** Related: Ars. Canth. Pul. Urt-ur.

APOCYNUM.

REGION.	WORSE.
URINARY ORGANS.	COLD { WEATHER. DRINKS.
Digestive Tract.	Uncovering. Lying.
Heart. Uterus.	

Tendency to weakness and dropsy. Irritation of digestive tract and kidneys. Great thirst, but water distresses and is vomited; with scanty discharges. Sinking at stomach. Loose bowels with dropsy. Uterine hemorrhage, followed by dropsy (Chin.). Rough, dry skin.

Related: Ars.

ARANEA DIADEMA.

REGION.	WORSE.
NERVES.	COLD DAMPNESS. BATHING.
Blood.	EXACT PERIODICITY.
Bones.	BETTER.
	Smoking.

Can't get warm. Feels cold to the very bones (Calc-c.). Every damp day chills. SENSE OF ENORMOUS ENLARGEMENT, **or numbness of parts.** Hemorrhage. Periostitis.——Violent pains in all the upper teeth at once, on retiring. Enlarged spleen. Malaria.

Related: Cedron.

ARGENTUM MET.

REGION.	WORSE.
Nerves.	USING VOICE. **Mental Strain.**
Cartilages Mucous Membranes { LARYNX. Throat. Joints. Genito Urinary.	**Noon. Cold Damp.** Coughing.
Left Side: Ovary. Testis (r).	BETTER.
	Motion. Wrapping Up.
	Coffee.

Slow, low grade processes. **Thickened secretions,** cartilages, eyelids, etc. **Gray or tenacious mucus. Sore rawness.** Increasingly violent pains, suddenly ceases; < touch; with polyuria. Arthralgia. **Loss of power;** mental, over limbs, etc. Epilepsy then rage.——Talkative and **forgetful.** Whirling vertigo. Emptiness or crawling in head. Itching canthi, eyelids or earlobes. Exhaustingly profuse coryza. **Pale, sallow and weak.** Croaking in abdomen (1). Emissions. Chronic urethritis (Alu. Sul.). Foul leucorrhœa (Kali-ar. Kali-p.). **Easily raises gray, gelatinous or**

starchy mucus; < laughing. Hoarseness. Aphonia. Weakness in chest (1). Heart stops, then trembles and throbs; > inspiration. Swelled ankles. Diabetes. Shocks on falling asleep.

Related: Sele. Stan. Zin.

ARGENTUM NIT.

REGION.

MIND. NERVES { Sensory. **ABDOMINAL.** Brain. Spine.

MUCOUS MEMBRANES { **STOMACH.** Bowels. **Eyes. Larynx.** **Throat.** Urethra.

Bones.

Left Side.

WORSE.

EMOTIONS { ANXIETY. SUSPENSE.

IN ROOM. SUGAR.

Brain Fag.

Drinking. **Light.** Crowds.

Night. Lying on Right Side.

BETTER.

COOL { AIR. Bath. **Open Air.**

Motion. **Hard Pressure** (bandage).

Looks old and dried up. Parts seem enlarged or bound. Aching or numb spots. Uncertain gait. **Deep sticking,** like a splinter (Hep.) or sharp radiating pains, like lightning; causing starting (Lyc.). **Ulceration, with much pus** (Calc-c.)——Strange ideas or emotions. **Anxious fear;** with weakness (Ars.); of ordeals, passing a certain point (Gel. Kali-br.), etc. **Impulsive and hurried,** yet timid. Faltering speech. VERTIGO. Compressive or deep head pains; he loses his senses. Migraine. Eyeballs feel too big (Guai. Mez. Nat-m. Par. Rhus-t. Spo.). **Swelled carunculæ;** chemosis. Photophobia. Violent ophthalmia. Dilated pupils. Sickly, **gray**ish-muddy color. Painful, red tip of tongue. Bitter-sour taste and vomitus. As of a rough stick (Phyt.) or splinter in throat; > cool drinks. CRAVES SUGAR, which disagrees. Gastralgia. Alcoholic gastritis. Belches up the ingesta. FLATULENCE; **as if abdomen would burst** (Lyc.); **loud explosive belching** (Coca.) **or noisy stools. Emotional diarrhœa. Shreddy, mucous stools,** turning green (Sanic.); < drinking. Cutting in urethra with painful priapism. Gonorrhœa. Painful coition (Lyc. Nat-m.). Palpitation < lying on r. side (Alu. Lil-t.). **Craves fresh air.** Laryngitis. Throbbing or weakness in spine. Trembling limbs. Weakness, rigidity or twisting in calves. Blueness. Chilly if uncovered, yet smothers when wrapped up.

Complementary: Nat-m. Related: Lyc. Pul.

ARNICA.

REGION.

BLOODVESSELS.
BLOOD.
NERVES.
Muscles.
Digestive Organs.

WORSE.

INJURY { BRUISES. **SHOCK.** Jar. CONCUSSION. OVEREXERTION. }

TOUCH. **After Sleep. Motion.**

BETTER.

Lying { **With Head Low. Stretched Out.** }

VERY PAINFUL EFFECTS. FEELS SORE. EASILY BRUISED; THE BED SEEMS TOO HARD (Psor. Pyrog.) **or as if full of lumps.** As of a lump in affected part. Crushing pains. RESTLESS AND PROSTRATE. Paralytic or suddenly shifting joint pains. INVOLUNTARY EVACUATIONS. FOULNESS. TYPHOID OR HEMORRHAGIC TENDENCY; soreness of bleeding part (Ferr.). Congestions.——Nervous, impressionable, sensitive, sanguine temperament. **Fearful; of being struck or approached** (Plb.).; of sickness; with horror of instant death; on awaking. Morose, repellant mood. Mentally apathetic, yet physically restless; **says nothing ails him.** Answers slowly and with mental effort. **Vertigo.** The brain feels tired.. **Blood shot eyes** (Aco. Nux-v.). Red, congested face; apoplexy, fever, etc. Foul breath. Bad taste. Eructations like bad eggs (Plant.). Retained or dribbling urine; after labor. **After pains;** $<$ suckling. Very painful cough; child cries, then coughs then cries. **Sore nipples** (Phyt.). **Many** very sore, but small boils (Sec-c. Tab.). Heart beat shakes the whole body. **Itching, crawling,** changing place when scratched. Dusky, mottled skin. BLACK AND BLUE SPOTS (Sec-c.). Petechiæ. Painful, symmetrical eruptions. Erysipelas. **Sopor;** drops to sleep as he answers. Troublous or frightful dreams. Awakes in terror. Coldness of part lain on. Thirst during chill.

Complementary: Calc-c. Nat-s. Sul-ac. Related: **Bellis. Rhus-t.**

ARSENICUM.

REGION.

MUCOUS MEMBRANES.
MIND.
RESPIRATION.
Nerves.
Blood.
Muscles.
SKIN.
Serous Cavities.
Organs.

WORSE.

COLD { ICES. DRINKS. / FOODS. **Air.** }
PERIODICALLY { **MIDNIGHT:** after. / AFTER 2 A. M. / **14 Days. Yearly.** }
VEGETABLES. EXERTION.
DRINKING. TIPPLING.
Eruptions { Undeveloped. / Suppressed. Quinine. }
Lying on **Painful Part.** **Tobacco.**

BETTER.

HOT { APPLICATIONS. / FOOD. **Drinks.** }
Motion. Walking About.
Company.
ELEVATING HEAD.
Sitting Erect.

Intense effects. PAINS BURNING, LIKE FIRE (Carb-v. Kre. Pho. Sul.); OF MADDENING SEVERITY; **exciting shortness of breath;** felt during sleep (Nit-ac.); like hot **needles** or wire (Ap. Spig. Vesp.); > **heat** (Alu. Carb-v. Lyc.). Neuralgias. IRRITABLE WEAKNESS (Cimi.). **REMARKABLY PROSTRATED. VERY RESTLESS.** ACRID, SCANTY WATERY SECRETIONS. PUTRID, CADAVERIC ODORS. MALIGNANCY. Infections. **Rapid emaciation. Baggy swellings.** Dropsy. Anæmia.——**Oversensitive. Fastidious. Faultfinding.** ANGUISH, **despair of recovery** (Aco.); AGONIZING FEAR; OF DEATH, **yet tired of living. Desperate. Destructive.** Self torture. **Suicidal impulses** (Nux-v.). **Congestion to head,** > cold (Bell. Glon. Zin.), but neuralgia > heat. **Pain alternating between head and body** (Cina. Gel.). **Restless head. Early** grayness (Lyc. Nat-m. Pho-ac.). Spasm of eyelids. **Burning tears.** Scrophulous ophthalmia. **Takes cold easily. Sneezing, with biting, watery coryza.** Sensitive smell; **can't bear odor or sight of food. Pale, anxious, sunken, haggard or distorted countenance; with cold sweat.** Toothache on retiring. **INSATIABLE, BURNING THIRST; FOR ICE COLD WATER** (Chin. Merc-c. Rhus-t.); **IT DISTRESSES THE STOMACH** (Nux-v.) **AND HE VOMITS AT ONCE. DRINKS LITTLE BUT OFTEN.** Gastritis. **Vomiting with purging.** Small, acrid, burning, black, mucous or lienteric stools. Scanty urine. Profuse, acrid leucorrhœa. SHORTNESS OF BREATH; felt in nose (Kre. Lach. Pul. Sul.); must sit up; < receding eruptions or ascending. **Asthma. Weak heart. Palpitation;** < slight causes. Bites the nails (Senec. Stram.). Alternate cutaneous and internal symptoms (Crot-t.). **Dry, rough, dirty, shrivelled or seared looking skin.** Free desquamation. Eczema. **Ulcerative tendency;** burning ulcers (Sil.). Phagedena. Shocks on dropping to sleep (Nit-ac. Op.). **Restless sleep.** External coldness with internal burning heat. Irregular chill, with thirst for hot drinks. Coldness in chest (Bry. Lach. Nat-c. Sul.). As of hot water in veins. Hectic. Sweat with insatiable thirst, dyspnœa and exhaustion. Incomplete malaria.

Complementary: Nat-s **Pul.** Thu. Related: Ver-a.

ARSENICUM IODATUM.

REGION.

MUCOUS MEMBRANES { **NOSE.** DIGESTIVE TRACT. **Lungs.** }

Glands. **Heart.** Nerves. Skin.

WORSE.

DRY Weather. Exertion.

Cold { Wind. Weather. }

Profuse catarrhal, mostly acrid, burning, corrosive discharges; thin in acute or thick (Hyds.) in chronic affections. Sense of rawness. Scrofula. Consumptiveness (Tub.). Debility.——**Dull, heavy headache, < in occiput** Acrid, foul otorrhœa. **Persistent but unsatisfactory sneezing; discharge** reddens the upper lip. **Shortness of breath. Air hunger.** Postnasal catarrh. Hay fever. Psoriasis. Rapid, irritable pulse. Night sweats.

Complementary: Kali-io. Related: Kali-bi.

ARUM TRIPHYLLUM.

REGION.

Mucous Membranes { THROAT. **Larynx.** }

Kidneys. Blood. Brain. Skin.

WORSE.

TALKING. Heat.

IRRITATION. PAINFUL SORENESS, RAWNESS, (Arg.) **AND BURNING,** CORRODING DISCHARGES.——Excessive crossness (Tub.). **PERSISTENT BORING INTO NOSE, OR PICKING AT LIPS** (Kali-br. Taren.) **OR AT ONE SPOT** (Hell.), **UNTIL IT BLEEDS** (Cina. Pho.). **Acrid, fluent coryza.** Raw, cracked lips (angles) (Psor.). Mouth painfully inflamed. Aphthæ. **Painful clearing of throat; grasps it or wants to scratch it.** **Diphtheria.** **Stools like cornmeal.** **Hoarseness. Voice breaks (Sep.).** Itching of fingers and toes. Pemphigus (Cop. Manc. Ran-b.).

Complementary: **Nit-ac.** **Related: Ars. Merc-c.**

ASAFOETIDA.

REGION.
NERVES. DIGESTIVE TRACT.
BONES { Tibia. Nose. Ear.

WORSE.
NIGHT. **In Room.** At Rest.
Eating. Noise. **Suppressions.**
Mercury.
BETTER.
Motion in Open Air.

Full, rugged persons, but who are intolerably nervous and oversensitive. Clavus. Globus. Hysteria. **Pains extend outward, are associated with numbness** and change their place or are eased by touch. **Sharp stitches.** Terrible throbbings. **Boring** pains. Foul, thin, acrid secretions.——**Face** is **puffy** and purple, as if heated. **Greasy taste.** **Spasm of œsophagus and stomach.** RANCID OR EXPLOSIVE ERUCTATIONS (**Arg-n.**). **FLAT-ULENCE**; pressing upward. **Reverse peristalis.** **Wind colic.** **Foul, dark,** watery diarrhœa. Indigestion. **Spasmodic tightness of chest (Ign.).** **Full, distended feeling at heart.** **Dark, red swellings.** **Bluish ulcers (Lach.) with thick edges.** **Burrowing pus** (Sil.). Caries.

Related: Sumb.

ASARUM.

REGION.
NERVES.
MUCOUS MEMBRANES.
Female Genitals.

WORSE.
PENETRATING **SOUNDS.**
Dry Cold. **Emotions.**
BETTER.
Cold Bathing of **Face.**

EXCESSIVE NERVOUS SENSIBILITY; **scratching on silk, the rattle of paper, etc., is unbearable** (Cop. Lil-t.). **Lightness; as if floating on air** Violent vomiting. **Shreddy** mucous stools. Lientery.

Related: Arg-n. **Castor.**

ASCLEPIAS TUBEROSA.

REGION.

SECRETIONS { SKIN. **Serous.** Mucous.

CHEST. Muscles.

WORSE.

Breathing deeply. Lying.

Colliquative states (Agar.) **SWEATING; with pleuro-pneumonia or diarrhœa.** Stools smell like rotten eggs or burn like fire. **Pleurodynia.**

Related: Ant-t.

ASTERIAS RUBENS.

REGION.

CIRCULATION. NERVES.

Female { **Genitals.** Mammæ. Rectum.

WORSE.

Heat. Menses. Contradiction.

Lancinating pains. Cancer.——Weeps from the least emotion. Congestion in head; it feels surrounded by hot air (Flu-ac. Plant. Pul. Ver-a.). **Pimples about mouth.** Stools of brown gushing water. Sexual excitement.

Related: Sep.

AURUM.

REGION.

MIND.

VASCULAR SYSTEM { HEART. CIRCULATION.

Bones { **Nasal.** Patellæ. Joints.

Glands. Liver.

WORSE.

EMOTIONS { DEPRESSING. DISORDERED. AFFECTIONS.

Mental Exertion. COLD.

NIGHT. Sunset to Sunrise.

BETTER.

Cool { Open Air. Bathing.

Becoming Warm. Walking.

Vaso-motor mobility, with strong ebullitions and venous congestions, especially to head and chest. Vascularity. **Weakened,** but sensitive to pain. Wandering pains that impel motion and finally attack the heart (Lach.). Boring, cutting osteocopic pains. Mercurio-syphlitic dyscrasia. Indurations. Hard glands. Necrosis. As of air blowing on part.——INTENSE AND HOPELESS MENTAL DEPRESSION (Lyc. Sul.). **Brooding melancholy;** alternating with irritability. Praying and self condemnation. SUICIDAL ANGUISH; starting from the heart. **Vexed mood; enraged by** the least contradiction (Helo.). Rapid questioning. Afraid of the least noise. Violent confusing headache. Sore orbitis. **Congested, bluish red** face. Tearing in zygomæ. Red, knobby nose. **Ozœna** (Calc-c. Cad-s. Nit-ac. Thu.). Foul breath. Bulimy. Soreness over liver (Aur-mur.). Hepatitis. Jaundice of pregnancy. Liver, with heart symptoms. **Crushing weight under sternum,** < ascending (Am-c.). **Dyspnœa. Oppression** at heart; as if it would stop, then gives one hard thump. **Violent palpitation;** at puberty. Cardiac hypertrophy. **Angina pectoris.** Sweat about genitals.

Related: Merc.

BAPTISIA.

REGION.

BLOOD. **MIND.** Nerves.

Mucous Membranes { **Digestive Tract.**

WORSE.

Humid Heat. Fogs. **In Room.**

On Awaking. Pressure.

RAPID PROSTRATION. **Restless and sore; the bed is too hard, yet he feels too sick to move.** VERY FOUL DISCHARGES. Zymoses. **Typhoid states.——Dull and confused.** Sense of duality; **parts of body seem scattered about** or too large. Eyes feel swelled. DUSKY, BESOTTED COUNTENANCE (Crot-h. Gel. Op.). Fetor oris. SORDES. Aphthæ. Tongue feels thick, is heavily coated or has a dark stripe down the center (Ver-v.). Viscid saliva. Nausea and vomiting. Sore over gall bladder. Slaty or dark, horribly foul, painless, **diarrhœic stools.** Awakes oppressed for air. **Drowsy, stupid and languid.** Hyperpyrexia.

Related: Arn. Mur-ac.

BARYTA CARB.

REGION.
MIND.
GLANDS. { THROAT. / Prostate. }
HEART.
Bloodvessels.
Nerves.
Lungs.

WORSE.
COMPANY. **Cold** { Damp. / To Head. / Changes. }
LYING ON PAINFUL PART.
Suppressed Footsweat.
Thinking of it.
BETTER.
Warm Wraps.

Torpid, dwarfish (Med. Syp.); **develops poorly in infancy or becomes senile early** (Calc-c.). Adenopathies. Scrophula. Isolated effects (Con.). Numb single parts; in mouth, of genitals, fingers and toes, etc. Vascular softening and dilatation. **Paralytic effects.** Apoplexy. Too tired to eat. Wants to lie down. Takes cold easily.——**SLOW, INAPT AND BACKWARD.** Childish, thoughtless behavior. Groans from every little thing. **Beclouded mind. Bad memory.** Irresolute and fearful. Mistrustful. **Shy of strangers.** Brain feels loose; > cool air. Heavy pressure over eyes (Bell.). Baldness. **Old, sickly, weazened look.** Crusts behind ears. Hazy cornea. Weakness of tongue (Caust. Con.). Burning, soreness or vesicles on tip of tongue (Berb.). **Throat (tonsils or parotids) is affected by every cold. Chronic quinsy** (Calc-c. Psor. Sil. Sul.) or sore throat; with the menses. Sore spot in stomach (Arg-n. Bis. Kali-bi.). Diarrhœa, with lumbar backache. Spasm of œsophagus. Flabby genitals. Paralytic loss of voice. Chronic bronchial catarrh. Heat and bruised feeling in soles at night. **Cold, foul foot-sweat.** Glands indurated (Con.) or cervical swelled like knotted cords (Aeth.). Cysts (Sil.). Fatty tumors. Warts.

Related: Kali-p. Med. Sil.

BELLADONNA.

REGION.

BRAIN. NERVE CENTERS.
BLOODVESSELS.

Mucous Membranes { EYES. **MOUTH. THROAT.**

SKIN.
Organs.
RIGHT SIDE.

WORSE.

HEAT { **In Sun.** Becoming Heated.

AFTERNOON (3 P. M.)

DRAFTS { **On Head.** Having Hair Cut.

After Taking Cold.
CHECKED SWEAT.
LIGHT. NOISE. JARRING.
MOTION. HANGING DOWN.
Pressure on spine, excites other symptoms.

BETTER.

Rest in Bed. Light covering. Bending Backward. Letting Hair Down.

Young or full blooded persons. **VIOLENT THROBBING. CUTTING** (Aco.), **STABBING, SUDDEN SHOOTING OR CLAWING PAINS; of maddening severity** (Aco. Ars. Calc-c.). **JERKING OR TWITCHING. Nervous excitability** (Aco.). **Spasms. FULNESS, SWELLING, BURNING HEAT, BRIGHT REDNESS**—in streaks (Pho.)—**AND GREAT PAINFULNESS. DRYNESS; scant or hot discharges** (Kre.). ACTIVE CONGESTION. Inflammation.——**Excited and overactive.** RESTLESS, WILDLY DELIRIOUS, FEROCIOUS (Aco.) OR NOISY. **Tries to escape. Mania** (Vera.). THROBBING HEADACHE; < IN TEMPLES (Aco.); every motion hurts; > letting hair down (Cina. Ferr. Pho.). CONGESTION TO HEAD. The brain seems to rise and fall in waves. **Rolling of head.** Meningitis. Sunstroke. **WIDELY DILATED PUPILS.** PROMINENT, SPARKLING EYES (Canth.). **Red sclerotic. Lurid, terrifying hallucinations,** < closing eyes (Calc-c.). PHOTOPHOBIA. **FIERY RED, TURGID, HOT FACE** (Bry. Coff.), or alternately, red and pale. Toothache, > clenching teeth. **DRY, HOT MOUTH AND THROAT** (Pho. Rhus-t.). Swollen tongue (Aco. Ap. Ars. Merc.). Strawberry tongue (Tub.). **Urging to swallow, with spasm of throat.** DRINKS IN SIPS. Craves lemonade. Pain from liver to shoulder and throat, < lying on it. Distended transverse colon. Clawing in abdomen (Lyc.). Downward forcing in abdomen. Stools contain chalky lumps. Enuresis nocturna. **Early, profuse, red, hot, gushing** (Ham. Ip. Sec-c.) **menses.** Barking voice (Canth.). **Red streaks in**

mammæ (Pho.). Back feels broken (Lyc. Nat-m. Pho.). **BRIGHT, GLOSSY RED, PAINFUL SKIN.** Intense dermatitis. Scarlatina. Erysipelas. **Sleepy, but can't sleep. JERKS DURING SLEEP** (Kali-c.). Frightful dreams; of quarrels, fire, etc. **HOT HEAD AND COLD LIMBS (Arn. Bry.** Cact. Fer. Gel. Glo. Lach. Mur-ac. Sul.). Hot sweat.

Complementary: Calc-c. Related: Glon. Hyo. Stram.

BELLIS PERENNIS.

REGION.
- BLOODVESSELS. **Muscles.**
- **Spleen.**
- Joints.
- Left side.

WORSE.
- INJURY. **Sprains. Bruises.**
- **Becoming Chilled While Heated.**
- COLD BATHS. Wet.

BETTER.
- Continued Motion.

BRUISED SORENESS. Squeezing pains. Tired, fagged feeling. **Deep traumatisms and septic wounds; especially abdominal,** pelvic, uterine, etc. Bleedings.——Impulse to move. **Fulness about spleen.** Falls on the coccyx. Boils. **Wakeful;** too early. Sensitive to cold.

Related: Arn.

BENZOIC ACID.

REGION.
- **URINE** { **Kidneys. Bladder.**
- **Bowels.**
- JOINTS. Heart.

WORSE.
- Change of Weather. **Cold.**

BETTER.
- Profuse Urine.

Strong urinous odor about the patient. **Changing or gouty pains, especially about the heart or alternating with urinary symptoms.** Painful, gouty nodes.——Salty vomit. **Copious, grayish stools; like soap suds; of a pungent urinous odor;** very foul; white. STRONG, DARK-BROWN URINE; **FOUL OR SMELLING LIKE HORSE URINE.** Gravel. **Cracking in joints; in knees.** Profuse sweat without relief.

Related: Calc-c.

BERBERIS VULGARIS

REGION.

Liver, } KIDNEYS.
Urinary and } Bladder.
Digestive Tract } Spermatic Cord.
Lumbar Region (Hips).

WORSE.

Motion { **Jarring.** **Stepping Hard.** Rising from Sitting.

Many changeful symptoms with a tendency to form calculi. Lithæmia. **Pains shoot about or radiate from a single point (Dios.),** lower spine **(Laur.), etc.** Sticking. Exhausted; sweats easily. Soreness. Gurgling (Rhe. Scil.). Numbness.——Earthy complexion. Sticky mouth. **Foamy, cottony saliva** (Ap. Bry. Dulc. **Ign.** Kali-bi. Nux-m. Pho. Pho-ac.). **Bilious or nephritic colic; the pain follows the uretus or arrests the breathing.** Pale smarting stools. Fistula ani. **Reddish, sandy, mealy or mucous sediment in urine.** Numbness in small of back. Lumbago. General chilliness or **coldness in single parts.**

Complementary: Mag-m. Related; Pul.

BISMUTH.

REGION.

STOMACH.
INTESTINES.

WORSE.

Eating.

BETTER.

Cold { Drinks. Applications.
Bending Backward. **Motion.**

Apathetic and prostrated. **Tearing, pinching pains.** Internal heaviness. ——Headache attending or alternating with gastric symptoms. **Craves cold drink which is vomited at once or in great quantities when the stomach becomes full** (Grat.). Vomits liquids only. Atrophia ablactatorum (Kre. Ox-ac.). Foul belching. Food presses like a load on one spot. Gastralgia. Prostration after stool. Chlorea infantum, when the body remains warm. Black ulcers.

Related: Ars.

BORAX.

REGION.

NUTRITION { NERVES. **MUCOUS MEMBRANES.**

MOUTH. **Skin.** Kidneys. Bladder.

WORSE.

DOWNWARD MOTION.

Sudden Noises. Cold.

Nurslings. Children. Fruit.

BETTER.

11 P. M.

Poorly nourished, soft, flabby persons of **aphthous-catarrhal tendencies.** Heat in single parts; mouth, vagina, palms, etc. **Clear, thick, hot, biting discharges.** Shrivelled skin or mucous membranes (Ars.). Stitching. Marasmus.——**Nervous, anxious and fidgety.** FEAR OF FALLING, OF DOWNWARD MOTION, etc. (Gel. Sil.). **Starts at sudden sounds.** Frowsy, tangled hair (Psor.). **Infants cry and scream when nursing and before passing stool or urine.** Entropion. Mouth is dry, tender and aphthous (Mag-c.). Nausea when thinking hard. **Stools like boiled starch** (Arg-n.). Mucous diarrhœa. Hot, acrid, smarting urine. **Nephritis.** Cystitis. Membranous dysmenorrhœa. Albuminous leucorrhoea. **Averse** to coition. Mouldy expectoration. **Pain in opposite breast when the child nurses.** Mothers milk is thick and tastes badly. **Itching on back of hands.** Eczema. DRY SKIN; which festers easily.

Related: Bell.

BOVISTA.

REGION.

CIRCULATION { HEART. **Uterus.** Kidneys.

SKIN.

WORSE.

During Menses. Morning.

Getting Warm. Washing.

BETTER.

Eating.

Hemorrhagic-herpetic diathesis.——Lax and awkward in speech and action; inattentive, stutters, drops things, joints feel loose, easy indentation (Caps.), etc. **General puffiness.**——Weak memory. **Head feels big. As of** a wedge pressing into occiput. As of a lump of ice in stomach. **Colic,** $>$ eating. Bloating; flatulence. **Diarrhœa before and during menses** (Am-m. Pul. Ver-a. Vib.). **Early menses; more at night; less when in motion; flows**

between periods. Corroding leucorrhœa. Visible palpitation. **Itching eruptions;** oozing and forming thick crusts or **scabs.** Eczema.

Related: **Ap. Ustil.**

BROMIUM.

REGION.

LARYNX. **Respiration.**
Heart.
Circulation.
Glands { **Parotid.** Ovaries. Mammæ.

Left Side.

WORSE.

WARM { DAMP WEATHER. **Overheating.** Sitting in Room.

Dust. Drafts. Until Midnight.

BETTER.

Nosebleed { Vertigo. Head. **Chest.**

At Sea. Motion.

Suited to scrophulous blonds. Spasmodic constriction, glandular indurations or membranous formations. **Weak and easily overheated, then sweaty and sensitive to drafts.**——Burning coryza. Nosebleed. **Flatus** from vagina. Inhaled air seems full of smoke (Bar-c.), cold or raw. **Lungs** feel coated with down. **Wants to take a deep breath,** but it excites cough. Suffocating fits; he starts up choked. Spasm of glottis (Chlor.). **Suffocative, croupy or wheezing cough.** Diphtheritic croup. Asthma. Nervous palpitation. Cardiac hypertrophy. Slow glandular enlargement. **Boring** in bones.

Related: **Lach. Samb.**

BRYONIA.

REGION.
- **BLOOD.**
- **CIRCULATION.**
- SEROUS MEMBRANES { **HEAD.** **CHEST.** JOINTS. ABDOMEN. Liver.
- **Motor Apparatus** { Nerves. **Muscles.**
- Right Side.

WORSE.
- **MOTION** { **RAISING UP.** Stooping. **EXERTION.** **DEEP BREATHING.** COUGHING.
- HOT { BECOMING. ROOM. Weather.
- Drinking While Hot.
- EATING { Vegetables. **Acids.**
- VEXATION. TOUCH.
- **Suppressions.** After Taking Cold.

BETTER.
- **PRESSURE** { LYING ON PAINFUL PART. **Bandage, etc.**
- **QUIET.** COOL AIR.
- **Drawing Knees Up.**
- Heat to Inflamed Part.

Forcible effects, in unyielding tissues. **BURSTING, STITCHING, shooting or sore heavy pain; going backward** (Phyt.). **AVERSE TO MOTION;** even of distant parts (Ap.). DRY MUCOUS MEMBRANES. **Scanty, adherent secretions.** Effusions (Ap. Hell. Ran-b. Sul.). **Congestion. Inflammation.** Bilious-rheumatic type.——Determined, taciturn and ugly (Nux-v.). **Wants to be let alone, or go home** (Op. Pho-ac.). Dullness. **FAINT ON RAISING UP** (Aco. Merc-i-f. Phyt. Ver-vir. Vib.). HEAVY OR SPLITTING HEAD-ACHE; fronto-occipital; < motion of eyes (Bell.), **coughing** (Merc. Nat-m. Nux-v. Pho. Sul.), straining at stool (Mang. Rat.), etc. Sensitive scalp; every hair pains. Sore eyeballs (Cimi.). Nosebleed. Chewing motions (Hell. Lyc.). **Dry mouth.** Tongue rough; coated along center. Soapy saliva (Ign. Kali-bi. Pho-ac.). BITTER TASTE. **Thirst for much water.** Craves what he can't relish (Ign. Mag-m. Pul.). Loathing. Sensitive epigastrium (Ars. Chin. Lach. Nux-v.). Heavy or sore liver, > lying on right side (Sep.). Peritonitis. LARGE, DRY, VERY HARD STOOLS, as if burnt. Constipation. Gushing diarrhœa on rising; after cabbage (Petr.). Vicarious menstruation. Stony hard mammæ; before menses. Milk fever. DRY, VERY PAINFUL COUGH (Aco. Eupat.); as if from stomach. Blood streaked expectoration. Pneumonia (r). **SHARP STITCHES IN CHEST.** Pleurisy. Pain from between scapulæ to epigastrium or from l. toward heart (Sul.). Laborious delirium (Rhus-t.), **FULL, QUICK, HARD PULSE.** Jaundice. Chill, with hot head and red face; < warm room. Dry, burning heat; with < of all symptoms; the blood seems hot. **Painful, continued fevers; after suppressions,** typhoid, catarrhal, etc. Sour or oily sweat.

Complementary: Alu. Related: Phyt. Rhus-t.

BUFO.

REGION.	WORSE.
HEART { **Blood.** / Circulation.	In Room. Sexual Excitation (Onanism). During Sleep.
Skin.	BETTER.
	Bleedings.

Burning and ebullitions of heat. Flushings. Festering sensation.——**Moral depravity.** Childish or silly; talks nonsense and gets angry when not understood. Fears animals or strangers. Feeble mindedness. Duplicity (Op.). Heart seems to float in water (Bov. Pip-n. Sumb.). **Red streaks under skin.** Lymphangitis. Panaris. Dropsy. Bullæ. Sexual epilepsy (Bar-c. Calc-c.).

Related: Bar-c.

CACTUS GRANDIFLORA.

REGION.	WORSE.
HEART.	LYING { ON LEFT SIDE; / on occiput.
CIRCULATION.	**Exertion. Periodically.**
Chest.	10-11 A. M. or 11 P. M. Night.
Circular Muscles.	BETTER.
	Open Air. Pressure on vertex.

CONSTRICTION. Body feels tight. **Violent congestion. Irregular circulation. Localized pulsations;** behind stomach. HEMORRHAGE.——As of a weight on vertex or chest. **Red face.** Menses cease on lying; black; lumpy. Dyspnœa. **THE HEART SEEMS ALTERNATELY CLUTCHED AND RELEASED** (Lil-t.). **BY AN IRON HAND** or seems to turn over.—(**Crot-h.** Lach. Rhus-t. Sep.). Palpitation. Endocarditis. Irritable heart. Intermittent heart beat. Chest seems constricted by an iron band. Constriction about neck. Numbness of left arm (Alo. Rhus-t.). Fingers tingle. Chill, not > covering. Periodical neuralgias.

Related: Aco. Coc-c.

CADMIUM SULFAT.

REGION.	WORSE.
STOMACH.	**Raising Up. Least Motion.** Cold.

Craves cold water, which is immediately vomited (Ars.). Must lie still to avoid vomiting. Nausea. Faintness on rising (Bry.).

Related: **Zin.**

CALADIUM.

REGION.	WORSE.
GENITALS.	**Sexual Excesses. Motion.**
NERVES.	Sudden Noises.
Skin.	On Falling to Sleep. Tobacco.
Mucous Membranes.	BETTER.
	Cool Air. Short Sleep. Sweating.

Sense of dryness: food eaten seems dry. Inclination to lie down. **Dreads to move.——Nervous excitation.** Fear. Vertigo as if rocked. Crawling as of a fly or cobweb on face. Flaccid, sweaty genitals. Spermatorrhœa (Pic-ac. Sele.). Impotency; after gonorrhœa. PRURITIS VULVÆ; with burning. Violent sexual erethism. Respiratory, alternating with skin symptoms. Coldness of single parts. Heat during sleep which ceases at once on awaking. Sweet sweat which attracts the flies. Low fevers.

Related: Caps.

CALCAREA FLUORICA

REGION.	WORSE.
GLANDS. VEINS.	Rest. Beginning Motion.
Bones.	Change of Weather. Sprains.

Indurations; of stony hardness (Kali-bi. Merc-i-r.). Nodes. Periostitis. Fissures. Exostoses. **Vascular dilatation.** Varicose veins. Hæmorrhoids. **Cataract. Lumbago. Dry, hard skin of alabaster whiteness** (Ars.). **Bursitis.** Chronic synovitis. Stinking pus. Cold wrists and ankles.

Related: **Hekla-lava.**

CALCAREA OST.

REGION.

NUTRITION { **GLANDS.** / BONES. / **Skin.**

BLOOD.
CHEST.
HEART.
CHILDREN.

WORSE.

COLD { **DAMP** OR RAW AIR. / BATHING. / **Change of Weather.**

EXERTION { **Mental. Physical.** / **Ascending.** / **Eyestrain.**

DENTITION.
PRESSURE OF CLOTHES.
MILK. **Awaking. Anxiety.**

FAT, FLABBY BLONDES WHO SWEAT EASILY, < ABOUT HEAD, OR CHEST DURING SLEEP. Malnutrition. **Faulty bony development; OPEN FONTANELLES.** TARDY TEETHING AND WALKING. Curvatures. Rickets. Lack of endurance; easily sprained. **Parts lain on go** to sleep. Torpid, scrofulus habit. Calculous tendency. **PROFUSE, OFTEN SOUR DISCHARGES, SWEATS,** etc. **Cold, moist air chills him through and through** (Am-c. Aran. Cimi. Cist. Elap. Mos.). Takes cold easily; in chest.——**Fears;** anxious; being observed; insanity (Lil-t. Nux-v. Sep. Ver-a.). Confusion. Misplaces words. Sadness. Sudden aversion to work. **Vertigo. BIG HEAD AND LARGE, HARD ABDOMEN** (Bar-c. Sil.). Deep head pains—beating, shattering, etc.— < wind, > dark; with eructations. Migraine. **Scalp itches;** on awaking. **DILATED PUPILS.** Sees things on closing eyes (Bell. Bry. Thu.). Coryza with polyuria. **Swelled upper lip** (Bar-c. Sul.). Swelled tonsils (Merc-i-fl.). Lost appetite; from overwork. Craves eggs or coarse things (Ant-c.). Sour or curded vomit (Nat-ph.). **STOMACH LIKE AN INVERTED SAUCER.** Biliary colic. Chalky or grayish stools. Lienteria. Foul or strong urine. Hydrocele. Gushing, thick, milky leucorrhœa. Painless hoarseness. Everything puts him **out of breath. Weak heart.** Palpitation. Sore chest; **breasts before menses. Chapped hands.** Arthritic nodes. ENLARGED GLANDS. Warts. Cysts. Polypi. **Thick, foul milk crust** (Sul.). **Nightmare.** SLEEPLESS; from rush of ideas. **Icy coldness on vertex.** Internal heat with external coldness and sweat. Heat of head from mental exertion. Clammy hands (Sul.). **COLD, DAMP FEET** (Bar-c.).

Complementary: Lyc. Sil. Related: Bar-c. Sil.

CALCAREA PHOSPHORICA.

REGION.

NUTRITION:
- **BONES**: PERIOSTEUM. **Cartilage.** Sutures.
- GLANDS.
- Nerves.

ABDOMEN. **Vertex.**

WORSE.

MENTAL EXERTION.
DENTITION.
Change of Weather to: Cold Moist. East Wind. Melting Snow.
Drafts. Touch. **Getting Wet.**
Puberty. **Loss of Fluids.**
Fruits. **Cider.**

Tall, scrawny children and youths, with dirty brown skin. **Debilitated;** by every exposure. Crawling. Numbness. Shifting pains. **Anæmia, as** a sequel. Rheumatism.——**Peevish and fretful.** Headaches; go down spine (Bry.); of school children (Nat-m.). Thin skull bones. **Open fontanelles** (Calc-c. Sil. Sul.). Hydrocephalus. Teeth soft, come late **and** soon decay. Adenoids. Mycosis tonsilaris (Kali-m.). Craves fat bacon (Mez, Rad. Tub.). FLABBY, SUNKEN ABDOMEN. **Festering navel** (Abrot. Lyc. Thu.). Diarrhœic tendency. Menses every two weeks **(Trill.).** Crawling about genitals. Exalted sexual instinct. **Sense of** weakness or aching in uterus. Albuminuous leucorrhœa; after menses. Child loses its breath on being lifted up. Cough > lying (Psor.). Cavernous phthisis. Neck or chest pains from drafts. **Weak, thin neck;** the head bobs about. Weak thro hips (Trill.). **Pains along sutures or edges of nails. Slow ossification.** Nonunion (Symph.). Rickets (Pho. Sul.). Potts or hip joints disease. **Swollen glands.** Easily **chilled.** Sickly sweat.

Related: Carb-a. Nat-m.

CALCAREA SULPHURICA.

REGION.

CONNECTIVE TISSUE.
Mucous Membranes.
Skin.

WORSE.

Heat of Room. Touch.

BETTER.

Open Air.

Everything turns to pus; thick, yellow, lumpy. Persistent, profuse suppuration. Ulceration of cornea. Bloody nasal discharge of infants (Sil.). Pyeletis. Many boils. **The skin won't heal. Dry** heat at night; **kicks** off the covers. Starts from sleep as if wanting air.

Related: Hep.

CALENDULA.

REGION.
SOFT PARTS. **Spine.**
Liver.

WORSE.
Weather {Damp. Cloudy. During Chill.

Excessively painful, open, torn, cut, **lacerated, ragged** or suppurating **WOUNDS.** Hemorrhages, in scalp wounds or after drawing teeth, etc. Prevents pus.——Yellow vision. Curdy stools. Bruised pain at angle of right scapula. Jaundice.

Related: Arn. Bellis.

CAMPHOR.

REGION.
DIGESTIVE TRACT.
Cerebro-Spinal Nerves.
Urinary Organs.
Nose.

WORSE.
Cold. **When Half Asleep.** (Mag-p-au.).
Suppression. Inattention.

BETTER.
Sweat. Thinking of it.

Bluish, old, pinched look. ICY COLDNESS OF BODY, WITH AVERSION TO BEING COVERED; or wants covers on then off; with internal burning heat. **Cold and anxious. Sudden weakness,** (dry collapse). Cholera. **Scanty or retained discharges.** Violent tonic spasm.——**Insensibility or anxiety.** Head feels knotted up. Hammering in occiput. **Coryza; in the** aged (Am-c. Ant-c.). Retraction of upper lip (Nux-m. Nux-v.). Cold tongue. Burning thirst. Burning in stomach. Strangury. Hematuria. Hoarse squeaking voice. Asphyxia neonatorum (Ant-t.). Cold breath. Thumbs cramp backward. Cramp in calves. Erysipelas. **Very sensitive to cold air and to taking cold.** Desires covers during hot stage only. Sudden inflammatory fevers with rapid alternation of heat and cold; followed by rapid prostration. Corrects spoiled cases and antidotes most remedies.

Related: Carb-v. Cup. Opi. Sec-c.

CANNABIS.

REGION.
EMOTIONS.
MIND. **Nerves.**
GENITO-URINARY ORGANS.

WORSE.
URINATING. DARKNESS.
Exertion. Talking. Walking.

Extreme psychic mobility. EXCESSIVE EXALTATION OF ALL NATURAL IDEAS AND PERCEPTIONS, WITH GREAT MENTAL EXCITE-

MENT. **Wonderful hallucinations;** of ecstatic pleasures; of heavenly calm; of agonizing terror or pain; destroying the sense of proportion (Plat.), of time and space (Onos. Stram.). Mania of grandeur. Levitation (Nux-m. Pho.). Parts seem enlarged. Loquacity. Gayety. Violence. Delirium tremens. **Trickling sensations;** at heart. **Vertex seems to open and shut.** Weak vision. Corneal opacity. **SCANTY, BURNING URÍNE, PASSED DROP BY DROP** (Canth.); with pain going backward. Swelled prepuce. Priapism. Gonorrhœa (Pul.). Nephritic colic. Profuse menses with great pain. Can't control voice. Dreams of the dead (Thu.).

Related: Anahol. Cocain. Nux-m.

CANTHARIS.

REGION.		WORSE.
SEROUS AND MUCOUS MEMBRANES	BLADDER. **Kidneys. Throat. Pleura. Brain. Lower Bowel.**	URINATING. DRINKING.
		Bright Objects.
		Sight or Sound of Water.
		Touch; of Larynx.
Skin. Right Side.		Heat.

Burning; as if raw or sore. **Smarting-biting pains.** Shooting burning. ACUTELY VIOLENT OR RAPIDLY DESTRUCTIVE INFLAMMATION. Serous inflammations. Discharge of bloody, acrid water. Gangrene.—— Amorous frenzy. Rage. Yellow vision. Swelled, tremulous tongue; raw on edges. Throat and larynx constricted, and as if afire. Burning thirst, with aversion to liquids. Violent retching and vomiting. **Sensitiveness over stomach and kidneys.** Cutting colic. SHREDDY STOOLS, **with burning at anus and tenesmus of bladder and rectum.** Dysentry. **BURNING, SCALDING URINE, WITH CUTTING, INTOLERABLE URGING AND FEARFUL TENESMUS OR DRIBBLING** (Dulc. Rhus-t.). **Bloody urine. Strangury.** Dysuria. Nephritis (Dulc. Rhus-t.). Cystitis. Pulls at penis. **Sexual irritation. Priapism.** Pleurisy. Vesicular erysipelas; turning dark (Ran-b.). Bullæ. Chill during stool. Urinous sweat; on genitals

Related: Ap. Ars. Merc-c.

CAPSICUM.

REGION.
MUCOUS MEMBRANES.
THROAT.
Kidneys.
Bones. Mastoids.

WORSE.
DRAFTS. COLD AIR.
Uncovering. Dampness. Bathing.
Empty Swallowing. **Drinking.**
Eating. Drunkards.
BETTER.
Continued Motion.

Lax, lazy, fat, red, clumsy or unclean persons, who react poorly and dread the cold. Old age. **SORENESS, BURNING-SMARTING. Constrictions.** Dark, red, spongy mucous surfaces, or oozing bloody mucus. **Sprangling, threadlike pains** (Cep.). Neuralgias. Deep abscesses.——Changeable. Capricious. Homesick. Splitting headache, > heat. **Mastoiditis (Pho.).** NOSE AND FACE RED, BUT COLD. Vesicles or flat, painful ulcers in mouth. **Burning tip of tongue.** Craves stimulating, pungent things; wants a bracer. Dipsomania (Ars. Nux-v.). Small, burning, mucous stool, with tenesmus; also of bladder; then thirst and lumbar pain; < drinking (Arg-n.). Dysentry. Urging to urinate. Strangury. **Burning** in prostate. Cough causes distant pain or raises a foul air (Dros. Lach. Sang. Sep.). **Chilly; with the pains;** begins in back, with violent thirst, but shivers from every drink (Eupat.); with excruciating backache. Coldness of affected parts. **Sweats easily;** cold on thighs.
Complementary: Nat-m. Related: Canth.

CARBO ANIMALIS.

REGION.
GLANDS.
VEINLETS.

WORSE.
Slight Causes { Small Depletions. Lifting. Sprains. Taking Cold. }
WHILE EATING. **Dry, Cold Air.**
Shaving (Ox-ac. Rad.). Old Age.
BETTER.
Laying Hand on Part.

Weakly, susceptible persons who are ready to take cold, easily sprained, affected by small losses, etc. Venosity. Induration (Con. Plb.). Slow painful processes that burn like fire, take on stony hardness or threaten malignancy. Sense of looseness. **Foul, acrid discharges.** Hemorrhage.—— **Brain feels loose or as if the crown would split open, > eating.** Can't tell whence sounds come (Arg-n.). Hard, red, swelled nose (Aur.). Gone feeling in stomach when child nurses. All foods distress the stomach. **Right ovary seems a heavy ball.** Neglected bubo. Dark menses; in morning only; then great weakness. Soreness and moisture at **anus** (**Carb-v.**). Indurated os (Sep.). Suffocation on closing eyes. Nervous **dyspnœa.** Hard painful nodes in breasts (Phyt.). **Bluish skin; cheeks, lips, affected** parts, etc. Coppery eruptions; on forehead. **Hard, swelled glands.** Surgings or hot flashes. Foul, exhausting sweats; at night; **staining yellow.**

Related: Calc-fl. Grap.

CARBO VEGETABILIS.

REGION.

MUCOUS MEMBRANES { DIGESTIVE TRACT. **STOMACH.**

HEART { **VENOUS CIRCULATION. Blood.**

Occiput.

WORSE.

WARMTH. DEPLETIONS.
EXHAUSTING DISEASES.
HIGH LIVING. DISSIPATION.
Overlifting. Pressure of Clothes.
Weather { **Extreme Temperatures. Cold; frosty or Warm, moist.**
Air. Wind on Head. Suppressions.

BETTER.

ERUCTATIONS. Cool Air.
Elevating Feet.

Low, grave, depraved or cachectic states. Failing reaction, or obstinate sequalæ. WEAK, PALE, COLD AND SHORT OF BREATH; WANTS AIR, **to be fanned or thirsts for cold water.** Fainting. Collapse. **Aching, burning pains.** FOULNESS. **Ulceration** (aphthous). **Hemorrhage** (dark, oozing). Sepsis. Thick, acrid discharges. Old catarrhs. BLUENESS. **Overfulness.** Venosity. Numbness; of parts lain on.——Slow, anxious and irritable. Dull, heavy (leaden) headache; < occiput; < overheating; < pressure of hat. Head colds go downward. PINCHED OR DUSKY FACE. **Loose** teeth. Scorbutic gums. Small, painful aphthæ. Black tongue. **RANCID BELCHING** (Asaf. Pul. Thu.). **EXCESSIVE FLATULENCE;** obstructed or distending; < upper abdomen; all food turns to gas. Dyspepsia. Colic. Burning in rectum. Itching at anus. Sore, hot, itching, swelled vulva. Hoarse in evening. Spasms of choking cough with headache and vomiting; < cold and in bed; expectorates with retching (Sil.). Whooping cough. Heavy, sore or weak chest; on awaking. Senile asthma. Continuous, anxious palpitation. Thready pulse. As of a plug in back. Weak fingers (Rhus-t.). **Raw** or mottled skin. **Varicosis.** Horrors during sleep. ICY COLDNESS; **of knees; legs; at night;** of breath (Colch.), tongue, unilateral, etc. Warm head, cold limbs. **Internal heat.** Sweats easily; takes cold; sour; cold on face.

Complementary: Chin. Kali-c. Related: Am-c. Ars. Colch. Grap. Lyc.

CARBOLIC ACID.

REGION.

MUCOUS MEMBRANES { **Throat.** STOMACH. **Bowels.** **Lungs.**

HEART. **Blood.** Respiration. **Skin.**

WORSE.

Jarring. **Reading.** **Pregnancy.** Combing hair. (Bry. **Chin.** **Ign.** Sele.).

Painlessness, languor and prostration. FOULNESS. Malignancy. Low fever. Prickling-burning or sudden pains.——Acute smell. **Dusky face.** **Whiteness about the mouth and nose (Pho.).** **Fetor oris.** Vomiting. Flatulence. Shreddy stools. Passes mucus from anus when urinating. Urine scant, green or dark. **Sopor.** Coma. Thready pulse. Collapse. Bloody exudations, vesicles or pustules. Erysipelas. Cold **sweats.**

Related: Kre.

CARDUUS MARIANUS.

REGION.

Liver.
Spleen.
Veins.

WORSE.

Lying on Left Side. Beer.
Eating. Motion. Cellars.

BETTER.

Bleeding.

Fatigue. Lateral hepatic enlargement. **Blood stasis;** varicose veins, bleeding, etc.; from hepatic engorgment. Knotty clayey stools. **Asthma.** Dropsy.

Related: Calc-a.

CASTOREUM.

REGION.

NERVES.
Female Generative Organs.

WORSE.

Emotions. Cold. During Menses.

BETTER.

Pressure.

Weak and lacks reaction. Nervous and spasmodic effects of uterine origin. Fibrillar twitchings. Hysteria. **Irritability.**——Twitching in tongue.

Abdominal symptoms with yawning. **Colics with sudden weakness,** > pressure. Summer diarrhœa of green mucus stools (Asar.). Violent cutting dysmenorrhœal pains, then **cold sweat.** Exhausting sweats after fevers.

Related: Mos.

CAULOPHYLLUM.

REGION.

FEMALE SEXUAL ORGANS.
MUSCLES. **Small Joints.**

WORSE.

PREGNANCY. Open Air. Afternoon. Evening. **Night.**

Muscular exhaustion. ERRATIC, DRAWING PAINS. Internal trembling. ——Suppressed menses. UTERINE PAINS THAT FLY ABOUT (to breasts), ARE TOO WEAK (Caus. Kali-c. Op.) OR IRREGULAR. **FALSE LABOR PAINS. Eases labor** (Cimi. Vib.). After pains (Cimi.). Uterine atony. **Miscarriage.** Dysmenorrhœa. Vaginal spasm. Profuse, acrid leucorrhœa of little girls (Calc-c. Merc.). PAINFUL NODES ON FINGER JOINTS (Abrot. Benz-ac. Calc-c. Clem. Kali-m. Led.). **Aching and soreness** of lower limbs, before menses. Rheumatism. Chloasma.

Related: Cimi. Pul. Sep.

CAUSTICUM.

REGION.

NERVES { **Motor.** / **Sensory.**
MUSCLES { **BLADDER.** / **LARYNX.** / Limbs.
Respiration.
Skin.
Right Side.

WORSE.

Air { **DRY COLD.** / WINDS. **Drafts.**
Cold { **Taking.** / **Bathing.**
Extremes of Temperature. Suppressions. **Coffee.**
3-4 A. M. OR EVENING.

BETTER.

A COLD DRINK. Washing.
Warmth; of Bed.
Gentle Motion.

Weakness, increasing uncertainty of control, stumbling, etc., **finally** PARALYSIS; **of single parts.** Atony. Anesthesia. **Stiff** joints. Deformities. Jerks of single muscles. Trembling. Burning. **Soreness. Rawness.——Mental tire. Anxious forebodings** (felt in head); < in **twilight.** Emptiness behind forehead. Tight scalp (Bar-c. Vio-o.). To and fro or nodding motions (Chin. Ign. Pho-ac. Sep. Ver-a.). **Heavy, drooping eyelids.** Diplopia; < looking to right. Profuse, acrid tears. Much foul earwax. Echoing in ears (Bar-c. Colo. Pho.). **Tinnitus. FACIAL PARALYSIS**; < opening mouth. **Urging to swallow** or swallows **the wrong** way. **Stool,** difficult; glistening (Alo.); **passed > standing. Insensible** rectum or urethra (Kali-br.); even for a solid stool (Alo.). **URINE SPURTS ON COUGHING** (Fer-ph. Nat-m. Pul. Rum.), dribbles or passes slowly (Arn. Hep. Lyc. Sep.); > **sitting. Menses more by day,** leucorrhœa by night. Cough, < heat of bed or cold air, > sips of cold water (Coc-c. Tab.). Can't cough deep enough, **the sputum slips back again** (Arn. Con. Seneg.). Hoarse in A. M.; speakers; > **talking** (Rhus-t.). **Sore** streak in larynx. Aphonia. Sore chest; the vest seems tight. Hamstrings feel short (Nat-m.). Cramp in calves, feet or toes. **Deep burns and their effects.** Warts on eyelids, tip of nose, hands or fingertips. Coldness, not > warmth; causes paralysis, cough, diarrhœa, etc. Sweat about 4 A. M.

Complementary: Carb-v. Grap. **Lach.** Stap.

Related: **Gel.** Kali-bi. **Pho. Rhus-t.** Sep.

CEANOTHUS.

REGION.
Spleen.

WORSE.
Cold Weather. Lying on Left Side.

Dyspnœa, diarrhœa or leucorrhoea with pain in left side. **Enlarged spleen.** Green urine.

Complementary: Nat-m.

Related: **Chin.**

CEDRON.

REGION.
Nerves. Blood.

WORSE.
Periodically. At the same hour. After Sleep.

EXACT PERIODICITY. Periodical orbital neuralgia (r) (Chin-s. Nat-m.). Brow ague. Excitement before the chill. Malaria. Numbness.

Related: Aran.

CEPA.

REGION.

MUCOUS MEMBRANES { **NOSE.** EYES. **Larnyx.** **Bowels.**

Nerves.

WORSE.

WARM AIR. IN ROOM.
Getting Feet Wet. Spring.
Singing. North East Winds.

BETTER.

Open Air. Motion.

Acute catarrhs and neuralgias. Shooting pains, as fine as a thread. (Ars. Bell. Caps. Plan. Syph. Tell.).——Frontal headache extending to eyes and face, > during menses (Lach. Zin.). FREQUENT VIOLENT SNEEZING. **ACRID FLUENT CORYZA, with burning, smarting, watery eyes.** Sensitive to odors. Rawness in throat. Noisy flatulency; foul flatus. Wind colic. Painless diarrhœa. **Copious urine. Hacking, tickling cough that threatens to tear or split the larynx and compels grasping it. Painful** talking. HOARSENESS. Senile bronchitis.

Complementary: Pho. Related: Euphr. Gels. Kali-io.

CHAMOMILLA.

REGION.

MIND. EMOTIONS.
NERVES.
DIGESTIVE MUCOUS MEMBRANES { STOMACH. **ABDOMEN. Liver.**
CHILDREN.

WORSE.

DENTITION. ANGER. NIGHT.
WIND. CHECKED SWEAT.
Taking Cold. Cold Air.
COFFEE. Narcotics. Opium.

BETTER.

BEING CARRIED.
Mild Weather. **Heat.**

OVERSENSITIVE. QUICKLY DRIVEN TO DISTRACTION OR PROSTRATED BY PAIN. Tosses about, cries out and insists upon instant relief. Colicky, neuralgic or gouty-rheumatic subjects. Pains followed by numbness.——CROSS, PETULENT, SNAPPISH AND UNCIVIL. **Averse to being spoken to or touched. WANTS TO BE CARRIED.** Nervous walking about in distress (Ars.). Sensitive to wind about the ears (Mez.). Sticking earache, > warmth. **Swelling or REDNESS OF ONE CHEEK.** Toothache, < warm drinks. Bad breath. Bitter taste. **Yellowish tongue.** Eructations like bad eggs. Distended abdomen. **Cutting or wind colic;** < night (Chin. Cyc.). ACID, GRASS-GREEN, SLIMY, HACKED OR UNDIGESTED STOOLS; WITH COLIC; **smelling like bad eggs** (Stap.). Irregular labor-like pains; going down thighs (Cimi. Kali-c. Ox-ac.).

Cramps when child nurses (Pul.). Dark, lumpy menses or lochia. **Arms go to sleep when grasping objects.** Jaundice. **Disturbed sleep, by pain,** starting up, etc.; in nervous women or children. **Chilly, yet easily overheated, hence takes cold.** Coldness of one part with heat of another; < **uncovering.** Alternate chill and heat. **Hot and thirsty or hot sweat with the pains.** Hot coryza; hot stools. Feverish from suppressed discharges. Sweat on head.

Complementary: Bell. Mag-c. Sanic. Related: Nux-v. Stap.

CHELIDONIUM.

REGION.

MUCOUS MEMBRANES.

RIGHT SIDE { **LIVER. GALL BLADDER. LUNGS** (Lower).

Bowels. Occiput.

Kidneys.

WORSE.

MOTION. Coughing. Touch.

Change of Weather.

4 A. M. 4 P. M.

BETTER.

HOT FOOD. Eating (dinner).

Milk. Pressure.

Symptoms (gastro-abdominal) **due to hepatic disturbances.** Jaundice. Catarrhs. Pain as if part were broken. Numbness. Horror of **motion.** ——Despondency. Headaches (r) extending backward. Heavy occiput. **Sallow or jaundiced face.** Bitter taste. Thick yellow coat on tongue; with indented edges (Hyds.). Choking; as from too large a morsel. Craves milk or hot things (Lyc.). Gnawing, scraping pain in stomach, > eating. PAIN FROM BORDER OF LIVER BACKWARD TO (Merc.), OR FIXED UNDER LOWER ANGLE OF RIGHT SCAPULA (to right shoulder and occiput—(Nux-v. Sep.). Gall stones. As of a string or band about abdomen (Caus. Plb. Pul.). Stools clayey, **bright yellow or of hard balls.** Cough as from dust. Conjoined symptoms of the right lower lung and liver. Bilious pneumonia (Merc.). Itching > eating. Lethargic drowsiness. **Icy coldness in nape and occiput.** Inclined to sweat, but without relief.

Complementary: Lyc. Related: Bry. Kali-bi. Merc.

CHIMAPHILA.

REGION.

BLADDER. **Prostate Gland.**

Kidneys.

Liver.

WORSE.

Cold Damp. Standing. Sitting.

BETTER.

WALKING.

ROPY **or muco-purulent, foul, scanty urine. Feels as if sitting on a ball,**

in the perineum (Cann.). **Fluttering in kidney region** (Brach.). **Acute inflammation in urinary tract. Gravelly urine.**
Complementary: Kali-m. Related: **Berb. Cocc-cac. Sabal.**

CHINA.

REGION.
BLOOD. CIRCULATION.
SECRETIONS — **DIGESTIVE. ORGANS. Liver.**
Nerves.
Spleen.

WORSE.
VITAL DEPLETIONS. TOUCH.
Wind. Jarring. Noise.
Periodicity. — **ALTERNATE DAYS.**
Cold — Open Air. DRAFTS. Mental Exertion.
Eating — Fruit. Milk.

BETTER.
HARD PRESSURE.

INTERMITTENCY. PROFUSE, EXHAUSTING DISCHARGES, **hemorrhages, etc. Weak, oversensitive and nervous;** everything upsets him; light, noise, odors, etc. **Touch is painful, but hard pressure relieves** (Lach.). **Bursting pain.** Neuralgias. Anæmia. Dropsy.——Stubborn, disobedient children. Bursting-throbbing or loose swashing in head (Ars. Bar-c. Nux-m.); the brain feels bruised (Ign. Mur-ac. Nux-v. Phyt.); < temples. **Sensitive scalp** (Mang. Merc. Nit-ac. **Nux-v.** Rhus-t. Sil.); < moving **hair.** Hot, red ears. **Tinnitus** (Euc.). Deafness. Pale, sickly look; with blue circles about eyes. Throbbing toothache; < as child nurses. Acute or **bitter taste.** Craves dainties, relishes or condiments. Anorexia. **Loud belching without relief** (Arg-n.). **Flatulent bloating.** Tympanites. Slow digestion. Sore stomach. Gall stones. Swollen liver and spleen. Pains from rectum into genitals (Lil-t.). **LIENTARY; dark, foul, watery, painless stools; < eating** (Ars. Pod.); at night. Dark, profuse, clotted menses. Rattling respiration. Every motion excites palpitation and takes his breath. Suppurative phthisis (Hep.). Painfully sensitive chest and spine (Cimi.). Heavy pressure between scapulæ (Calc-c. Rhus-t.). As of a band about legs. Swollen veins (hands, face). Clearly staged chill, heat and sweat. Marked prodrome. Thirst follows the chill. Red, hot face with cold hands. **Hectic** (Fer. Iod. Lyc. Pho. Sang.). DRENCHING SWEATS; AT NIGHT; **from least exertion,** etc.
Complementary: Carb-v. Fer. Kali-c. Related: **Carbo-v.**

CHININUM SULF.

REGION.
NERVES.
CIRCULATION.
Dorsal Spine.

WORSE.
EXACT PERIODICITY. Cold.
Turning or leaning head to left.
BETTER.
Yawning.

Nervous and sensitive. Neuralgias.—**As of a net, fog or black speck before eyes.** Tinnitus. Deafness. Brow ague (Ced.). **Urine has a granular,** brick red sediment. **Spine (cervico-dorsal region) aches or is tender** (Hyper.). **Anticipating chills.** Delirium during the heat. **Profuse sweat, which relieves, but exhausts. Thirst in all stages.** Clear apyrexia. Typical malaria. Itching. Petechiæ.

Related: Chin.

CHIONANTHUS.

REGION.
LIVER. **Head.**

WORSE.
Cold. Motion. Walking.
BETTER.
Lying on Abdomen.

Bilious, sick headaches. Soreness; of eyeballs; of liver. Gall stones. Bilious colic. Clay-colored **stools. Jaundice.**

Related: Bry.

CHLORAL HYDRATE.

REGION.
BRAIN. HEART.
Muscles. Liver. Skin.

WORSE.
Alcohol. Night. Exertion.
BETTER.
Open Air.

Muscular prostration.——**Cerebral excitement;** hears voices (Aco. Cham.). **Mania.** Bileless stools. **Bed-wetting.** Wants to be fanned. **Dyspnœa.** As of a weight on chest. Weak heart. **Urticaria.** Sleepless from over-fatigue. Night terrors.

Related: Ap. Cancer-flu.

CHLORUM.

REGION.

Respiratory Organs.
Mucous Membranes.
Nerves. Skin. Glands.

WORSE.

After Midnight. **Lying.**

BETTER.

Motion. Open Air.

Rapid emaciation.—Constrictions.——Fears going crazy or losing his senses. **Protruding eyes. Acrid coryza.** Putrid aphthæ. **Dry tongue. DYSPNŒA,** CAN'T EXHALE (**Meph.** Samb.). Asthma of hay fever (Ars. Naj. **Sep.**). Spasm of glottis. Laryngitis. Laryngismus stridulus. Sensitive skin.

Related: Ars-io. Iod. **Meph.**

CICUTA.

REGION.

BRAIN.
NERVES.
Skin.

WORSE.

CONCUSSION OF BRAIN.
Injury. Jarring. Noise. Touch.
Dentition. Cold.

VIOLENT CONVULSIVE PHENOMENA. Sudden shocks through **body.** Twitchings. Jerks. **Terrific spasms moving downward** (reverse Cup.) or coming with sudden rigidity; **with staring, jerking eyes, OPISTHOTONOS and frightful contortions, then utter prostration.** Epilepsy.—— Childish. Suspicious. Rashness. Delirium. Congestion to head with vomiting and purging (Ver-v.). **Vertigo.** Meningitis. Squint. Red, sweaty face. Grinding of teeth. Trismus. Spasm of gullet. Craves chalk, coal, etc. **Loud hiccough.** Oppressed breathing. Thoracic spasm (Stry.); alternating with hiccough. Tremulous palpitation (**Stap.**). Heart seems to stop. Turns feet inward. Turns big toes upward during the spasm. Pustules coalescing into thick, yellow (loose), massive crusts; < head and face. Impetigo.

Related: Cup. Stry.

CIMICIFUGA.

REGION.

Mind.

Nerves. (Cerebro Spinal) — **Occiput. Eyes.** **Back (Lumbar).** OVARIO-UTERINE. **Muscles (belly of).** **Heart.**

Left Side.

WORSE.

Cold; damp. Drafts.

Menstruation. Pregnancy. Labor.

BETTER.

Open Air. Continued Motion.

Pressure.

An irregularly acting, depressing irritant, causing exhaustion and **low spirits,** combined with supersensitiveness; < during pain (Nux-v.). **Heavy, aching soreness,** with a sick feeling (Serp.). **Pains shoot about, from nape,** eyes, lumbar spine (Kali-c.) or from side to side in ovaries or chest. Myalgias. **Reflex utero-ovarian pains. Tremblings,** twitchings; tongue, fingers when writing, etc. Fidgets. Chorea; of heart. Nervous, hysterical or rheumatic females.—**Gloom.** Forebodings of insanity, death, etc. Melancholia. **Illusions;** of rats (Calc-c.). Mania; puerperal or alcoholic. Waving in brain (Glo.). Vertigo. Head seems to open and shut, or vertex to fly off (Cann. Syp.). Cold draft or heat on vertex. **Eyeballs ache,** feel big or heavy. Pale, hot face. Uneasiness in teeth. Hawks tough, coppery mucus. Nausea; **in A. M.;** felt in bowels; < pressure on spine. Vomits green, holds the head and groans. Ovaralgia. Much clear urine; it weakens her; contains yellow sand. Heavy inert uterus. **Menses irregular in time and amount** (Coc-c. Ign. Nux-m.); more flow, more pain (Cann. Tub.). Slow labor with nervous shivers. After pains. Incessant dry night cough, < speaking. Needle-like pain at heart; going backward (Kali-c.) or to left arm (Ars. Pul. Rhus-t.); it feels bound to side. Inframammary pain (1). Stiff, contracted neck, back (Agar.) or tendo Achilles. Pain at angle of left scapula (Chenop.). Pain—heavy or pulsative—in small of back, thro hips and down thighs. Lumbago. Cramps in limbs. Itching soles. Dizzy, drunken sleep, with arms across head or yawning. Weak, irregular pulse. Cold sweat on hands and feet.

Related: Caul. **Ign.** Lil-tig. **Pul.** Rhus-t.

CINA.

REGION.

NERVES { **ABDOMEN.** / **BRAIN.** / SPINE. }

Eyes.

Mucous Membranes.

Left Side.

WORSE.

WORMS. **TOUCH.** **Vexation.** **Looked at.** DURING SLEEP. Yawning. Staring.

BETTER.

Wiping Eyes. Motion. Lying on Abdomen.

Bruised soreness. **Stiffens out when crossed, looked at, during cough, etc.** (Cup. Ign. Jus.). Twitchings or spasms; worm spasms (Cic.); unilateral. ——TOUCHY. **Ugly, cross and petulent;** rejects everything offered; wants to be rocked. **Dilated pupils.** Squint. Colored vision. Eye fatigue, > rubbing. Wings of nose drawn in. **PICKS AND BORES AT NOSE** (Nat-p.). **Dark rings about eyes.** BLUISH-WHITE ABOUT MOUTH. **Sickly pale face;** during cough. **GRINDS THE TEETH.** Chews and swallows in sleep (Ign.). Drinks gurgle noisily downward. **Canine or gnawing hunger; after eating** (Merc. Pho. Stap.); after vomiting; alternating with anorexia. Hard, distended abdomen. Twisting at navel, > pressure. Whitish, watery stool. Bed-wetting. **MILKY URINE.** Choking cough, then gurgling down throat. Restless sleep; lies on abdomen; cries out; wakes in terror. Fever with pale face (Bry.). Cold sweat about nose and forehead.

Complementary: Calc-c. Dros. Related: Cham. Nat-p.

CINNABAR.

REGION.

BLOOD.

Bones.

WORSE.

Touch. Light.

BETTER.

Open Air.

Pain along orbital bones from inner to outer canthus; or at root of nose. Dry mouth awakes him from sleep. Hawks down stringy mucus. Indurated glands. **Fiery red** eruptions, ulcers, etc. Figwarts on prepuce.

Complementary: Thu. Related: Merc.

CISTUS.

REGION.

MUCOUS MEMBRANES { **Nose.** **Throat.** Lungs.

Glands; **of neck.**

Skin.

WORSE.

COLD { TAKING. **Drafts.** **LEAST AIR. Water.** INSPIRATION.

Mental { **Exertion.** Excitement.

Touch.

Painfully sensitive to cold (Mos.). **Coldness;** tongue, saliva, stomach, eructations, etc.; < sweating. **Suppurative tendency. Much thick, yellow or foul mucus leaving painful rawness** (Aesc. Ant-c.). Internal and external **itching. Burning.**——Headache from missing the noon meal, > eating (Lyc.). Colds affect the throat; it feels spongy, sandy (Bov. Colo. Thu.) or itches. Cough. Indurations; callosities. **Hard, swollen glands;** on neck. Crawling over body. Cracking tetters; canthi, lips, fingertips.

Related: Calc-c. Hep.

CLEMATIS.

REGION.

MUCOUS MEMBRANES { EYES. **Urethra.**

GLANDS { TESTES. Mammæ. Ovaries.

Skin { Scalp. Occiput.

Spermatic Cord.

WORSE.

HEAT OF BED. NIGHT.

GONORRHŒA (suppressed).

Washing in Cold Water. Waxing and Waning with the Moon.

BETTER.

Sweat.

Flaccid muscles. VERY HARD, PAINFULLY SWOLLEN GLANDS, (Carb-a.). Burning, itching, stinging or crawling pains. Neuralgia. Cancer. Rheumatism (gonorrhœal).——Chronic conjunctivitis. **Iritis.** Urine flows in fits and starts (Con. Tub.) or dribbles; strains to pass a few drops, then a full stream follows. Stricture (Con.). Mucus in the urine. SWELLED TESTES (r), **inguinal glands** or spermatic cord. Gonorrhœal orchitis (Pul.). Loathes coition. Full, heavy, sensitive breasts; outward darts in (Arg. Ol-ani.). Corroding eruptions; ending in eating ulcers. Vesicles. Pustules. Thick crusts; < on occiput. **Sleepiness.**

Complementary: Merc.

Related: Pho. Rhod. Stap.

COBALTUM.

REGION.
Spine (lumbar).
Kidneys. Genitals.
Bones.

WORSE.
Sexual losses. Sitting.
Heat of Bed or Sun.
BETTER.
Hawking out Mucus.

Aching bones. **Sour,** taste, stomach, footsweat, etc.——Sense of guilt. Vertigo or head feels big, < stool. **Cracks across tongue.** Emptiness at navel (Flu-ac.). Yellow spots on abdomen. Sweet, foamy, lumpy expectoration. **Lumbar backache;** < sitting; with weak knees; <**atonic emissions;** can't straighten up.

Related: Eup-per.

COCA.

REGION.
NERVES { **BRAIN.** / **Respiration.** / Heart. }
Muscles.

WORSE.
Ascending. High Altitude. **Cold.**
Mental Exertion.
BETTER.
Quick Motion in Open Air.
After Sunset.

Dizzy, short of breath and exhausted (Ars.).——Mental prostration. Timid. Craves solitude. Sense of impending death. Loquacious excitement, with blissful visions. **Like a band across forehead** (Ap. Carb-ac. Coccl. Lac-c. Merc. Sul.). Migraine. Carious teeth. Aphonia. Something under skin moves when touched. Palpitation. Sleeplessness. Crawling and numbness of arms.

Related: Cann.

COCCULUS INDICUS.

REGION.
CEREBRO SPINAL AXIS { **OCCIPUT.** / **Lumbar Spine.** / Muscles. }
SENSORIUM.
Female Sexual Organs.
One Side.

WORSE.
MOTION { CARS. / CARRIAGE, Boat, etc. }
SLIGHT CAUSES { **Loss of Sleep.** Noise. / **Night Watching.** / **Exertion. Pain.** / Touch. Emotions. }
ANXIETY. COLD. Open Air.
After Eating. During Menses.

Active senses, with heaviness and **paralytic muscular relaxation; too weak**

to hold up head, stand or even speak (Alu. Dig. Fer. Hep. Stan.). Trembling. Spasms. **Benumbed.** Paralysis. EMPTY, HOLLOW FEELING. Hysteria. **Sensitive to cold.**——Dazed; things seem unreal. Slow comprehension. Sad. Easily offended. VERTIGO; **with nausea;** with palpitation; <raising head. Heaviness in head. Ache in occiput, < **lying on it** (Cac.); > bending backward. OCCIPUT SEEMS TO OPEN AND SHUT (Calc-c. Cann. Cimi.). Articulates or swallows with difficulty. NAUSEA; rising into head. Loathing. VOMITING. Sea sickness. **Abdomen seems full of sharp stones** (Colo.). Twisting (wind) colic, with salivation. Distending flatulence. Clutching in uterus. Depleting menses; < standing on tip toe; replaced by gushes of leucorrhœa. SPINAL WEAKNESS; < IN SMALL OF BACK, < walking. Paraplegia (Arg-n. Ars. Caul. Nux-v.). Limbs go to sleep, < grasping anything. Symptoms alternate between arms. Clumsy gait. Drowsiness. Low fever. Sweatiness.

Complementary: Petr. Related: Gel. Ign.

COCCUS CACTI.

REGION.

MUCOUS MEMBRANES: **FAUCES.** Throat. **Larynx.** Chest. Genito-Urinary Organs.

WORSE.

IRRITATING FAUCES.
Heat (of Room, Bed. Exertion).
Exposure to Cold (Wind). **Lying.**
Periodicity. On Awaking.

BETTER.

Cold Drinks. Cool Room.

Catarrhal, spasmodic, hemorrhagic or uric acid effects. Dark blood. **Intolerable internal tickling. General sensitiveness,** skin, vulva, etc. **Pulsations.** As of a fluid forcing its way (Glo.).——**Sadness, on awaking at** 2-3 A. M. (Lyc.). SENSITIVE FAUCES; **hawking, cleaning teeth, etc. causes cough, retching or vomiting** (Dig. Euph. Stap.). Constricted throat. **Urging to urinate;** > clots of blood from vagina. Urine scanty, thick and heavy; mucous, bloody or **dark red, sandy sediment.** Nephritis. Nephritic colic. Menses flow more at night. Uterine hemorrhage, of large, black clots < lying (Kre.). REGULARLY RECURRING VIOLENT PAROXYSMS OF RACKING, TICKLING COUGH WHICH END IN RAISING OR VOMITING MUCH CLEAR ROPY MUCUS (Kali-bi.), WITH A PURPLE RED FACE **and internal heat,** > cold air or drinks. Whooping cough, etc. Soreness or stitches in apices of lungs. Coldness in back. **Burnings;** as of pepper in nostrils, at tip of tongue, etc. (Lach.).

Related: Ap. Lach. Pho.

COFFEA.

REGION.
NERVES.
CIRCULATION.
Sexual Organs.

WORSE.
NOISE. **Touch.** Strong Odors.
Air (Open. Cold. Windy).
Mental { Emotions (Joyous). Exertion.
Alcohol. Overeating. Night.

BETTER.
Lying Down.

OVERACTIVE, EXCITABLE AND ACUTELY SENSITIVE, EVEN TO PLEASURE; CAN'T BEAR PAIN OR NOISE, which may even excite pain (Therid.).——Rush of ideas. **Weeping, lamenting and tossing about.** Now joyous, now gloomy. Faints easily. Brain seems torn, shattered or crushed. Clavus. Bright eyes. Acute hearing; overhears distant sounds (Chin. Nux-v. Op.). Face-ache (r). **Toothache; > ice cold water** (Clem.); pain to fingertips; during menses. Stomach feels overloaded. Hot itching genitals. After pains. Nervous palpitation. Trembling hands. **Painfully sensitive skin.** NERVOUS SLEEPLESSNESS, from mental activity (Calc-c. Hyo. Nux-v.); awakes at or hears every sound. (Op.).

Complementary: Aco. Related: Coca. Ign.

COLCHICUM.

REGION.
DIGESTIVE TRACT.
MUSCLES.
HEART.
Circulation. Kidneys.
Tissues { **Fibrous.** **Serous.** Small Joints.

WORSE.
MOTION. **Touch. Night.**
WEATHER { **Cold Damp.** **Changing. Autumn.**
Checked Sweat. Strong Impressions. Receding Gout. Stretching Legs.

BETTER.
Warmth. Sitting. **Doubling Up.**

RAPID SINKING; COLD AND WEAK BUT RESTLESS. Moist collapse. Creepings. Small, rapidly shifting areas of pain. Dropsical or gouty-rheumatic.——**Very irritable and sensitive; every little hurt pains terribly.** Unequal pupils. Acrid tears. Dark nostrils (Hell.). ACUTE SMELL; **odors nauseate even to fainting,** etc. Pinched, sunken face. Mouth hangs open. Flow of saliva with a sense of dryness (Alu. Kali-c. Lyc. Mag-m. **Merc.** Nat-m. Plb.). Glossitis. **LOATHES THE SMELL OR SIGHT OF**

FOOD (Ars. Cocel.); > lying quietly. NAUSEA. **Burning or icy coldness in stomach** (Ars. Bov. Caps. Caus. Chin. Epip.). **Tympanites. Choleraic** or shreddy, gelatinous, mucus stools, then tenesmus or spasm of anus. Black urine (Lach.). Nephritis. Chest seems squeezed, by a band (Cup.). Cutting or stinging at heart. Weak heart. Cold limbs. Heat on rump. Sweating; cold on face.

Complementary: Ars. Spig. Related: Ars. Carb-v. Ver-a.

COLLINSONIA.

REGION.

PELVIS { RECTUM. **Uterus.** Bowels. }

HEART.

Pharynx. Liver.

WORSE.

PILES { During. Suppressed. } **Night.**

Pregnancy. Emotions. Cold.

CONGESTIVE SYMPTOMS ORIGINATING IN, OR COMBINED WITH HEMORRHOIDS; **especially if cardiac** (Lycops.). **Congestions and constrictions.**—Speakers sore throat. Colic. Light, knotty stools. **Constipation.** Rectum seems full of sticks (Aesc.) or sand. Prolapsus uteri. Pruritus ani or pudendi. **Palpitation.** Rheumatism.

Related: Nux-v.

COLOCYNTH.

REGION.

NERVES { **ABDOMINAL.** TRIFACIAL. SCIATIC. }

INTESTINES.

Ovaries. Kidneys.

Left Side.

WORSE.

EMOTIONS { INDIGNATION. **Chagrin. Anger.** }

Food or Drink.

Night in Bed. Rest. **Pain.**

Taking Cold. **Drafts.**

BETTER.

HARD PRESSURE.

Heat. Gentle Motion.

Passing Stool or **flatus.**

Sudden paroxysms of atrocious cramping of griping pains which make him twist, turn or cry out; with nausea or diuresis. **Cutting, pinching, clamping, gnawing or boring pain;** then numbness. Parts seem too short. **Constriction.** Neuralgia.——**Anger. Easily vexed;** < pain. Tearing head pains, < moving eyelids. Faceache (1) (Bell. Mag-ph.). Distorted face. Persistent bitter taste. **WAVES OF VIOLENT GRIPING OR CLUTCHING AB-**

DOMINAL COLIC DOUBLING HIM UP (Aco. Colch.); > hard pressure (Stan.). Cutting abdomen (Nit-ac. Pul. Sul.); at navel (Nux-v.). **Intestines feel squeezed between stones** (Ant-t. Cocl. Scop. Stap.). **Ovaralgia.** Gelatinous, shreddy, sourish or **yellow, frothy, watery stools with colic and gas.** Dysentry. Slippery bubbles escape from anus (Nat-m). Gelatinous, sticky urine. **Cramps in hips.** Screwing, band like, or shooting pains down the sciatic nerve, < night, rotating it (Bry. Cocl. Kali-c.), > lying on painful part. The limbs are drawn up like a hedgehog. Urinous sweat.

Complementary: Caus. Related: Stap.

CONIUM.

REGION.
- NERVES. MUSCLES.
- GLANDS {MAMMÆ. Ovaries.
- **Sexual Organs.**
- Respiration.

WORSE.
- SEEING MOVING OBJECTS.
- ALCOHOL.
- **Night. After Exertion. Injury.**
- **Cold; Taking. Continence.**
- **Old Age.** Lying; Head Low.

BETTER.
- Letting Part Hang Down.

Languid and exhausted; < in lower limbs; early in bed, after walking in open air, etc. Progressive debility, as of old age; clothes distress him, faints after stool (Cocl. Pod.); difficult articulation; **uncertain gait; trembling,** etc. Cachexy. **As of a lump;** in brain (Arn. Chel. Cocl.); in epigastrium (Arn. Chel. Cup. Lach. Nat-m. Pho.). Ascending symptoms (Grind). Sudden sick attacks; with **numbness,** etc. Paralysis. Stabbings. Tearings.——Slow. Shy of people, yet averse to being alone (Clem.). Weak memory. WHIRLING VERTIGO; **on lying, turning over** (Hyds.), **moving eyes or head** (Bry. Calc-c. Gel. Kali-c.), etc. **Eyes feel crossed** (Bell. Op. Pul.); **lids droop,** < outer side. **Photophobia.** Pulpy earwax. Cold flatus. Urine passes fitfully, > standing. **Cutting; as** semen passes; in ovaries, uterus, etc. Prostatic dribble; < stool, emotions, etc. Emissions from mere contact (Arn. Gels. Nat-c. Pho.). **Acrid leucorrhœa.** Palpitation from exertion, drinking, at stool, etc. Tormenting tickling cough. **GLANDS SWELL, HARDEN AND GET SORE.** Congested breasts, before menses. Sticking in mammae (Iod. Nit-ac.). Too much milk. Foul eruptions. Greenish discoloration. Hebetude. **Heat or sweat on dropping to sleep** (Pul. Sil.); at night.

Complementary: Pho. Related: Arn. Bar-c. Calc-fl. Caus. Gel.

COPAIBA.

REGION.	WORSE.
MUCOUS MEMBRANES { **GENITO-URINARY.** **Bronchi.**	Morning.
Rectum. Skin.	Taking Cold.

BLENORRHŒAS; of a foul odor. Stools covered with mucus. Pulsation in penis (Coc-c.). Catarrh of bladder. Offensive bronchorrhœa (Phel.) Urticaria. Purulent gonorrhœa.

Complementary: Sep. Related: Tere.

CORALLIUM RUBRUM.

REGION.	WORSE.
RESPIRATORY ORGANS.	AIR { Change of. **Inhaling.**
NERVES.	Eating. Toward morning.
MUCOUS MEMBRANES.	

Almost continuous paroxyms of extremely violent, spasmodic cough, which begin with gasping for breath (Meph.), are accompanied by a purple face, and **followed by exhaustion** (Ant-t.) and vomiting of stringy mucus. A minute gun cough. Coughs as soon as he eats. Whooping cough. Very red, (flat) venereal ulcers. Too hot if covered, but chilled by uncovering.

Complementary: Sul. Related: Coc-c.

CORNUS.

REGION.	WORSE.
Blood. Liver. Spleen.	Night. Taking Cold.
Digestive tract.	

Weak and depressed. **Liver symptoms, with aching eyeballs** (Chio.). Dark, foul stools, with burning at anus. Diarrhœa. Sallow skin. Sleepy before the chills, with the heat and after meals. Old malarias.

Related: Eupat.

CROCUS.

REGION.	WORSE.
MIND.	**Motion.** Reading. Pregnancy.
NERVES. **Circulation. Eyes.**	Heat.
Female Sexual Organs.	BETTER.
	Open Air.

Rapidly changing or alternating symptoms; of opposite moods; of sides;

of mind and body, etc. Twitching of single muscles; upper eyelids, etc. Chorea. **As of something alive jumping about internally.** DARK, STRINGY HEMORRHAGE (Merc. Ust.).——**Impressionable, affectionate and moody.** Involuntary laughter; < music. Hysteria. Climacteric hemicrania; > pressure; instead of menses. Dry burning in eyes as after weeping (Aru-t.) or as if in a cool wind. Winks or must close eyes tightly. **Lachrymation** when reading. Nosebleed (Merc. Plat.), with faintness and cold sweat on forehead. Sexual excitement. **Dark**, foul, stringy (Lac-c.) menses. Threatened abortion. Narcotic sleep.

Related: Ign. Taren.

CROTALUS HORRIDUS.

REGION.
- BLOOD.
- **LIVER.**
- **Right Side.**

WORSE.
- **Lying on Right Side.**
- Warm weather. **Spring.**
- **Falling to Sleep.**

BETTER.
- Light.

Deathly sick, tremulous and weak. MALIGNANCY; TENDENCY TO SLOW HEMORRHAGE, **of dark, thin blood, putridity and rapid decomposition. Sepsis.** Dark or bluish parts. Petechiæ. Gangrene.——Torpid. Forgetful. Mistakes in writing (Am-c. Lach. Lyc. Thu.). **Occipital headache**; in waves from spine. Distorted face on awaking. Epilepsy. **Dark,** besotted face (Bapt). Grinds the teeth. Mouldy breath (Rhus-t.). Swelled tongue. Craves pork. Bilious vomit. Anxious, labored breathing. Heart seems loose, tremulous or sensitive to lying on left side. Jaundice. Blood boils. **Horrible dreams**; of the dead.

Related; Lach. Sul-ac.

CROTON TIGLIUM.

REGION.
- **MUCOUS MEMBRANES** { **INTESTINES. Eyes.**
- **SKIN** { SCROTUM. FACE. **Scalp.**

WORSE.
- DRINKING. **Eating.**
- Receding Eruptions.
- Washing. Motion.

Eyes or nipples feel drawn backward (Croc. Par.). Pressure excites pain in rectum or a stool. **Gurgling or swashing as of water in bowels; then** SUDDEN, PROFUSE, GUSHING STOOL OF YELLOW WATER, <

DRINKING (Arg-n. Pho.), then prostration. Diarrhœa. Cholera infantum. Can't inhale deeply enough. Pain from nipple to back as child nurses (Phel.). Itching, tense, burning, red skin; sore if scratched, > gentle rubbing. **Vesiculo-pustular eruptions** (Sep.), < genitals, temples and crown of head. Eczema. Zoster.

Related: Rhus-t.

CUBEBAE.

REGION.

Mucous Membranes { URETHRA. Bladder. **Vagina.**

WORSE.
Night, in Bed.
BETTER.
Walking About.

Burning rawness. Violent inflammation, then acrid, yellow or green, offensive discharges. Catarrhs. Gelatinous, cold stools; with grains like rice. Cold stools.

Related: Cist. Cop.

CUPRUM.

REGION.
CEREBRO-SPINAL AXIS.
NERVES. MUSCLES.
DIGESTIVE TRACT.
Blood.

WORSE.
Suppressions. Overtax. Motion, Hot Weather. **Vomiting.** Touch. Loss of Sleep. Raising arms.
BETTER.
COLD DRINKS.

Convulsive phenomena. **Groups of violent, but similar effects. Convulsive, jerking or cramping;** begins at a single point, fingers, etc., then deathly exhaustion. **The muscles draw into knots** (Phys.). Epilepsy. Radiating pains. Latency. **Relapses easily.**——Impulsive. Nervous. **Piercing shrieks.** Delirium. Can't hold head erect. Meningitis. Eyeballs oscillate behind closed lids (Agar. Coccl. Gel.). **Bluish face.** Grinds the teeth. **Metallic taste** (Rhus-t.). Spasm of glottis. **Nausea.** Tormenting vomiting. Painful transfixing cramp. Hard pressure in epigastrium. Lies on abdomen and jerks the buttocks up. Tense abdomen. **Frightful colic,** > pressure. Spurting stools; of bloody, greenish water. Cholera. Suppressed urine. Cramps prevent coition (Grap). After pains. Paroxysmal or whooping cough. **Dyspnœa;** can't bear anything near mouth (Lach.); < coughing or laughing. Constriction of (lower) chest (Coccl. Plat.). Jerks in hands and feet. Clenches thumbs into palms. CRAMP IN CALVES

OR SOLES (Colo. Sul.). Repercussed or undeveloped eruptions or discharges (Zin.). Icy coldness. Cold, viscid sweat. Collapse.

Complementary: Calc-c. Related: Ver-a.

CUPRUM ARSENICUM.

REGION.	WORSE.
DIGESTIVE TRACT.	Touch. Pressure. Damp Weather.
Muscles. Nerves.	

Violent colics. Icy cold body, with cramps and obstinate hiccough. Visceral neuralgia. Garlicky urine. Uræmic convulsions. Cold, clammy, intermittent sweat.

Related: Cupr.

CYCLAMEN.

REGION.	WORSE.
Cerebro-Spinal Axis. Sensorium.	COLD. Evening. Sitting. **Fats.**
FEMALE SEXUAL ORGANS.	BETTER.
DIGESTIVE TRACT. **VISION.**	Motion. During Menses.

VISUAL EFFECTS **or vertigo due to menstrual** or gastric disorders. Dreads open air.——Dull, sad and morose. Silent weeping. Brain feels wrapped up. **Pain in left temple.** Migraine. Convergent squint. FLICKERING, GLITTERING OR BLACK VISION. Loss of smell. Taste lost or salty. Nausea in throat. Craves lemonade (Bell. Sabi.). Chlorosis. Quick satiety. **Excessive menses,** early, dark, clotted. Dysmenorrhœa. Air seems to stream from nipples. Swelled breasts. Milk in breasts of virgins. Weakness, < in knees. Chilliness. Offensive sweat.

Related: Pul.

DAPHNE INDICA.

REGION.	WORSE.
Muscles. **Bones.**	Cold Air. **Waning Moon.**
Left Side.	Evening in **Bed.**

Part—head, arms—seems separated from body (Bapt. Psor.). **Bruised** pain. **Fetor.** Exhaustion.——Sad. Head feels big. **Tongue coated on one side only** (Irid. Rhus-t.). Sleepless; from **bone aches.** Clammy sweat.

Related: Rhus-t.

DIGITALIS.

REGION.
HEART.
CIRCULATION { LIVER. **Lungs.** Stomach.
Genito-Urinary Organs.

WORSE.
Motion. **Rising Up.** Exertion.
Lying on Left Side. Excesses.
Smell of Food. Cold; drinks.
BETTER.
Lying Flat on Back.

SLOW, WEAK OR IRREGULAR PULSE. **Venous stasis. Attacks of great weakness;** can hardly talk.—Anxious solicitude. **Dizzy.** Yellow, inflamed conjunctiva. Seething in ears. **Bluish lips; or tongue** (Ars. Gym. Rad-b.). Thick, flabby tongue. Much thirst, little appetite. Nausea. Deathly sinking at pit of stomach (Staph.). Sore liver. Liver with heart symptoms. White, putty like stools. Teasing to urinate; must walk about. Throbbing in neck of bladder. Dropsy. Atonic, night-losses. Gonorrhœa of glans (Jacar.). Slow breathing. Cough with pains in shoulders and arms. **Heart threatens to stop** (Cimi. Gel. Lob. Vib.). Heart sprain. Palpitation. Numbness or weakness of left arm. **Drowsy.** Dreams of falling; awakes with a shock. Flushes of heat, then **great weakness.** Cold, clammy sweat.

Related: Glo. Spig.

DIOSCOREA.

REGION.
NERVES { ABDOMINAL. Sciatic.
Gall Bladder. **Navel.**

WORSE.
Doubling Up. Tea. Eating. Lying.
BETTER.
Stretching out or Bending Back.
Hard Pressure.

Pains; in regular paroxysms, dart about or radiate, to distant parts, arms, etc. (Berb. Cup. Plb.). UNBEARABLE, CUTTING, TWISTING OR GRINDING PAIN. Abdominal colic. **Eructations.** Flatulence. Darting from anus to liver (Lach.). Piles like a bunch of red cherries. Atonic emissions, then weak knees (Cob.). Felon. Sciatica (r) < motion. Cold, clammy sweat.

Related: Colo.

DIPHTHERINUM.

REGION.
Blood.
Mucous Membrane of THROAT.

WORSE.

Marked weakness; malignancy. Low temperature. Fetor. **PAINLESS DIPHTHERIA;** thick membrane. Relapses. Dark red spot back of tip of tongue.

Related: **Carb-ac.**

DROSERA.

REGION.
RESPIRATORY ORGANS.
Larynx.
Chest.

WORSE.
After Midnight. On Lying Down.
Warmth. **Talking.** Cold Foods.
Laughing. After Measles.

BETTER.
Pressure.

Spasmodic, catarrhal and hemorrhagic effects.——Desire to drown himself. Painful sneezing. Putrid taste. PERIODICAL FITS OF RAPID, DEEP BARKING OR CHOKING COUGH, TAKING AWAY THE BREATH (Cup. Ip. Sep.), **compel holding the sides** (Bry. Eupat. Nat-s. Pho. Sep.) **and end in retching, vomiting, nosebleed or cold sweat.** Typical whooping cough Tickling like a feather or crumb in larynx. Bloody expectoration. **Hoarse, toneless voice.** Constriction of chest. Stitches below axillæ. Writers cramp.

Complementary: Sul. Related: Coc-c. Cor-r.

DULCAMARA.

REGION.
MUCOUS MEMBRANES { BRONCHI. BLADDER. Eyes.
BACK { **Muscles. LOINS.**
SKIN.
Lymphatic Glands.

WORSE.
BECOMING CHILLED or Taking Cold { **Cold wet;** rains. **WHILE HOT. CHANGE OF TEMPERATURE. Uncovering.**
SUPPRESSED DISCHARGES { SWEAT. **Eruptions.**
Autumn. Night. Rest.
Before Storms. **Mercury.**

BETTER.
Warmth.

Excessive secretion of mucus. Catarrhal, rheumatic, herpetic tendency.

Stiff, numb and sore. Tearing pains. Paralytic effects.——**Confusion. Depression. Scolding.** Difficult speech. Easily becomes delirious. Occiput feels large (Bry. Cocl.). Ringworm of scalp. Aching in nose. Stuffed coryza. Swelled tongue. Tenacious, soapy saliva. Cutting at navel; then painful, green, slimy stools. Diarrhœa. **Every cold affects the bladder** (Pul.), bowels or respiration (Sul.). **Cloudy, slimy or foul urine.** Cystitis. Dropsy. Watery menses. **Eruptions;** scaly, thick, crusty, moist, bleeding or herpetic; < before menses. **Large fleshy warts. Coldness;** in occiput; in lumbar region; in bones; icy, of paralyzed part. Pruritus.

Complementary: Bar-c. Nat-s. Related: Rhus-t.

ELAPS.

REGION.	WORSE.
BLOOD.	COLD. **Drinks** or Food. **Night.**
Right Side.	Wet Weather. In Room.

Black discharges. Internal coldness. Oscillatory motions.——Black rings before left eye (Calc-c.). **Deafness; at night. Stuffed feeling in naso-pharynx.** Green yellow crusts in nose. Ozœna. Nosebleed. Red spots on face. Drinks feel like ice in stomach. Stools of black frothy blood. Air hunger. Pain at apex of right lung. Weak arms.

Related: Crot-h.

EPIPHEGUS.

REGION.	WORSE.
NERVES.	**FATIGUE; Nervous.** Eyestrain.
Stomach.	BETTER.
Liver.	Sleep.

Confusion.——Pressure like fingertips into **temples.** Compressive, (r) headache, spreading backward; < until 4 P. M., then >; with **spitting of viscid saliva** (Helo. Plan.) and nausea. **Neurasthenia.**

Related: Iris. Ign.

EQUISETUM.

REGION.	WORSE.
GENITO-URINARY TRACT.	**At Close of Urination.**
	Pressure.

Aching, full, tender bladder (Tereb.). Cystitis. **Prickling,** burning or cutting in urethra. Dysuria. **NOCTURNAL ENURESIS;** with irritable bladder. Dribbling urine. **Mucus in urine.**

Complementary: Sil. **Related: Canth.**

ERIGERON.

REGION.
Genito-Urinary Tract.
Joints.

WORSE.
Rainy Weather.

Hemorrhage; bright, gushing. **Congestion. Smarting-burning.** Hard aching.——Tympanites. Anus seems torn. Vesico-rectal tenesmus. Aching in bladder (Tere.). Sticky sweat on genitals.

Related: Tereb.

EUCALYPTUS.

REGION.
Mucous Membranes.
Respiration. Muscles.

WORSE.
Periodically.
Night.

Aching, stiff and weary; feels as if had taken cold. Grippe. Migraine. **Profuse catarrhal discharges;** acrid; foul.——Burning in eyes. Tinnitus. Tension across nose (Ham.). Watery coryza. Pasty tongue. Throbbing in stomach. Weight in bowels. Slow digestion with putrid gas. Diuresis. **Bronchial asthma.** Chill ends in nausea and vomiting. Scanty sweat. Old malaria.

Related: Chin. Dulc.

EUONYMUS.

REGION.
Liver. Kidneys.

WORSE.
Eating.

Vertigo, as if drawn up and pitched forward (Calc-c.). Pressure over brows, as if to compress eyes. Engorged liver. Gall stones. Pain about navel. Profuse stools; varying in color. Albuminuria.

Related: Rhe.

EUPATORIUM.

REGION.
BONES. LIVER.
Occiput. Stomach. Bronchiæ.
Muscles: **Chest. Back.** Limbs.

WORSE.
MOTION. COLD AIR.
PERIODICALLY: 7-9 A. M.; Every 3rd or 7th day.
Lying on Part. Coughing.
Food: Sight or Smell of.

BETTER.
Vomiting Bile. Sweating.
Lying on Face.

BREAKING BONE PAINS (Pyro. Rut.). **Bilious effects; yellow eyes,**

face, vomit, etc. Restless, chilly and sore, with nausea. Colds. Grippe (prophylactic).——Vertigo, swaying to the left; > vomiting. Sore throbbing head pains, < occiput; alternating with gouty pains. Migraine. Sore eyeballs (Bry. Cimi. Gel. Onos.). Thirsty, but drinks excite vomiting (Ars.) or < the chill (Caps.). Whitish stools. Hoarse in A. M. Raw and sore in chest and bronchi. Bruised pain in calves (Staph.). Dropsy of legs. Painful gouty nodes. **Thirst or nausea, then violent shaking chill**; begins in small of back. **Bitter vomiting after chill** or during heat. Burning heat. Scanty sweat. Malaria. Catarrhal fevers.

Complementary: Nat-m. Sep. Related: Bry. Nux-v.

EUPHORBIUM.

REGION.	WORSE.
Mucous Membranes.	**Sitting.** Rest. Beginning Motion.
Skin. Bones. Teeth.	Mercury.

Slow inflammation. Paralytic weakness in joints. **Internal burning.** Caries. Much secretion, with a sense of dryness.——Mouth feels coated with rancid grease (Iris.). Brittle, crumbling teeth. Stitches from epigastrium into sides of chest on coughing. Erysipelas bullosum; with high fever.

Related: Nit-ac. Sul.

EUPHRASIA.

REGION.	WORSE.
MUCOUS MEMBRANES { **EYES.** NOSE. Chest.	**SUNLIGHT. WARMTH. WIND. ROOM.** Evening.
	BETTER.
	Winking. Wiping Eyes. **Open Air.**

Free, acrid, watery secretions. Acute catarrhs. Acrid pus.——WATERY EYES (Saba. Thu.); as of a hair before them, wants to wipe them (Croc.). **ABUNDANT ACRID OR HOT, SMARTING TEARS, WITH BLAND CORYZA;** < open air, lying down or coughing (Chel.); leaving a varnish-like mark (Grap.). Photophobia; with spasm of lids. Pressive cutting eye pains. Sticky eyegum (Kali-bi.). Red, burning-itching tarsi (Sul.); violent injection. Chronic sore eyes. Chemosis. Conjunctivitis. Gushes of fluent coryza (Agar.). Loose cough with easy expectoration in daytime only (Pho.) > lying down at night (Mang.). Measles.

Related: Cepa.

FERRUM.

REGION.
VASO-MOTOR NERVES.
CIRCULATION.
BLOOD.
Spleen.

WORSE.
REPOSE. VIOLENT EXERTION.
NIGHT (Mid.). **When Sweating.**
Loss of Vital Fuilds. Eating.
Heat and Cold. Quinine.

BETTER.
GENTLE MOTION. Heat.
Leaning Head on Something.

Erethistic, yet internally weak and must lie down. **Excited, surging circulation; pulsations, hemorrhages** (bright or with small clots), dilated veins, etc. False plethora. Red faced old men. Exophthalmos. Pressure upon chest, in stomach, etc. Pale, dry mucous membranes (Pho.); food tastes dry (Calad.), dry vagina, etc. Rapid emaciation. Anæmia. Cachexy.—— Excited; < contradiction. **Hammering, throbbing headache;** starts in temple; < coughing or stooping; > letting hair down. Puffy eyelids. Face feels bloated. **Nosebleed.** FACE REDDENS FROM THE LEAST THING (Amy-n. Ign.). Toothache, > ice water. Averse to meat. Easy vomiting. Spits up his food. Painless lientery; < while eating. Enuresis. Pale menses. Acrid, milky leucorrhœa. Dry, tickling cough. Blood spitting (streaked). Constriction of or flying stitches in chest. Sudden cramps or tearing, boring in limbs. Omodynia (1). Swelled hands and feet. Varicoses; < during menses. Chill with red face and thirst. Heat with distended veins.

Complementary: Chin. Related: Arn. Mang.

FERRUM PHOSPHORICUM.

REGION.
Vaso-Motor Nerves.
Venous Circulation { LUNGS. Ears. Eustachian Tube.

WORSE.
Night (4-6 A. M.)
Open Air. Jarring.
Checked Sweat.

Passive febrile congestion, FULL, SOFT, FLOWING PULSE **and weakness. Bloody** (streaked or meat water) **discharges.** Pneumonia; intercurrent.—— Talkative. Headache, > **nosebleed or cold. Face red and pale alternately.** Suffused eyes. Earache. Otitis media (Sul.). **Frequent stools of bloody water.** Threatening hydrocephalus. Enuresis. Early menses with heavy pain on vertex. Heavy or sore chest. Omodynia (Mag-c.). Heat with sweaty hands (Am-c. Nit-ac.).

Related: Gel.

FLUORIC ACID.

REGION.

FIBROUS TISSUES { **VEINS.** Skin.

BONES. Mastoid.

WORSE.

HEAT; of Room. Night. Alcohol.

BETTER.

COOL BATHING. RAPID MOTION (walking). Short Sleep. Bending Head Back. Eating.

Pale, miserable and broken down. Slow, deeply destructive effects. Puffy, indurated or fistulous tissues. Felon. Palmar abscess. Caries. Bed sores. Ulcers. Oedema. Secondary syphillis, etc. **Thin, foul, acrid** (or salty) **discharges. Always too hot; wants to bathe in cold water.——Impulse to walk rapidly** (Kali-iod.). Lecherousness (Pic-ac.). Stunning headache; > urination. Brittle, tously hair. As of a cold wind on eye (Syp. Thu.). Lachrymal stricture (Grap.). Deafness, > bending head back. **Puffy glabella.** Thin enamel. Teeth decay rapidly; < at roots (Mez. Thu.). Gnawing hunger; for pungent or cold things. Stale eructations. Itching or burning at anus. Upward drawing in urethra (down Merc.). Profuse, acrid leucorrhœa. Sexual erethism. Distorted nails. Varicose veins. Dry, harsh, itching, cracked skin; seeming to emit a hot vapor. Scars, surrounded by pimples. Ebullitions of heat; with pain in bones. **Acrid, eroding sweat,** excites itching. Oily, pungent sweat on genitals. Sweat on hands and feet.

Complementary: Sil. Related: Pul. Sul-ac.

FORMICA.

REGION.

Spine. Liver. Kidneys. Vision.

WORSE.

COLD. Wet. Before Snowstorms.

Sudden rheumatic or gouty pains. Takes cold easily. Hyperplasia.——Light, foaming stools. Hives in flat plaques. Profuse sweat without relief.

Related: Rhus-t.

FRAXINUS.

REGION.
UTERUS. **Nerves.**

WORSE.
Injury. **Sprains. Lifting.**

Nervous females with enlarged or prolapsed wombs.——Throbbing in occiput. Burning heat or dryness on top of head. Sensitive left ovary. Cramps in feet.

Related: Vib.

GAMBOGIA.

REGION.
Stomach and BOWELS.
Liver.

BETTER.
AFTER STOOL.
Motion in Open Air.

Burnings.——Itching eyelids; he rubs them. Sneezing. **Gurgling, pinching in bowels, then yellow or green,** THIN STOOLS COMING OUT IN PROLONGED GUSHES, **with burning at anus** (Ars. Merc-s. Nat-c. Scop. Sul.) **and much relief.**

Related: Crot-t.

GELSEMIUM.

REGION.
BRAIN. CORD { **OCCIPUT Base. Neck.**
MOTOR NERVES { **MUSCLES.** Knees. EYES { LIDS. VISION.
MUCOUS MEMBRANES { Nose. Gall Ducts.
Right Side.

WORSE.
EMOTIONS; DREAD. Surprise.
Weather { SPRING. Foggy. HUMID. Muggy.
Heat. Periodically. Tobacco.

BETTER.
Profuse Urination. Sweating. Shaking. Alcoholic Drinks.

HEAVY ACHING. WEAK, DIZZY, DROWSY AND DULL OR RELAXED, TIRED AND SORE. **Wants to lie quietly; in half reclining posture (Sang). Nerve exhaustion.** Grippe. **Facial neuralgia.** FULNESS. **Passive congestion. PARALYTIC EFFECTS;** in eyes, throat (Caus. Cocc. Lach.), anus, genitals, etc. **Trembling;** chin, tongue, etc.——DAZED, CONFUSED, STUPID. **Fears falling** (Bor.). **VERTIGO; felt in occiput** (Ib. Petr. Sil. **Zin.**). **Heavy headache;** from nape to eyes. Throbbing, tender occiput. Basilar headaches (Cimi. Ver-v.). Meningitis. Apoplexy. **HEAVY, DROOPING EYELIDS** (Caus. Cocc. Rhus-t. Sep. Zin.). Aching, suffused eyes. **Diplopia.**

Full, dusky-red face; as if drunken. **Sneezing. Thin, acrid coryza.** Heavy, tremulous tongue; **thick speech.** Pains go into ears on swallowing. **NO THIRST.** Copious yellow stools. Painless psychic diarrhœa (Aco. Arg-n. Coff. Hyo. Op. Pul. Ver-a.). Clear, watery urine (Ign.). Alternate pelvic and head symptoms. Seminal losses. **Heavy, sore feeling in uterus.** Labor pains go up, backward or down thighs. Rigid os (Caul.). Congestion to chest; tiresome breathing. Heart threatens to stop, > motion. Dull pains up and down spine; > walking. Heavy lower limbs (Rhus-t.). **Weak knees** (Chin. Coccl. Lach. Nat-m. Nit-ac. Sep. Stap.). Can't direct his legs. Yellowness. **Moist skin. DROWSINESS. Full, soft pulse.** Visual disturbances then chill. **Chills, with languor** (Sil.); **mingled with heat.** Chilly along back (4-5 P. M.). **Heat with sopor and absence of thirst.** Malaria. **Bilious, remittent type.** Cerebro spinal fever.

Complementary: Sep. Related: Bell. Con. Mur-ac. Sep. Ver-v.

GLONOIN.

REGION.

BRAIN.

VASO-MOTORS { **CIRCULATION.** / **HEAD** (forehead) / HEART.

Respiration.

WORSE.

HEAT { **ON HEAD,** Overheating. / **OF SUN,** Lamp, etc. / **WEATHER.**

MOTION { SHAKING JAR. / Injury.

Suppressed Menses.

Weight of Hat.

BETTER.

Open Air. Elevating Head.

Cool Things.

PULSATION; general (Fer. Grap. Kali-c.). Violent congestion or ebullitions. SUDDEN UPWARD RUSHES OF BLOOD. **Full distended or enlarged feeling.**——Bewildered; loses himself. Falls unconscious. Sunstroke (Aco. Ver-v.). Apoplexy. **WAVES OF TERRIBLE, BURSTING, PULSATING HEADACHE;** as if standing on head (Elap. Pho.), it were expanding and contracting (Calc-c.) or the blood was surging back and forth from the head to the heart; < sunshine (Nat-c. Nux-v.); < damp days. Cracking snapping (Ars. Dig. Kalm.), shocks through (Pho. Zin.) or soreness in brain. Swelling of veins of temples (Ars.). Protruding, staring or dry eyes; lids stick to balls. Blind spells. **Bluish face.** Heavy tongue. Heavy breathing. As of a load on chest. **Violent palpitation.** Pain from

heart to arm (Alu. Kali-n. Nat-m. Pho. Plb.). Neck feels full and stiff. Trembling hands. **Awakes fearing apoplexy. Heat on crown of head and** along spine.

Complementary: Bell. Related: **Amyl-n.** Bell.

GNAPHALIUM.

REGION.
NERVES { **SCIATIC.** **Crural.** Abdominal.

WORSE.
Walking. Lying.
BETTER.
Flexing Limbs. **Sitting.**

Intense sciatic pains; alternating with numbness (Colo.). Offensive diarrhœa with colic, < in morning.

Related: Colo.

GOSSYPIUM.

REGION.
UTERUS. **Ovaries.**

WORSE.
Motion.

Uterine reflexes. Ovarian pain, extending toward uterus. **Uterine torpor.** Cervical pains. Sensitive womb. Menses late, scanty and **watery.**

Related: Ustil.

GRAPHITES.

REGION.
NUTRITION.
SKIN { FOLDS. ANGLES. FLEXURES. **Nails.**
Circulation. Eyes. Glands.
Mucous Membranes.

WORSE.
COLD. **During Menses.**
Suppressions. Warmth of Bed.
Light. Scratching. **Fats.**
BETTER.
Open Air; After Walking in.
Eating. Touch. Noise.

THICKNESS AND HARDNESS; **skin,** tarsi, nails, scars, callosities, stools, crusts, etc. EXCORIATIONS, CRACKS OR FISSURES; **in angles** (Merc.); of mouth, canthi, fingertips, nipples (Caust. Rat.), anus, etc. **Emaciation;** of affected part. **Foul, corrosive secretions.** Watery hemorrhages. Sense of burning, numbness or deadness. **Fat, chilly and costive.**——Sad, fearsome and irresolute. Music brings tears. **Brain** feels numb. **Burning** spot on vertex. Wens. Matted, brittle or falling hair. Milk crusts. Inflamed or scaly tarsi (Mag-m.). Ingrown lashes (Tell.). **Photophobia.**

Briny otorrhœa, Tinnitus. Hears > in a noise (Jab.). **Eruption and moisture behind ears.** Dryness in ears and nose (Nit-ac. Petr.). Acute smell. Acne before menses. Barbers itch (Lith-c.). Rotten taste. **Hunger.** Averse to meats and sweets. Alternate digestive and skin symptoms (Ant-c.). Gastric pains that necessitate eating. Can't have pressure about waist. **Flatulence. Intestinal torpor. Large, knotty, difficult, slimy coated stools** or loose. brown and very foul. Itching of anus and pudendum. Sexual exhaustion. Averse to coition. Menses irregular; late, scanty, etc. Gushes of irritating leucorrhœa; instead of menses. Foot sweat. **IRRITABLE, DRY SKIN THAT BREAKS EASILY AND EXUDES A GLUEY MOISTURE** (Mez.) **WHEN ABRADED; < in the folds—and is slow to heal** (Lyc.). MOIST, CRUSTY ERUPTIONS. Eczema. Wandering or recurrent erysipelas (Rhus-t.). Eruptions < from heat. **Supersensitive to cold; it < bone pains, coryza and stomach.**

Related: Ars. Calc-fl. The. Carbons. Kali-bi. Pul.

GRATIOLA.

REGION.
Gastro-Intestinal Tract.
Mind. Sexual Organs.

WORSE.
Drinking too Much Water.
Summer. Coffee. Dinner. Motion.

Coldness.——Weak will. Emptiness after eating. As of cold water or a loose, heavy load in stomach. **Profuse, gushing, watery or frothy, yellow-green, exhausting stools, then relief** (Gamb.). Nymphomania. Coccygeal pain. Limb gives away with sciatic pain.

Related: Mag-c.

GRINDELIA.

REGION.
Respiration. Bronchiæ.

WORSE.
Falling to Sleep.

Profuse secretions.——**Smothers on falling to sleep.** Asthma. Tenacious expectoration. Bronchorrhea. Cutting and soreness about spleen.

Related: Lach.

GUAIACUM.

REGION.

SECRETIONS { GLANDS. TONSILS. **Skin.**

FIBROUS TISSUES { **Ligaments.** Joints.

WORSE.

HEAT. Touch. Motion. Exertion. Mercury.

BETTER.

Cold (Locally). Apples.

Arthritic symptoms. FREE, FOUL SECRETIONS; sweats, expectoration, etc. **Impending suppuration;** quinsy, old bronchitis, etc. **Burning heat;** in affected parts. Sticking or gnawing pains. **Muscular soreness.** Contractions; distorting (Caus.); between scapulæ. Nodes. Pain from head into neck (Bry.). Eyeballs seem too big for the lids. Burning in throat. Red, swelled tonsils. Tonsilitis. Averse to milk. Stoppage in epigastrium; causes cough, dyspnœa, etc. Dry cough with heat of face and burning fever. Sticking in apex of left lung. Phthisis. Recurrent pleurisy. Aching soreness of neck; one side stiff. Tense, short thigh muscles. Yawning and stretching. Sweat on single parts; face, etc. Nightsweats.

Related: Kali-bi. Kre. Phyt.

GYMNOCLADUS.

REGION.

Urinary Organs.
Circulation.
Sensations.

WORSE.

Cold. Walking.

BETTER.

Rest. Leaning Against Something.

Lividity. Numbness.——Slow grasp. Head feels bound. Pain under brows and into nose. Out pushing in eyes; wants to rub them. Crawling on (1) face. Teeth sensitive to cold air. BLUISH TONGUE. Hot, sour belchings. Burning spot in stomach.

Related: Op.

HAMAMELIS.

REGION.

VEINS { Rectum. Genitals. Throat. }

Abdominal and Chest Walls.

WORSE.

INJURY. Bruises. Pressure.

Air { Open. Warm. Moist. Cold. }

Motion. Jar.

LOCALIZED, BRUISED SORENESS. CONGESTIVE FULNESS. DARK HEMORRHAGES; which relieve or cause undue weakness (Hydr.). **Painfull varicose conditions** (Pul. Thu.).——**Irritable and chilly.** Hammering in temples. Bloodshot eyes. Taste of blood. Pain and heaviness back of stomach. Soreness in abdomen. Piles. Orchitis. Neuralgia of testes. Varicocele. Profuse, dark menses. Scapular pains. Dull ache about kidneys. Phlebitis. Ecchymoses.

Complementary: Fer. Flu-ac. Related: Arn. Pul. Vip.

HELLEBORE.

REGION.

MIND. BRAIN.

NERVES { SENSORY. MOTOR. }

MEMBRANES { **SEROUS.** MUCOUS. }

Muscles. Serous Exudations.

WORSE.

COLD AIR. Dentition. Puberty.

Suppressed Eruptions. Exertions.

Evening (4-8 P. M.)

BETTER.

Strong Attention.

Gradual onset with **blunted senses and sluggish responses**; muscles obey feebly (Crot-h. Gel. Kali-br. Phys.); slow answers, drops things (Ap.), staggers, etc. Automatic acts (Lyc. Zin.). Lies on back with knees drawn up. Feeble and delicate.——**Stupid, obtuse or apathetic.** Blank despair. Won't eat or speak. Fixed ideas. Things look new. Heavy, numbing headache. **Rolls the head** or bores it into pillow (Zin.). Hydrocephalus. **Stupid, staring or tired look. Eyes half open.** Dark, sooty nostrils. **Pale face.** Chewing motion. **Fetor oris.** Numb, dry, trembling tongue or covered with yellow ulcers. Ptyalism. Distended abdomen. Stools watery or gelatinous. Scanty urine. with dark flecks or sediment. Small, soft pulse. Sopor; with **cries or starts.** Dropsy. Amenorrhœa. Coldness.

Complementary: Zin. Related: **Bry. Op.**

HELONIAS.

REGION.
- FEMALE ORGANS.
- **Kidneys.**
- **Mind.**
- **Muscles.**

WORSE.
- **Fatigue** { After Labor. Abortion. Stooping.
- Pressure of Clothes.

BETTER.
- **When Busy. Mental Diversion.**
- **Holding Abdomen.**

Exhausted females. Uterine reflexes. Aching-burning; in **muscles.** Aphthæ.——**Deep gloom.** Irritable, wants to be left alone. Heat or upward pressure in vertex. **Dull ache and heat in region of kidneys** (Phyt.). Excessive urine. **Heavy** (Pall.), **sore, tender, ulcerated or prolapsed womb.** Dark, foul blood from uterus. Foul or **curdled, lumpy leucorrhœa** (Merc. Psor. Rad-b.). Inflamed, itching aphthous vulva. **Heavy dragging in pelvis. Squeezing in chest.** Aching between scapulæ (Pho.). Sore pain in outside of thighs. Anæmia. Hot when tired.

Related: Senec. Sep. Tril.

HEPAR.

REGION.
- **NERVES.**
- **CONNECTIVE TISSUES.**
- **Respiratory Membranes.**
- **GLANDS.**
- Skin.

WORSE.
- COLD { AIR (dry). WINTER. DRAFTS. WIND. PART BECOMING.
- LEAST { UNCOVERING. TOUCH. EXERTION.
- **LYING ON PAINFUL PART.**
- **Mercury.** Night.

BETTER.
- **HEAT { WARM WRAPS; TO HEAD.**
- **DAMP WEATHER.**

Lax, chilly and sensitive; can't stand pain; faints easily. SWEATS EASILY, **but dare not uncover** (Cham. Nat-c. Zin.). **As of wind blowing on part.** Always taking cold. SORE, STICKING, LIKE SHARP SPLINTERS (Arg-n. Nit-ac.). SUPPURATION, EVERY HURT FESTERS (Merc.); **much thick pus.** Abscess. **Secretions profuse; sour. foul** (like old cheese—Bry. Sanic.).——**Hasty, irritable and dissatisfied. Fall-**

ing hair. Photophobia. Chronic otorrhœa. Nose is stuffed and painful. Hawks much mucus. Rough sticking in throat; as of a fish bone or crumb (Arg-n. Ign. Kali-c. Nit-ac.). Quinsy (Lyc. Sil.). **Weak stomach.** Craves acids, condiments and stimulants. Eating refreshes, but causes heaviness. Stool difficult, altho soft (Anac. Chin. Nux-m. Psor. Pul.). Very foul leucorrhœa (Kali-p.). Whistling breathing; must bend head back. Croup. Asthma; from suppressions. **Barking or loose, choking, croupy cough;** < cold drinks or in A. M. **WEAKNESS AND MUCH RATTLING IN CHEST** (Sil.). **Much expectoration** (Kali-bi.). Skin is sensitive to cool air. Moist, foul eruptions. Torpid, pulsating ulcers; surrounded by pimples. smaller ones or boils (Lach. Mez. Pho.). **Low** fevers. Nightsweats.

Complementary: Sil. Related: Merc.

HYDRASTIS.

REGION.	WORSE.
MUCOUS GLANDS { Post Nasal. STOMACH. Gall Ducts. **Intestines.**	AIR { **Inhaling Cold.** Open. Dry Winds.
Muscles. Uterus.	Washing. Old Age.

Catarrhal or ulcerative-hemorrhagic tendency; with **thick, yellow, acrid** (Sanic.), **ropy secretions.** Sense of raw-burning. Weakness.——Post nasal catarrh. Thin, yellow, sunken face. Cachexia. **Dirty, yellow, slimy, flabby, indented tongue** (Nat-p.). Taste, bitter; burnt. Aphthæ. Loathing. **Raises quantities of thick yellow, tenacious mucus.** "Goneness" at stomach (Sul.). Indigestion. Lumpy stool, coated or mixed with yellow mucus (Grap.). Constipation. Tenacious mucus in urine. Ulcer of cervix. Leucorrhœa. Palpitation; with weakness. Heat; alternating with chilliness.

Related: Kali-bi. Pul.

HYDROCYANIC ACID.

REGION.	WORSE.
Heart. Respiration. Epigastrium.	Suppressions.

Lighting like jerks pass from head to feet. Spasms. Paralysis. Prolonged faints. Evacuations suddenly cease (Cam.). **Cholera. Pale, bluish** face. Noisy swallowing. Slow, **gasping, irregular** breathing. Dry, tickling night cough. **Failing pulse.** Icy coldness. Collapse. Heart failure.

Related. Laur.

HYOSCYAMUS.

REGION.

MIND. BRAIN. NERVES.

Muscles { Face. Eyes.

Blood.

WORSE.

MENTAL EFFECTS { FRIGHT. Jealousy.

TOUCH. **Lying**. **Cold**. Sleep.

BETTER.

Sitting Up.

Congested nerve centers, with a pale face. Spasmodic effects, **tremor, jerking,** cramps, etc. or **active mania;** all alternating with or **ending in a depressive narcosis,** with angular or **clutching motions,** CARPHOLOGY, **subsultus,** etc. Zymoses. Eclampsia (Cic. Cup. Stry.).——**Many bewildering aberrations.** MANIA; **erotic, exposing the genitals** (Canth.); riotous; noisy, with laughter, singing, talking, quarreling, etc.; **silly,** with comical acts; **suspicous,** fears being alone, being poisoned (Lach. Rhus-t.), water, **wants to escape,** etc. First, can't think, then can **barely be aroused, then** profound relaxation with **muttering;** the lower jaw drops, he slides down in bed (Mur-ac.), has **involuntary**—bloody or yellow **watery—stools,** etc. Typhoid states. Pulsating headaches; the head shakes to and fro, > bending forward. Squint (Bell.). Averse to light. Spasmodic closure of eyelids (Merc. Nat-m. Rhus-t. Sil.). Grimaces. Stiff, dark, **red, cracked tongue. Elongated uvula** (Caps. Merc. Sul.). Spasms of dry, hacking, night cough; < lying, eating or talking. **Nervous wakefulness (Coff.).** Starts out of sleep. Low fever; with hot, pale skin. Warm sweat.

Related: Bell. Pho. Stram.

HYPERICUM.

REGION.

NERVES; SPINAL.

Vertex.

WORSE.

INJURY { JAR. **Bruises.** Punctures. Lacerations

Cold. FOGS. Damp. Motion.

BETTER,

Bending Backward.

BRUISED, LACERATED OR INFLAMED NERVES. Injuries of or reflected upon the brain and cord. **Very painful sore parts after injuries,** shots, having teeth pulled, fingers mashed, etc. **Violent, shooting pains;** toward the trunk or down sides of head or chest (Dulc. **Rhus-t.**); with numbness or **crawling. Shudderings.** Neuritis. Spasms. Tetanus.

——Heaviness or formication in brain. **Head feels drawn up to a point** (Stro. Ther.). **Bubbling at navel. Dry rectum. Heart seems to drop. Painfully sensitive spine (Agar.). Limbs feel detached (Bapt.). Cutting in fingertips. Feet feel furry. Gaping wounds. Laborious dreams.**

Related: Arn. Led. Rhus-t.

IGNATIA.

REGION.
MIND.
NERVES.
Cerebro-Spinal **Axis.**

WORSE.
EMOTIONS: **SILENT GRIEF.** Reprimands. **MORTIFICATION.** WORRY. FRIGHT.
AIR: **Open. Cold.**
Odors. **Coffee.** Tobacco.
Touch < but Pressure >.

BETTER.
Position: **Change of.** **Lying on Painful Part.**
Walking.
Profuse Urination. When Alone.

ERRATIC OR CONTRADICTORY, often very violent effects; with rigidity, twitches, trembling, spasms, etc. **Sense of sharp pressure or of a plug or foreign body.** Clavus; globus. Hysteria (Pul.). Pain in one spot (Lil-t.), < close attention. Symptoms pass off with a profuse flow of urine.——ALERT, SUPERSENSITIVE AND NERVOUS. **Emotional** (Nat-m.), **capricious,** moody. **Changeful;** SIGHS; weeps or laughs by turns. Unhappy love (Aur. Hyo. Pho-ac.). **Faints easily. Brooding grief. Alternate headache and backache** (Melil.). Eyelids seem dry. Nose is sensitive to inspired air (Am-c. Brom. Cist. Cor-r. Hep. Hyds. Sep.). Sneezing attacks. **Redness of one cheek.** Face twitches, jaws snap shut (Plat.), bites inside of cheek, tongue, etc. (Nit-ac.). **Indurated** tonsils, with little ulcers (Nit-ac.). **Must swallow over a lump;** > solids. **Hiccough;** with eructations (Dios.). Hunger with nausea. **Craves** raw foods. **Empty sinking or spasmodic aching in stomach;** > eating. Difficult or painful stool, although soft; then, constriction of rectum. **Pains shoot up rectum. Prolapsus recti.** Piles > sitting. Irregular menses. TAKES DEEP BREATHS (Coca. Dig. Ran-b.). **Choking** (Chel. Con. Lach.). Spasm of **glottis** (Calc-c Gel. Mos. Samb.). **Dry cough, as from dust or sulfur fumes;** < coughing (Bell.

Mar. Stict.). Constriction of thorax (Nux-v.). Heavy feet. **Painful** skin, > pressure. **Violent, spasmodic yawning.** Chill with thirst, > heat. Heat with aversion to uncover, but no thirst.
Complementary: Aur. Nat-m. Pho-ac. Related: Cimi. Nux-v. Sep.

IODUM.

REGION.

GLANDS { THYROID. **Mesenteric.** Mammæ. Testes.

MUCOUS MEMBRANES { LARYNX. Lungs (Apices).

HEART. Skin.

Connective Tissue.

WORSE.

HEAT { OF ROOM. Air. Wrapping Head.

Exertion { Ascending. Talking.

Fasting. Night. At Rest.

BETTER.

COLD { AIR. **Bathing.**

Motion. **Eating.**

Weak and losing flesh. ALWAYS TOO HOT. **Hot, corrosive or watery discharges. Hard, heavy, enlarged glands; later dwindling away.** Emaciation. Scrofula. Acute exacerbations. Local torpidity (little pus). Internal tickling. General pulsation or local throbbings.——**Dejected or angry, and restless.** Sudden, dreadful impulses (Ars.); > if busy, but motion < and soon exhausts. Prominent eyes (Chlor.). Pain at root of nose. Fluent, hot coryza, < open air. Miserable, withered, sallow or dusky look. Increased saliva; soapy; foul. **Hungry, yet emaciates rapidly** (Calc-c. Nat-m. Psor. Sul.) **or variable appetite.** Frothy, wheyey, fatty, cheesy or lienteric stools. Hydrocele. Wedgelike pain from ovary (r) to uterus (Gos.). Menses flow; with weakness (Carb-a. Grap. Sep.); after every stool. Leucorrhœa eroding the thighs and linen (Kre. Pho. Sul-ac.). DRY, CROUPY COUGH. PAINFUL, CHOKING HOARSENESS. Larygitis (Pho.). **Diphtheria** invades the larynx. Rough voice. Short breath. Pneumonia. Heart feels squeezed. Palpitation. Heavy mammæ (Lac-c.). Hard goitre. Dry, rough, dirty skin. Restless feeling in blood prevents sleep (Aco.). **Hyperpyrexia** or external coldness, with anxiety or **stupor.** Sweats easily. Early morning sweats, with relief.
Complementary: Lyc. Related: Ars. Pho. Spo.

IPECAC.

REGION.

MUCOUS MEMBRANES: DIGESTIVE. **Stomach.** RESPIRATORY. Lungs.

Nerves: **Pneumogastric.** Spinal. Cutaneous.

WORSE.

WARMTH; **Damp.** Room.

Overeating: Ices. Pork. Veal. Mixed or rich foods.

Periodically. Quinine.

Heat and Cold. Recessions.

BETTER.

Open Air.

Affections accompanied by PERSISTENT NAUSEA, **shortness of breath, increased secretions,** sudden faintness or BLEEDING. PROFUSE, BRIGHT RED HEMORRHAGE; rapidly clotting. **Foamy discharges.**——Cries, screams and is hard to please. Crushing pain—downward—in cranium. Migraine. Pain in occiput and nape; < vomiting, during chill, etc. **Gushes** of tears. Conjunctivitis. Sneezing. **Pale face;** blue about lips; white linea nasalis (Aeth.). **Clean tongue.** NO THIRST. HORRID NAUSEA; not > vomiting. Bilious vomit. Repugnance to food. Miserable sinking or loose feeling at stomach. Griping, clawing or cutting at navel; toward uterus. Brown, grass green or **bloody stools. Dysentry. Urging to urinate.** Bloody urine. Gushing, uterine hemorrhage. Larynx and chest seem tight, < least motion. Asthma. **Paroxysms of shaking, incessant or suffocative cough;** with every breath; stiffens out (Cina.), turns red or blue and finally gags or vomits; < stepping into open air, > warmth and repose. Whooping cough. LOOSE (coarse) RATTLE WITHIN CHEST (Mos.); WITHOUT EXPECTORATION. Broncho-pneumonia. Hæmoptysis. Pains from kidneys into thighs. Mixed intermittents; nausea in all stages. Short chill. Long heat; without thirst. Catarrhal or gastric fevers.

Complementary: Ars. Cup. Related: Ant-t. Lob.

IRIS VERSICOLOR.

REGION.

GLANDS: **DIGESTIVE TRACT.** **LIVER.** **Pancreas.**

Right Side.

Nerves.

WORSE.

PERIODICALLY: **Weekly.** 2-3 A. M. After Breakfast. Spring and Fall.

Mental Exhaustion.

Hot Weather.

BETTER.

Gentle Motion.

Affections accompanied by rapid elimination. **Sour, acrid, burning excretions.**——**Nausea, acid vomiting,** urging to stool and profuse urine, with **periodic visual disturbances,** blindness, hæmiopia, etc. **Ophthalmic migraine** (r). Burning; < **along whole digestive tract;** not > by cold drinks. Profuse ropy or sweet (Iod. Saba.) saliva. Mouth feels greasy (Ol-ani.). burnt or scalded (Hyds. Mag-m. Phyt. Pul.). BILIOUS, WATERY, SOUR OR ACRID VOMITUS, WITH BURNING. Soreness over liver. ACRID, WATERY STOOL, BURNING LIKE FIRE (Ars. Asc. Gamb. Rat.). **Cholera morbus** (Ant-t. Pod. Ver-a.). Oily stool. Goitre. Zoster (r). The hip feels wrenched out. Shooting, laming pains along limb. Sciatica (l).

Related: Ars.

JABORANDI.

REGION.

GLANDS. Eyes.

WORSE.

At Start of Menses. Cold.

Exhaustion.

Tendency to sweat and take cold.——Eyestrain. Nervous deafness, > noise. Tension in salivary glands. **Salivation.** Mumps. Nausea on using eyes (Pul.) or looking at moving objects. Menses begin with coldness, throbbing in head and pelvis and backache. Night sweats.

Related: Agar. Ant-t. Ip.

JALAPA.

REGION.

Intestines. Stomach.

WORSE.

Night. Eructations.

Child is good all day, but screams and tosses about all night. Colic. **Stools watery,** muddy or sour and bloody.

Related: Colo.

JATROPHA.

REGION.
Stomach and Intestines.

WORSE.
Covering Up. Morning. Summer.
BETTER.
Hands in cold water.

Icy coldness. Vomiting; albuminous, easy. **LOUD GURGLING LIKE WATER FROM A BUNG HOLE IN ABDOMEN, THEN PROFUSE GUSHING STOOLS** (Alo. Crot-t. Gamb. Pod.). Violent cramps that draw the calves flat.

Related: Crot-t.

JUSTITIA.

REGION.
Cerebro-Spinal Nerves.
Respiratory Membranes.

WORSE.
Close Room. Dust.
Noise. Eating.

Sensitive.——Fits of sneezing with lachrymation and loss of smell and taste (Mag-m. Nat-m. Pul. Sil.). Fluent coryza. Stools seem too large. Long paroxysms of violent cough; as if chest would burst; **obstructing the breath;** with sneezing, stiffening out, trembling or convulsions. Whooping cough. Tough expectoration. Puffy hands and feet; in A. M Chiliness.

Related: Pul.

KALI BICHROM.

REGION.

MUCOUS MEMBRANES { **Air Passages.** **Pharynx.** **Stomach.**
JOINTS.
Circulation. Kidneys.
Skin.

WORSE.
COLD { Open Air. Spring. **Undressing.**
MORNING. BEER. 2-3 A. M.
Protruding Tongue (Cist.).
Suppressed Catarrh.
BETTER.
Heat. Motion.

Slowness. Deeply destructive effects; round perforating ulcers, of septum (Sil.) stomach, etc. Chubby and chilly or cachectic and **weak. YELLOW, THICK, LUMPY, TOUGH, STRINGY OR STICKY SECRETIONS** (Ant-t.). Plastic exudates. Chronic catarrhs. **Erratic pains;** attacking the stomach (Bism. Colch. Dulc. Lap.); in small spots. As of a hair on tongue (Ars Coc-c. Nat-m. Nat-p. Sil. Sul.); in nostril, etc. Cracking in joints.——Headache over eyes. Yellow eyes. Granular lids (Pul.). **Blindness, then migraine** (Iris. Lac-def. Pho. Pod. Psor.). Pressure at root of nose (Kali-io.). **Acrid, gluey nasal discharge** (Lyc. Merc-c. Nit-ac.) or of greenish clinkers (Pho.). Frontal sinusitis. Snifling (Pho.). Smooth, cracked, shiny tongue (Cist.); pains when protruded (Cocel. Cist. Phyt.). Sticky mouth (Chel. Lach. Myr.). Hawks sticky mucus (Arg-n. Cocc-c. Lach. Mag-m. Phyt.) must wipe it away (Lac-c.). Ropy saliva. Bladder-like œdema of uvula (Ap.). Dry burning in throat. Fissure in pharynx (Elap.). Craves beer. Sensations ascend from stomach; to chest (Nux-v.). Sore spot in stomach (Arg-n. Bar-c. Bis.). Peptic ulcer (Arg-n. Ars. Ura-n.). Contraction from liver to shoulder (Crot-h.). Gelatinous stools or gushes of brown frothy water, then burning tenesmus. A drop remains after urinating. Constriction at root of penis. **Acrid, adhesive leucorrhœa. Cough;** after eating, > heat. Pain from chest or sternum to back (Cimi. Kali-c. Nit-ac.). Asthma. **Weak** heart; it feels cold (Helod. Kali-n.). Sciatica > **bending leg.** Sore heels. Dark ulcers with overhanging edges. Skin symptoms > **in cool air. Absence of fever.**

Complementary: Ars. Related: Kali-c. **Merc.** Phyt. **Pul.**

KALI BROM.

REGION.
- MIND.
- **NERVES** { **Brain.** **Spine.** **Genitals.**
- **Skin.**

WORSE.
- **Mental Exertion.** Emotions.
- Periodically { Night. New Moon. Summer.
- Sexual Excesses. Puberty.

BETTER.
- When Busy.

General numbness, < occiput.——**Depressive delusions,** with suspicion; he fears people, yet can't be alone, the dark, etc.; looks on all sides; fidgets and fumbles with his hands (Taren.). Mania. Night terrors. **Melancholy;** remorse, wrings hands, bursts into tears, etc. Slow and hesitating; omits or mixes up words. Indifference. Hebetude. Poor memory. Numbness in head. Brain fag. Vertigo, as if ground gave away. Green, watery stool with rapid collapse. Depressed sexual power. Flooding of young women. Acne.

Related Calc-c. Con. Stram.

KALI CARB.

REGION.

MUSCLES { HEART. LUMBAR REGION. **Uterus.**

SEROUS SURFACES { CHEST (R. Lower). Joints.

Mucous Membranes.

BLOOD.

WORSE.

COLD { AIR. **Drafts.** **Water.** After Overheating. **Changes.**

TIME { WINTER. **Before Menses.** 2 to 3 A. M.

Lying; **On Painful** or Left **Side.**

Loss of Fluids. **After Labor.**

BETTER.

Warmth.

Old, soft, thin blooded and cold. WEAK; **given out feeling; wants to lie down.** Muscle exhaustion. Ruptured muscles. Acrid discharges. Catarrhs. Subacute affections. SHARP, STICKING PAINS. **Pulsation or sense of coldness in single parts,** abdomen, fingers, etc.——Peevish. Easily startled. **Anxious aversion to solitude. Weakness in eyes.** Spotted vision. LITTLE SACKS OVER EYELIDS—inner angle—(Coccl.). Outward stitches in ears. **Subject to head colds;** going to chest. Swelled, stuffy nose, > open air; yellow-green (Pho.) or crusty discharge. Pale, yellow, puffy face. Hawks up tough mucus in morning. **Difficult swallowing. Sensitive, distended stomach and abdomen. Fulness,** even after drinks; as if full of water. Impressions are felt in epigastrium, as an anxious throbbing (Pho.). Gastric pains radiate to chest, back, limbs, etc. **Flatulence. Large** (Ver-a.) **difficult stool,** then burning or torn feeling. Inflamed or bleeding piles; descend when urinating. **Irritating menses, preceded by colic.** Inefficient labor pains. Retching cough, ends in vomiting. Whooping cough. Stitches in chest (Nit-ac. Ol-jec.). Lungs seem to stick to ribs. Pleurisy. Weak heart; as if hanging by a thread. Palpitation. Valvular effections. **Soft, variable, intermittent pulse. Back and legs give out;** feel heavy. Lumbago. **Painful tips of toes or fingers. Sensitive soles.** Dry hair and skin. Sensitive skin. Sleepy from eating (Aur. Chin. Nux-v. Pho.). Internal burning.

Complementary: Carb-v. Nit-ac. Pho. Related: Calc-hypo. Lyc.

KALI IOD.

REGION.	WORSE.
Glands. Nose. Eyes.	**HEAT;** Room. Clothes.
Lungs {Upper. Lobe.}	Cold {Food. Drinks. Dampness. **Night.**}
Periosteum.	Mercury. Lying on Affected Side.
	BETTER.
	Cool Air.

Acrid, watery discharges, or copious, thick-green. Crushing pains. Sharp stitches, in periosteum; flying about heart, etc. **Weakness. Organic processes;** syphilitic or gouty-rheumatic; gummæ, nodes, œdema, etc.——**Despondency. Bad temper.** Cruelty. Bilateral headache. Burning, watery eyes. Raw conjunctiva (Arg-n. Lyc.). **Red, swollen nose.** Violent sneezing. **Coryza,** < in the open air. **Pain at root of nose** and tongue. Ozœna. Taste salty (Con.); bitter on awaking. Salivation. Squeaking in stomach. Corroding leucorrhœa; like meat washings. Dyspnœa, with flatulency (Zin). Awake strangling. Asthma. **Rawness** in air passages. **Croupy hoarseness.** Expectoration like suds (Ip. Sul. Zin.). **Pneumonia. Hives.** Chilly, as if in bones. Heat in evening. Profuse nightsweat **relieves.** Actinomycosis.

Related Iod. Sul. Syp.

KALI-MUR.

REGION.	WORSE.
Epithelium.	Heat. Fat or Rich Foods.
Mucous Glands.	Getting Wet. Motion.
Joints.	BETTER.
	Cold Drinks.

Whiteness. Toughness. **Thick, white, sticky discharges.** Catarrhs. Firm white exudates or hard deposits (Sul.). Swelled glands. **Shifting, cutting pains.**——Quietness. **Gray-white coat on tongue.** Aphthæ. Tonsilitis. Acrid stool and leucorrhœa. Dark, clotted or tarry menses. **Rawness in chest** (Carb-v. Nat-m. Nux-v.). Cutting bone pains. **Desquamation.** Mealy skin. **Blisters.**

KALI NITRAS.

REGION.	WORSE.
Vaso-motors { **BLOODVESSELS.** / **Heart.** / **KIDNEYS.**	WALKING. **Cold.** / Lying With Head Low.
Respiratory Organs.	BETTER. / Gentle Motion.

Internal burning. Hemorrhage. Sudden œdema. Throbbing. Dull stitches. **Numb;** as if made of wood.——**Faintness.** Nausea. Pain from epigastrium to arms. Dark, fluid stools. **Diuresis.** Profuse, inky menses. VIOLENT DYSPNŒA; can only drink in sips. Free, sour expectoration >. Asthma. Relapses during phthisis (Fer-p.). Hands and fingers feel swelled. **External coldness.**

Related: Glo.

KALI PHOS.

REGION.	WORSE.
NERVES { **Brain.** / Cord.	**Slight Causes** { **Pain.** / **Cold.** **Fatigue.**
Excretions.	BETTER.
One Side.	Gentle Motion.

Easily fagged. Putrid or golden yellow discharges. Paralysis.——Dread. Gloom. As if cranial bones would break and eyes be torn out. Yellow-gray, milky secretion from eyes. Canker sores. Tongue coated like liquid mustard. Hunger soon after eating. Watery, painless diarrhœa, then weakness and hunger. Horribly foul leucorrhœa. Aphonia. Prickling in hands and feet. Weak, intermittent, irregular pulse. Inactive skin.

Related: Cocci.

KALI SULF.

REGION.

EPITHELIUM { Respiratory Organs. **Skin.**

Glands.

WORSE.

Warmth; Room; Air. Noise.

BETTER.

Cool Air. Walking.

PROFUSE, YELLOW, PURULENT DISCHARGES. **Suppurations.** Stitching, tearing, festering **pains that shift about.——Hurried.** Yellow, slimy tongue. Oxaluria (Berb. Nitro-m-ac.). Pyeletis. Croupy **hoarseness. Rattling in chest** (Ant-t.). Rheumatism. Dry skin. **Desquamation (Ars.).** Ulcers ooze thin yellow water.

Related: **Pul.**

KALMIA.

REGION.

NERVES { SPINAL. **Eyes.** Face.

HEART.

CIRCULATION.

Joints.

WORSE.

MOTION { **Lying on Left Side.** Bending Forward. **Looking Down.**

Heat. Becoming Chilled.

With the Sun.

BETTER.

Eating. Cloudy Weather.

Tingling, numbness or paralytic weakness. Changing pains; shooting outward along nerves or dull tearing crushing, **moving upward, even to heart,** or alternating with cardiac symptoms (Visc.) or between upper and lower limbs (Val. Visc.). Neuralgia. **General aching, bruised stiff feeling.** Rheumatism. Trembling.——Vertigo. Cracking noise in head (Calc-c. Dig. Glo.). Shooting from nape to vertex and face. Stiff eyelids. Maddening supraorbital pain. Prosopalgia (r). **Pain at heart** or in chest; to left scapula or arm (Lach.); taking away the breath. Fluttering. Palpitation. **Very slow, weak pulse.** Cardiac paralysis. Brachialgia. Stiff skin.

Complementary: Benz-ac. Related: Aco. Dig. Rhus-t. Spig.

KREOSOTUM.

REGION.	WORSE.
Mucous Membranes { **DIGESTIVE TRACT.** GUMS. **Stomach.** Female Genitals.	DENTITION. **REST. Cold.** **After Eating. Lying.** Summer. 6 P. M. to 6 A. M. During Menses.
Teeth. BLOOD.	BETTER. **Warmth.** Hot Food. **Motion.**

Miserable and weak. **PROFUSE, ACRID, FOUL DISCHARGES; reddening the parts. Rawness. BURNING,** like coals (Ars.). **Hemorrhage;** of brown blood. **Pulsation;** general. Heaviness. **Tumefaction.** Scorbutus. Marasmus.——**Cross, wilful and obstinate** (Stap.). Yellow pallor, with red blotches (Iod.). **TEETH show black spots; SOON DECAY** (Mez. Stap.). **Puffy, bluish, painful, bleeding gums.** Painful dentition. Aphthæ. Frothy eructations (Canth. Mag-m.). Nausea. **VOMITING;** long after meals (Sabi. Sang.); of undigested food; sweetish; of pregnancy (Med.); reflex. Brown, watery or undigested stools (Psor.). Hurried urinating; involuntary when lying (Pul.). Diuresis. Profuse, lumpy, intermittent menses (Lac-c.). **Gushing leucorrhœa** (Mag-m.); like bloody water; **acrid.** Cough, with sore pain in larynx and chest. Anxious heaviness in chest. Dragging from back to genitals, as if to come out. Violently itching, moist or scurfy eczema; more on face and back of hands (Pix.). Ulcers break out and heal, repeatedly.

Complementary: Sul. Related: Aru-t. Carb-ac. Grap. Psor.

LAC CANINUM.

REGION.	WORSE.
NERVES. THROAT. **Female Generative Organs.**	TOUCH. **During Menses.** Jar. Morning of One Day and Evening of the Next (Eupat.).
	BETTER. Open Air.

SYMPTOMS CHANGE SIDES (Cimi. Pul. Stict.) or wander about. **Glistening** parts (Calc-fl. Syph.). Oversensitive.——**Full of imaginations;** horrid, of snakes (Tub.), etc. Every symptom seems a settled disease. Seems to be floating. **Throat looks glazed** (Kali-bi.) **or contains patches of china-like whiteness.** Tonsilitis. Diphtheria. Sore throat at menses (Calc-c. Mag-c.). Gushing menses. **Breasts sore and swelled before menses** (Bry. Con.). DRIES UP THE MILK.

Related: **Lach.**

LACHESIS.

REGION.

NERVES { **CUTANEOUS.** **VASO-MOTOR.** PNEUMOGASTRIC.

BLOOD { **HEART.** **CIRCULATION.**

LEFT SIDE { **THROAT.** OVARIES.

FEMALES.

Vertex.

WORSE.

AFTER SLEEPING. MORNING.

HEAT { SPRING. SUMMER. SUN. DRINKS. ROOM.

SWALLOWING { EMPTY. **of Liquids.**

SENSITIVE TO { **SLIGHT TOUCH.** **PRESSURE** **ABOUT NECK.** **Waist** (Ap. Bov. Grap.).

RETARDED DISCHARGES.

CLIMACTERIC. ALCOHOL.

BETTER.

OPEN AIR. Hard Pressure.

Rapid onset. **NERVOUS EXCITABILITY. EXCESSIVE PAINFULNESS. MUSCULAR PROSTRATION. BLUISH COLOR. EXCESSIVE FETOR. Malignancy.** Disintegration. Sepsis. Gangrene. **HEMORRHAGE;** dark, thin or with dark particles. Purpura (Pho. Sul-ac.). **HARD THROBBING. CONGESTIONS. RUSHES OF BLOOD. FLASHES OF HEAT** (Amy-n. Glo. Sang. Sep. Sul.). RISING SENSATIONS. Globus. Chorea. Epilepsy (Bell. Caus. Cic. Hep.). Apoplexy. CONSTRICTIONS.——**AIMLESS ROVING. LOQUACITY** (Arg. Cimi. Tub.). **Jealousy. Compelling delusións. Suspicion** (Cimi.). Feels filled with poison (Vip.). Indolence. Heavy or bursting headache; from nape; into nose (Calc-c. Cimi. Mez.). Sense of a skull cap (Aco. Berb.). Side of head (r) feels cut off. Pain from eyes to vertex (Cimi. Croc. Kre. Pho.). Blood and pus from nose. Rum blossom (Agar. Led.). Purple face or with netted veinlets. Fetor oris. Pasty saliva. **Tongue catches behind the teeth.** Peppery taste (Aco. Chin. Hyds. Mez. Sul.). Thick, blundering speech (Gel.). A lump descends and rises as she swallows (Chel. Lac-c.) or coughs. VERY PAINFUL SORE THROAT (Iod.); pains into ears (Hep. Phyt.); $<$ adhesive mucus in; drinks return thro nose. **CAN'T BEAR ANYTHING ABOUT THROAT.** Tonsilitis. Quinsy. Diphtheria; laryngeal. Thirsty, but afraid to drink. Dipsomania. **Soreness or cramp in epigastrium** (Vip.). Sore, festering feeling in liver (Croth-h.). Foul stools. Pain from anus to navel (Colo.). **Drawing or constriction at anus.** Piles, $<$ coughing. As of a ball in bladder or rectum. **Pain in left ovary. Scanty, dark, foul or vicarious**

menses. SUFFOCATES ON FALLING TO SLEEP (Am-c. Dig. Grind.). Membranous croup. Must take a deep breath. Tickling cough, < **touching neck** or auditory canal (Kali-c. Sil.); > a little expectoration. **Heart weak; seems to turn over;** feels too big (Bov.), etc. Carditis; metastatic (Aur. Colch. Kalm. Pho. Spig.). Trembling hands. Numb fingertips. MOTTLED, BLUISH OR LIVID SKIN (Ail. Pul. Sul.). **Eating ulcers; on** legs; with dark areolæ (Aesc.); fungoid. Frightful dreams. Ascending chills. **Heat on vertex.** Sweat about neck; during sleep; bloody; garlicky axillary.

Complementary: Calc-c. **Lyc.** Related: Caus. Sep.

LAC VACCINUM DEFLOR.

REGION.
NUTRITION. BLOOD.
Heart.
Head (left).
Thigh (outer).

WORSE.
COLD { **Least Draft.** Wet. / Hands in Cold Water. }
MILK. Weekly. **Loss of Sleep.**
BETTER.
Rest. Pressure; of bandage.

Great exhaustion. Despondency. Blindness then throbbing headache with much pale urine. Migraine. Photophobia. Painless swelling of face. Pale, sickly look. Anæmia. **Averse to milk. Sour vomiting. Large, painful stools.** Boring, sore pain in kidneys. Polyuria; < during pain. Scanty flow of milk. **Always chilly.** Cold fingertips. Skin is super-sensitive to cold.

Related: Nat-m.

LAPPA.

REGION.
Secretions. **Skin.**
Joints.

WORSE.
Violent Exertion. Shaking.
BETTER.
Cloudy Weather.

Heavy, sore aching. Constrictions—Weight on vertex. Redness about eyes and across nose. Vomits soured food. **Bruised soreness of uterus.** Front of thighs weak. Aching, numb calves. Itching spots. **Eruptions** of head, face, etc.; sticky. Sores about joints. Cold, foul axillary sweat.

LATRODECTUS.

REGION.
Vaso-motors.
Heart. Blood.

Nausea, then abdominal pain. Sinking at epigastrium. Gasps, fears to lose the breath and die. Apnœa. **Violent cardiac pain,** to shoulders or arms (1) (Bar-c. Cimi. Dios. Kali-c. Kalm. Spi. Tarent.); with numbness. **Angina pectoris.** Quick, feeble, thready pulse. Skin cold as marble.

Related: Tarent.

LAUROCERASUS.

REGION.
MIND. BRAIN.
NERVES.
Respiration.
Heart.

WORSE.
Before Eating. Exertion.

BETTER.
Lying With Head Low.
Open Air. Sleep.

Symptoms accompanied by SUDDEN LOSS OF MEMORY (Arg Arg-n. Hep. Lyc. Nux-m.), blunted senses (Calc-c.), cyanosis or **LACK OF REACTION.** Nerve exhaustion. **Sinking.** Spasmodic effects.——Blue or twitching face. **Drinks roll noisily downward** (Arn. Ars. Cina. Cup. Elap. Hell. Thu.). Spasm of gullet. Falling down feeling in abdomen (Nux-v. Plb. Pod.). Gurgling flatulence. **Suffocation;** unable to expand the **lungs;** holds hand over heart (Hyd-ac. Naj.). Short dry, **tickling cough,** < **lying;** blood flecked, gelatinous sputum. Small pulse. Cool, moist skin.

Related: Gel. Hyd-ac.

LEDUM.

REGION.
Fibrous Tissue { JOINTS (Small). Eyes. Heels.
Capillary Circulation { SKIN. Lungs.
Nerves. **Blood.**

WORSE.
Warmth { **Covers.** Bed. Stove.
Night. **Injury.** **Motion.**

BETTER.
Cold; bathing, etc.

Purple, puffy and cold, yet averse to heat. **Ascending effects;** from feet. Shifting, tearing pains. **Parts** become weak, numb, **cold and wither.** Torpid processes. Gouty-rheumatic. Nodes. Dropsy. **Hemorrhage; bright;** frothy. Petechiæ. Foul pus.——Raging, pulsating headache; < covers. Persistent nosebleed. Mottled or red pimply face. Much sand in urine.

Tormenting cough from tickling in larynx; < receding eruptions. Double inspirations. Hæmoptysis; alternates with rheumatism. Cramps over hips. Stiff back; < rising. Swelled, blotchy legs and feet (Solid.). Feet itch at night and are stiff in morning. **Punctured wounds,** from nails, stings, etc. **Coldness,** of part (Colch.), < limbs; with the pain; during fever; as if in cold water. Foul sweat.

Related: Arn. Bry. Rhus-t. Sec-c.

LEPTANDRA.

REGION.	WORSE.
LIVER. Right Side.	Cold Drinks. Motion.

TARRY OR BLACK, FETID STOOLS (Crot-h.); spurting out; with pain at navel. Burning or dull aching over liver (posterior) or gall bladder and down over bowels. Dysentry; after diarrhœa. Jaundice.

Related: Bapt.

LILIUM TIGRINUM.

REGION.	WORSE.
VENOUS CIRCULATION { **FEMALE ORGANS.** **Uterus.** Ovaries. **HEART.** Rectum. Bladder. Left Side. }	WARMTH; of **Room.** **Walking. Standing. Consolation.**
Nerves.	BETTER. **Cool, Fresh Air. When Busy.** Lying on Left Side.

Heavy, full feeling. **Utero-ovarian sagging with marked reflexes** (Con.); < **mental or cardiac** (r). Acrid discharges.——**ACTIVE, NERVOUS, HURRIED, snappish and erotic.** Wild, crazy feeling (Med.). **Dread;** fears insanity, is incurable, etc. Ache (over left eye) with vertigo and visual effects. Biting, burning in eyes when reading. Hungry feeling, as if along spine. **Stiff, tense** abdomen. **Early morning diarrhœa; with** tenesmus. **Dragging or heavy-outward urging in pelvis;** wants to hold the parts (Sanic.); **with dysuria.** Distress about left ovary; into limb. Free menses while moving only. Thin, brown leucorrhœa. Oppression, as of a load on chest; she takes long breaths. As of a rivet or ball between left mammæ and shoulder. Heart feels overfull; cold (Helod.); weak, etc. Palpitation. Pain from heart, (left nipple) to back. Bloating about hips. Nervous trembling in spine, knees, etc. **Chilliness, > in open air.**

Related: Alo. Plat. Pul. Spig.

LITHIUM CARB.

REGION.
Small Joints.
Heart.
Urine.

WORSE.
Bending Forward.
Menses; Suppressed; After.
BETTER.
Eating. Urinating. Motion.

Soreness, sourness and lithiasis. Heaviness. Gout. Rheumatism.——Dry eyes, after using them. Vertical hemiopia (r). Chunks of mucus drop into throat (Mar.). Gnawing in stomach with pain in left temple (Ars.). Urine has a red-brown sediment. Pain goes from heart to head; from mammæ to arms. **Heart pains.** Dry, harsh skin. Eczema.

Related: Kali-bi.

LOBELIA.

REGION.
RESPIRATION.
Secretions.
Heart.

WORSE.
Cold Bathing. Suppressions.
Tobacco.
BETTER.
Rapid Motion.

Weak, relaxed, sweaty and deathly sick all over. Sits with elbows on knees.——As of a lump in throat or stomach. **Deathly nausea;** with vertigo; < night and early morning, > eating or drinking. **Vomiting;** with sweat (cold on face.). **Weak sinking at stomach.** Deep red urine, with red sediment. **Dyspnœa;** nervous; with every labor pain; as from a wedge in larynx; > rapid motion (Bell. Brom. Coff. Fer. Pul. Rhus-t. Samb. Sep.); with general prickling. Asthma. Spasmodic cough; with sneezing, belching (Amb.) or gastric pain. Oppressive fulness in chest. Soft flowing pulse. Prickling in skin. Plaques of œdema (figurata); with ecchymoses.

Related: Ip. Tab.

LYCOPODIUM.

REGION.

Nutrition { **DIGESTIVE TRACT.** **Liver.** **Skin.**

URINARY ORGANS.

RIGHT SIDE { THROAT.
Then Left { Ovary.

Lungs.

WORSE.

PRESSURE OF CLOTHES.

WARMTH { AIR. Bed. Applications.

Cold Drinks. Eating.

INDIGESTION. Awaking.

4 TO 8 P. M. Rising from Sitting.

BETTER.

WARM DRINKS, Food, etc.

Motion. Exertion. **Urinating.**

Cool, Fresh Air.

Repeating or alternating symptoms; flexion then extension (Cup. Tab.), automatic motions, chill after chill, flushing then paling, etc. Pains that cause jerks. ACIDITY; sour taste, vomit, eructation, etc. **Calculous tendency;** gall stones, gravel, tophi. Gout. **Thin, withered and full of gas.** Poor circulation, limbs seem dead; numb spots. Descending symptoms; emaciation, etc. Threatening chronicity. Early senility. Dropsy. ——**Mentally active, but gets weaker.** Can't think. Miscalls or omits words, syllables. etc. **AWAKES IN ANGER,** sadness, anxiety (Ant-t. Psor. Tub.), etc. Hateful, cranky, **domineering** (Plat.), **exacting** (Ars.), reserved, despairing. Headache when heated. Falling hair; comes in gray. Eyes half open. Hemiopia (r). **FANLIKE MOTION OF WINGS OF NOSE** (Ant-t. Chel. Pho.). Stuffy nose. Acrid ozœna. Yellow-gray pale face. Wrinkled forehead (Hell. Stram.). Frowning. Twitching face Meningitis; tubercular. Hydrocephalus (Bell. Calc-c. Hell.). Sore lips, Mouth hangs open (Colch. Hell.). Yellow teeth. Stiff, heavy, swelled, trembling or cracked tongue A ball rises and sticks in throat (Calc-c.). **Sore throat (r).** Diphtheria. **Hunger with sudden satiety. A LITTLE FOOD FILLS HIM UP** (Bry. Chin.). Averse to soups. **Incomplete eructations.** As of a band about waist. **MUCH NOISY FLATULENCE;** < lower abdomen (Sul.). Brown spots on abdomen (Pho.) and chest. After stool the most seems to remain behind. Alternate diarrhœa and constipation (Chel. Nat-s. Pod. Pul.). **Suppressed urine. Cries before urinating** (Aco. Bor. Sars.). **RED SAND IN URINE** (Nat-s.). Pollutions. **Sexual exhaustion.** Impotency. Menses mixed with clots and serum. **Acrid leucorrhœa.** Painful coition. Gas from vagina (Sang.). Craves air but is chilled thereby. Short rattling breathing. Salty or foul expectorate. Unresolved pneumonia (Pho. Sul.). Stiff back. Fingers twitch during sleep (Rhe.). As of a stone under heel (Aur. Hep.). **Dryness;** of palms, vagina, etc. **Rawness;** in folds, nipples, anus, etc. (Carb-v. Caus. Cham.). Suppurating eruptions. Receding boils or erysipelas. Vascular swellings. Aneurysm. **Cold;** as from ice; it < the stomach, cough, throat and head. **One foot cold.** Chill, then sour vomit. Burning between scapulæ (Ars. Pho. Sul.). Foul axillary and footsweat.

Complementary: **Calc-c.** Kali-c. **Lach.** Related: Carb-v.

LYCOPUS.

REGION.
HEART. **Circulation.**

WORSE.
Heat. Excitement.
Suppressions. Exertion.

Symptoms associated with **RAPID AND TUMULTUOUS HEART ACTION** (Aco. Amy-n.) or **oppression** and pains at heart. Exophthalmos. Polyuria. **Hemorrhages;** bleeding piles; hæmoptysis, etc.——Nervous **hurry.**

Related: **Cact.**

LYSSIN.

REGION.
Nerves. Cord.
Throat.
Sexular Organs.

WORSE.
Running Water. Heat of Sun.
Glistening Objects. Drafts.

BETTER.
Bending Backward.
Gentle Rubbing.

Spasm. **Overacute senses.**——Fear. Rapid speech. Impatience and **violent temper.** Constant spitting; ropy, frothy saliva. Spasm of gullet. Can't urinate unless he hears water run. Sexual excitement. Sensitive womb (Helo.). Barking cough. Pain in neck, **Blueness.** Convulsions.

Related: **Lach.**

MAGNESIA CARB.

REGION.

DIGESTIVE TRACT { **Stomach.** Bowels. Liver.

NERVES { Facial. Dental.

WORSE.

NIGHT. **Rest. Noise.**

Cold { **Changes of Weather.** Wind. Drafts.

Food; Starchy; Milk.

Touch. Children. Nurslings.

BETTER.

Motion. Walking About.

Weak, flabby, flatulent and sour or nervous, ailing and worn out. **Emaciation.** Marasmus. **Sharp shooting along the nerves;** must walk about (Fer.). Numb, distended feeling. Neuralgia.——Heaviness in brain. Tearing, digging, boring face pains or toothache; < pregnancy (Chin. Kali-bi. Rat.); > cold. Waxy pallor. Nibbling appetite. Vomits bitter water. **Cutting colic.** GREENISH STOOLS, LIKE THE WATER AND SCUM OF A FROG POND (Sal-ac. Sanic.); or with gelatinous or fatty masses (Dulc. Pho.). Undigested or foaming stools (Colo. Kali-bi. Merc. Pod. Sul.). **Dark, tarry or viscid menses** more at night and on first rising; leaving a fast stain (Med. Pulex.). Takes cold, chilliness, coryza, toothache, sore throat, etc. before menses. Craves open air. Paroxysmal cough with difficult, thin, salty or bloody sputum. Weary, heavy feet. Chilly and dry.

Complementary: Cham. Related: Rhe.

MAGNESIA MUR.

REGION.

NERVES.

LIVER.

Digestion.

Pelvic Organs { **Uterus. Rectum.**

WORSE.

LYING ON RIGHT SIDE.

Night. Noise. Sea Bathing.

Eating. Salt Foods. MILK.

BETTER.

HARD PRESSURE. Cool, Open Air. Gentle Motion.

Hanging down.

Nervous, hepatic and pelvic symptoms. Darting. **Cramping. Burning.** Dryness. Dinner excites faintness, dyspnœa, etc. Globus.——Yellowish sclera. Acrid, crusty ozœna. Yellowish, scalloped tongue. **Pain from liver** to spine or epigastrium. Gastralgia. **Sore, enlarged liver;** it drags when lying on left side (Nat-s.). STOOLS DRY, KNOTTY OR OF LITTLE

BALLS; crumbling at anus. **Profuse, dark, lumpy menses,** with cramps, backache and pain in thighs. **Gushes of leucorrhœa follow each cramp or stool** (Stan.) Palpitation; > motion (Gel.) or lying on left side. **Bruised** or burning feeling in hips and back. Dead fingertips. Tense thighs and calves; must move limbs. Cutting in heels. Sweat on head and feet. Jaundice.

Related: Natr-m. Pul. Sep.

MAGNESIA PHOSPH.

REGION.	WORSE.
NERVES { Face. Head.	COLD { AIR. Uncovering. WATER.
Muscles.	**Touch. Night. Periodicity.**
Right Side.	**EXHAUSTION.**
	BETTER.
	WARMTH.
	Pressure. Doubling Up.

Nervous; subject to violent neuralgias, colics, cramps, **etc. Paroxysms of pain;** shoot like lightning; changing place; in waves; radiating, or squeezing the part; **excorting cries;** causing restlessness or prostration, etc. **Face-ache,** toothache, etc. **Twitchings.** Spasmodic effects. Hiccough. Chorea. Writers cramp, etc.——Photophobia. Cracks in angles of lips. Flatulent colic. Cough. > cool air. Irritable pulse.

Related: Colo. Dios.

MAGNESIA SULF.

REGION.	WORSE.
Intestines. Urine.	Morning on Awaking.
Female Sexual Organs.	BETTER.
	Rubbing. Walking.

Diarrhœa with diuresis. Greenish urine; with red sediment. Profuse, dark, intermittent menses. Much, thick leucorrhœa. As of a lump between shoulders. Back feels broken. Left arm and foot fall asleep. Crawling in fingertips (l). Warts.

Related: Nat-s.

MANCINELLA.

REGION.	WORSE.
Surfaces {Mucous. **Skin.** Mind.	Cold. **Puberty.** Climacteric. **Touch.**

Irritation. Burnings.——Depressed, with sexual erethism. Empty in head. **Foul saliva.** Craves cold water. Swelling at epigastrium. Colics. Cough on drinking. Desquamation of soles. Vesicles. Scarlet fever.

Related: Rhus-t.

MANGANUM.

REGION.	WORSE.
INNER EAR. LOWER LIMBS.	Varies with the Weather. **Touch.**
Larynx and Trachea.	**Cold. Damp. Night.**
Periosteum {**Joints. Shins.** Heels.	**Speaking. Feather Bed.**
Skin.	BETTER.
	Lying Down. Open Air.

Painfully sore; ears, bones, joints, etc. **Diagonal pains.** Yellow-green, lumpy or bloody discharges. Catarrh. Infiltrated joints. Festination. Motor paralysis.——Weak and nervous. Headache, < straining at stool, etc. **Everything affects the ears** (Plant.). Blowing nose is painful. Pale, sickly face. Anæmia. Cough, < reading or laughing; > lying (Arg. Euphr.). Rough, hoarse voice; < A. M.; chronic. Raw larynx. Late or pale first menses. Weak, uncertain legs. Digging in shin bones. Rough, cracked (flexures) or bluish skin. Dry, hard ulcers.

Related: Chin. Psor.

MARUM VERUM.

REGION.	WORSE.
RECTUM. NOSE. Lungs.	Weather; Changing; Damp.
Fingertips.	In Bed.
Toe Joints.	BETTER.
	Open Air.

Delicate and sensitive. **Crawling in nose; wants to pick it;** side lain on closes up. Lumpy discharge. Loss of smell. Atrophic catarrh. Polypi. Mouldy taste when hawking. **Itching at anus; prevents sleep.** Pinworms. Cough, < coughing. Ingrown nails (Mag-p-aus.).

Complementary: Calc-c. Related: Cina. Sil.

MEDORRHINUM.

REGION.

MIND. NERVES.

Mucous Membranes.

Cellular Tissues { **Lungs.** Pelvis. Joints. }

Kidneys. Left Ovary.

WORSE.

Daytime. 3-4 A. M. **Cold.**

Pregnancy. Thinking of it.

BETTER.

LYING ON ABDOMEN. Fresh Air. Seaside. Dampness.

Clutching Hands. Uncovering

SYCOTIC TAINT, **poor reaction and many pains. Stiff, puffy,** sore and rheumatic. Nephritis. Emaciation. **Profuse, acrid discharges; causing itching.** Small, very sore aphthæ, blisters, etc. Fetor. Fishy odors (Ol-ani.). Formication. Sense of trembling.——**Sensitive, nervous and hurried.** Feels far off or unreal. Tearful and fearful. Greenish face (Ars.). Yellow at edge of hair (Nat-m.). Craves stimulants. Vomiting of pregnancy. Heavy lower abdomen or prostate. Grinding colic (Dios.); must brace the feet. Dysmenorrhœa. Leans back to force a stool; then shivers. Cholera infantum. Fiery red, moist, itching anus. Scalding or ammoniacal urine. Leucorrhœa. Craves fresh air. **Cough > lying on face.** (Am-c. Bar-c. Eupat.). Sore, oozing or icy nipples. Heavy legs. **Tender, itching soles.** Skin is cold, but the blood feels hot (Sec-c.). Sleeps in knee-chest posture. **Easy sweating.**

Related: Bar-c. Nat-m. Psor. Thu.

MELLILOTUS.

REGION.

HEAD { Vaso-Motor Nerves. Circulation. }

WORSE.

Climacteric. Walking.

Weather **Changing,** Stormy, or Rainy.

BETTER.

Bleeding. Profuse Urine. Vinegar.

Congestions. Bright red hemorrhage.——Desires to escape. VIOLENT THROBBING HEADACHE; threatening his reason. FIERY RED FACE. **Profuse nosebleed** (Aco.).

Related: Bell. Glo.

MENYANTHES.

REGION.
Circulation.
Motor Nerves.

WORSE.
Walking. Ascending. Rest.
BETTER.
Hard Pressure. Stooping.
Twilight. Laying on of Hands.

ICY COLDNESS OF PROMINENT PARTS; nose (Ap. Med.), ears, fingers, knees, etc.; at night (Pho.). Visible jerks or twitches. Fidgets. Paralysing pains.——**Heavy pressure on vertex** (Cact. Fer-p. Glo. Lach. Lyc. Phel. Pho-ac. Tub. Zin.). Head pains ascend from nape. Misty vision. Frequent scant urination. Cramps from ankles to calves (r). Skin feels too tight. Vivid dreams. Shivering with yawning.

Related: Ver-a.

MEPHITIS.

REGION.
Nerves.

WORSE.
Night. Lying Down.
BETTER.
Cold Bathing, Weather.

Spasmodic effects.——Vivid fancies. Food goes wrong way. Chokes easily. Can't exhale. Asthma. **Violent spasmodic cough.** Whooping cough.

Related: Coral.

MERCURIUS.

REGION.
BLOOD.
GLANDS
- **SALIVARY.**
- **TONSILS. THROAT.**
- LYMPHATICS. **Liver.**
- MUCOUS.

Cellular Tissues.
Joints.
Bones.
Skin.

WORSE.
NIGHT. Night Air. **SWEATING.**
LYING ON RIGHT SIDE.
HEAT OF BED or fire.
SENSITIVE TO
- DRAFTS, to Head.
- Changing, Cloudy or **Cold Damp Weather.**
- Taking Cold.

Wet Feet. Firelight.
BETTER.
Moderate Temperature.

Weak, tremulous and sweaty. Sense of rawness. FREE SECRETIONS. **Suppuration. Thin, acrid, foul or greenish discharges. Glandular activity.** Catarrhs. Biliousness. Scrofula. Pains stick to one joint. Rheumatism. ——Nervous; hurried. Violent impulses (homicidal), etc. Forgetful. As of a band about head (Gels. Nit-ac.). Eyes draw together (Nat-m. Zin.). Swelled, scurfy tarsi. **Colds travel upward** (Brom.) or attack the eyes (Dulc.). Sees black specks. Heaviness in nose (Kali-bi.). Red, raw, dirty nostrils. **Swelled cheeks** (Plant.). Aching in jaws. Mumps Salty lips. Loose, hollow, black, **aching teeth; pain into ears.** Ragged, swelled gums. Gumboil (Sil.). Aphthæ (Bor. Iod.). Bad breath. **INCREASED SALIVA** (Stap.); flows during sleep (Bar-c. Lac-c. Lach. Lys. Nit-ac. Pho. Rhus-t. Syp.). **FLABBY, INDENTED TONGUE.** METALLIC TASTE. Sticking in tonsils. Enlarged tonsils. SORE THROAT. Weak bowels; must hold them. Swelled inguinals (Hep. Nit-ac. Sul.). Scanty, bloody or green slimy stools; then tenesmus or chill. WHITE STOOLS (Pod.). Frequent, scanty urine; then burning. Swelled glands or foreskin. Gonorrhœa. Chancre. Bloody emissions. Cough in double bouts; dry at night, yellow sputum by day. Milk in breasts; spoiled; instead of menses. Awakes with trembling heart. Cracked, peeling palms. Numb fingers. **Orgasms** (to head or chest), **erethism and restlessness; < lest exertion.** Tender, excoriated skin; like raw meat. Moist, crusty eruptions. Irregular, shallow, spreading, bleeding ulcers. Jaundice. Nightly bone pains (Lyc. Mang.); < near surface. Easily chilled or overheated. Alternate chill and heat. EASY, PROFUSE SWEATING; WITHOUT RE-

LIEF (Ben-ac. Chel. Form.); with the pains; oily or sour; staining yellow. Creeping chills. Catarrhal fever; after suppressions.

Complementary: Bell. **Related: Kali-io.**

MERCURIUS CORROSIVUS.

REGION.	WORSE.
RECTUM. BLADDER.	**AFTER** {**URINATING.** STOOL. **Swallowing.**
THROAT {Uvula. Palate.	**Night. Cold.** Acids.
Kidneys. Bones (flat).	**Autumn.** Hot Days; Cool Nights.

Violent effects. Inflammation with burning, swelling and constriction. EROSIVE DISCHARGES. Phagedena.——Anxious and restless. Acrid tears. **Photophobia.** Iritis. Keratitis. Red, swollen nose. **Fluent coryza.** Nightly **toothache** (Lyc.). Red. swollen uvula. **DYSPHAGIA.** Insatiable thirst. Vomiting slime and blood. Burning, **distended, sensitive** stomach. Gastritis. **Cutting colic. Continuous urging to stool and urine (Canth.** Lil-t. Sabi.). **SCANTY STOOLS OF BLOODY OR SHREDDY SLIME, WITH TORMENTING TENESMUS: "A NEVER GET DONE FEELING."** Dysentry (Aco. Nux-v. **Rhus-t.** Stap.). Spasm of rectum during coition. **HOT URINE PASSED DROP BY DROP.** Nephritis. Gonorrhœa. Hard chancre. Phimosis. Chordee. Cold skin. **Sweats; from every motion;** partial; < forehead and lower parts; **foul, at night.**

Related: **Ars. Canth.**

MERCURIUS CYANATUS.

REGION.	WORSE.
THROAT. MOUTH. Nose.	Swallowing. Speaking.

Rapid and extreme prostration; with coldness and cyanosis. Much **thick,** green or grayish membrane in throat. **Putridity.** Septic **diphtheria;** prophylactic of soft parts. Cutting pains: **in throat** (Nit-ac.) **Weak heart.**

Related: **Lach.**

MERCURIUS DULCIS.

REGION.	
Duodenum. **Eustachian Tube.**	
Bowels.	

Pallid, flabby and catarrhal. Biliousness. Eustachian catarrh (Petr.). Acrid, grass-green diarrhœa; of infants.

Related: Kali-m.

MERCURIUS IOD FLAV.

REGION.	WORSE.
THROAT.	Raising Up. Warm Drinks.
Glands.	Lying on Left Side.
Right Side.	BETTER.
	Open Air.

Faintness. Cornea looks scratched. Nasal catarrh. Increased saliva. **Moist tongue.** YELLOW COAT AT BASE OF TONGUE (Kali-bi. Nat-p. Nat-s. Phyt.). SORE THROAT (right then left). Swelled **tonsils** (Calc-c.). Tonsilitis. Yellow leucorrhœa of children. Soft glandular swelling. Syphilis.

Related: Lyc.

MERCURIUS IOD RUB.

REGION.	WORSE.
THROAT. **Glands.** **Left Side.**	Empty Swallowing.

Painfully heavy occiput. Chronic granulated eyelids. **Dark red fauces** SORE THROAT (left then right). Stiff **throat, base of tongue and neck** (Phyt.). Profuse, acrid, green leucorrhœa. Hard chancre. Stubborn, suppurating buboe. **Hard glandular swelling.** Moist cracks in **palms.** Wandering pains.

Related: Lach.

MERCURIUS PRECIP RUB.

REGION.	WORSE.
Mucous Membranes. Skin.	Lying. Falling to Sleep.

Burning. Patchy tongue. Coat like old cheese on mouth and throat. Mucous patches (Arg-n. Merc-i-fl. Nit-ac. Pul.). Suffocation when lying or falling to sleep.

Related: Lach.

MEZEREUM.

REGION.	WORSE.
SKIN, **Nerves**, **Bones** { **Head.** **Face.** Jaws.	NIGHT. **Suppressions.**
	WARMTH OF BED, Fire, etc.
	Cold Air; Drafts; Damp.
Mucous Membranes { Mouth. Stomach.	Motion. **Touch.** Mercury.
	BETTER.
One Side.	Wrapping up. (Nerves. Bones)
	Eating. Open Air.

Irritative, smarting, burning. Rawness. Effects of suppressed eczema capitis. As in a cool breeze (Med. Mos.). **Pain then chilliness,** soreness or numbness. Neuralgia; after shingles (Kalm. Zin.). Emaciation of part (Carb-v. Grap. Led. Pul.). Gouty-rheumatic-syphlitic dyscrasia.—— Head pain (l) into eyes, malar bones, neck, etc.; with lachrymation. Painful skull. Eyes seem dry. Ears feel open to cool wind (Cham. Lach. Sep.). Deafness. Dry, dark red mouth (Phyt.). Blunt teeth. Toothache; into temples; > cool air. Sore throat in winter. Gastric pain > milk (Grap. Merc.). Constricted, prolapsed rectum (Lach.). Glistening particles in stools (Cina. Pho.). Cough excited by hot things; unto vomiting. **Intolerable itching;** changing place on scratching. Pruritis senilis (Alu. Ars. Mucun.). Eruptions ooze acrid, gluey moisture (Grap.), form thick crusts with pus beneath or are chalky white (Ars.). Milk crust. Bones seem enlarged. Periostitis. Chilly; limbs feel cold. Heat of one hand.

Related: Ars. Guai. Kali-io. Merc.

MILLEFOLIUM.

REGION.

CAPILLARIES { LUNGS. **Nose.** Uterus.

WORSE.

Injury. **Violent Exertion.**

BETTER.

Bleeding. **Discharges.**

Bruised soreness. Congestion. Painless, bright, red, fluid hemorrhage; nosebleed, hæmoptysis (Aco. Led.), etc. Spasms after suppressed menses (Abs.). Flatulent colic. Oppression of chest, with palpitation.

Related: Arn. **Led.**

MOSCHUS.

REGION.

NERVES { SENSORY. **Genital.**

Respiration. Circulation.

WORSE.

Excitement. Cold. Suppressions. Suppressed Menses.

BETTER.

Open Air.

Poor reaction. Spasmodic, nervous effects, laughter, hiccough, etc. Twitchings. **Chokings. Faints.** Globus. Hysteria.——**Hurried,** **tremulous and awkward.** Anger; talks excitedly or scolds until she **faints.** Fears noise, dying, etc. Imaginary sufferings. Headache with coldness, faintness and profuse urine. One cheek red but cold (Fer.), other pale and hot. Blue lips. **Sudden, nervous suffocation or anxious palpitation;** wants a deep breath. Cramp in lungs. Sleepy by day; nervous and sleepless at night. **So sensitive cold air** makes him shudder. Shivering **on** scalp. **Cold skin.** Burning heat with restlessness.

Related: Castor. **Ign.** **Nux-v**

MUREX.

REGION.

FEMALE SEXUAL ORGANS.

WORSE.

Touch. Sitting.

Sinking at stomach. Urging in bladder. Sore spot in pelvis. **Painfully sore uterus.** Pain from genitals into breasts. Bearing down pains; **must cross limbs. Frantic desire.** Copious menses. Leucorrhœa alternating with mental symptoms. Lumbar pain impels walking, which <.

Related: Lil-t. **Sep.**

MURIATIC ACID.

REGION.

BLOOD. **MUSCLES** { HEART. **ANUS.** }

Mucous Membranes { **Digestive Tract.** **MOUTH.** }

Brain.

WORSE.

Touch. Wet Weather. Walking. Cold Drinks; Bathing. Sitting. Human Voice.

BETTER.

Motion. Warmth. Lying on l. Side.

SORE, RESTLESS AND ERETHISTIC, BUT SOON PARALYTIC WEAKNESS FOLLOWS; he slides down in bed (Ars. Colch.), eyes fall shut, lower jaw drops. etc. **Bluish parts;** tongue, piles, ulcers. Tearing in limbs. BURNINGS. Dry. bleeding, cracked or **deeply ulcerated parts.** Thin, foul, acrid discharges. Decomposition. Typhoid or scorbutic states.——**Sad and taciturn. Muttering. Persistent, loud moaning.** Vertigo, if lies on right side. Brain feels bruised. Periodical pain over left eye. Occipital pains; leaden heaviness. Deafness. Nosebleed. **Dark or glowing red face with cold hands,** but no thirst. **Dry mouth and throat.** Sordes. **Tongue heavy** (Nat-c.). stiff, shrunken or burnt looking. Aphthæ. **Averse to meat.** Profuse, involuntary stool or prolapse of bowel; when urinating or passing flatus (Alo.). **Very sore piles** (Grap.), > heat. Atony of bladder, must press until the rectum comes down. Red, swollen, burning fingers and toes. Scurfy eruption on dorsæ of hands (Nat-c. Pix-l.). Ulcers throb on walking. Sparse scarlatina, mixed with petechiæ (Ail.). Pulse drops every third beat (Nat-m.). Cold in bed in early morning. **INTENSE BURNING HEAT, WITH AVERSION TO COVERS.**

Related: Bapt. Bry.

NAJA.

REGION.

NERVES { HEART. **Respiration.** Throat. }

Left Side { **Ovary.** Temple. Arm. }

WORSE.

Lying on Left Side.

After { Sleep. Menses. } Air { **Cold.** Drafts. }

Pressure of Clothes. Alcohol.

BETTER.

Riding in Open Air. Sneezing.

Nervous and cardiac effects; often reflex. **Trembling.** Parts seem drawn together (Par.).——Suicidal brooding. Shootings in head. As of a blow on occiput and neck (Ap. Lach. Tab. Taren.). PAIN FROM LEFT OVARY TO HEART (Cimi. Lach. Sabal.). Suffocative choking; **grasps** the throat. Puffing breathing (Chin. Op.). Asthma or cough; cardiac (Laur. Spo.). Palpitation. Stitches at or **weakness of heart.** Pain from heart to shoulder or scapula. Dryness or emptiness in lung (1). The ribs feel broken (Kali-bi.). Cramps in shoulder, nape or thigh. Numb left arm. Terrifying racking in marrow of thigh (Am-c.). Puffy or sweating hands and feet. Itching cicatrices. Pulse changes force (Dig.). Internal heat < chest (Aco.).

Related: Cimi. Lach.

NATRUM CARB.

REGION.
- DIGESTION. **Nerves.**
- Skin.
- Hands (dorsæ).
- Heels.

WORSE.
- **HEAT** { SUN. **Sultry Air.** / WEATHER. Gaslight.
- **Dietetic Errors. Milk. Drafts.**
- **PERIODICALLY** { **Summer (Head).** / **Winter** (Body). **5 A.M.**
- Mental Exertion.

BETTER.
- Motion. Mental Exertion.

Puffy, relaxed and easily exhausted; by summer heat. OVERSENSITIVE; **to open air, music, noise, dietetic errors, etc.** Pains cause trembling, cold sweat, anxiety, etc.——Lively, yet fearful; during thunderstorms. Averse to company. Vertigo from wine. Head pains go thro' eyes (Ign.). Dazzling flashes or stars before vision. Swelled or peeling nose (Pho.). Violent sneezing. **Post nasal discharge**. Pale, wilted face. **Acidity, flatulence and lithiæmia. Weak digestion.** Stools like orange pulp. Pollutions. Cough on entering a warm room. Purulent, salty sputum. Boring at tip of left scapula (Hypher.). Heavy legs. **Weak ankles.** Blisters on small joints (Ars. Bor. Sep.); tips of toes or fingers. Milky, watery or dry, rough skin. Cold between scapulæ. Burning wrists and ankles. **Sweats easily.**

Complementary: Sep. Related: Lyc. Nat-m.

NATRUM MUR.

REGION.	WORSE.
NUTRITION { **Digestive Tract.** BRAIN. BLOOD. MUSCLES.	**PERIOD-ICALLY** { 9-11 A. M. **With the Sun.** After Menses.
MIND. HEART.	HEAT. **Sun.** Summer.
GLANDS { MUCOUS. Spleen. Liver.	**Exertion;** Eyes; Mental. **Puberty. Sympathy.** Nitrate of Silver.
Skin.	BETTER. **Open Air.** Cool Bathing. Sweating.

Lean undeveloped or poorly nourished; < neck (Mag-c. Sars.); **descending** emaciation (Lyc.). Anæmia. Malarial cachexia. **Tremulous, easily exhausted; takes cold.** Violent emotions <. Nervous erethism. DRYNESS. **Thick, white or clear, acrid discharges.——Sad, reserved** and likes to be alone. Angry when consoled. Scattered thoughts or an idea clings, prevents sleep, inspires revenge, etc. Apprehension. **Maddening bursting or hammering headache;** with disturbed vision or numbness; < motion, even of eyes. Migraine. Heaviness over eyes, as from loss of sleep (Tell.). Falling hair. Blurred vision (Pho.). Letters run together. **Lachrymation;** with sneezing on coughing, etc. Alternate fluent and dry coryza. Pale, muddy or greasy color (Merc.). HERPES ABOUT LIPS (Rhus-t.) or at edge of hair; pearly. Dry mouth and throat, but hawks much mucus (Merc.). **Mapped tongue,** or beaded along edge. Blunted taste and smell. THIRST. Hunger without appetite. Averse to bread. CRAVES SALT. Tense abdomen (Ap.); < groins (Am-m.). Dry, hard, crumbling stool (Am-m. Mag-m.); tears anus or causes burning; on alternate days (Calc-c. Cocc. Kali-c.). Chronic diarrhœa. Constriction of rectum. Herpes about anus. Averse to coition or it is painful; then backache, weak legs (Calc-c.), depression, etc. Cough excited by **a dry spot in throat** (Cimi. Cist. Con. Lach.) or tickling in epigastrium. Soreness at heart (Ap. **Arn.** Flu-ac. Spig.). **Palpitation;** fluttering; shaking the body (Rhus-t.); < emotions, lying on left side or motion. Bruised backache; > pressure (Rhus-t. Sep.); < coughing. Sobs during sleep. **Awakes feeling weak. Dreams of robbers.** Dry, dirty, unhealthy skin, given to chaps and **herpetic eruptions.** Cold hands and feet; at heart (Helod. Petr.). Morning chill with thirst. Sweat at edge of hair; on nose (Cina. Tub.); on face while eating (Cham.). Profuse sweat relieves.

Complementary: Ign. Sep. Related: **Pul.**

NATRUM PHOS.

REGION.
- Mucous Glands.
- Duodenum.

WORSE.
- **Children. Mental Exertion.** Sugar. Milk. Thunderstorms. Gaslight.

BETTER.
- Eating. Cold.

Debility. Deep yellow discharges. SOURNESS; acid stomach; sour sweats, etc.——**Mental weakness.** Itching of nose, about mouth and at anus. **Child picks nose.** Worms. **Pale face;** or red on alternate sides (Chel. Lach. Pho.). YELLOW CREAMY COATING AT BASE OF TONGUE. As of a hair on tongue. As of a lump in throat. Noisy flatulence. Eruptions about joints (Sep.). Itching ankles. Awakes frightened.

Related: Cina. Kali-s. Rhe.

NATRUM SULPH.

REGION.
- **OCCIPUT.**
- **GLANDS** { **LIVER.** Intestinal.
- Chest { **Left.** Lower.

WORSE.
- **DAMP** { Weather. Spring. **Night Air.** Cellars.
- **Injury to Head. Light.**
- Time; **Late Evening;** Morning.

BETTER.
- Dry Open or Cool Air.
- Change of Position.

Sudden, violent effects. **Fulness.** Sourness. Biliousness. **Lithæmia.** Sycosis. **Stitches;** thro' ankles; back thro' left lower chest; < **rising or** sitting down.——Sensitive and suspicious. Sadness, < **music or subdued** light. Dire (suicidal) impulses. Vertigo; > head sweat. **Crushing** or gnawing in occiput. Meningitis. **Photophobia.** Yellowish face. **Greenish-yellow pasty tongue;** feels burnt at tip (Colo.). Bitter taste. Slow digestion. Concomitants to nausea. Sore, heavy liver; < lying on left side (Ptel.). Clawing in gall-bladder (Lyc. Med.). Colic > rubbing abdomen (Pod.). RUMBLING IN BOWELS, THEN A SUDDEN, GUSHING, NOISY (Arg-n.), SPLUTTERING STOOL; after rising. White sand in urine.

Dyspnœa. Sycotic asthma (Sil.). **Loose, but violent cough; must hold the sides. Run-rounds** (Syph.). **Hang-nails. Moist pimples. Chilly, can't get warm in bed** (Ars.). **Burning below knees. Warty nodules.**
Complementary: Ars. Thu. Related: Colo. Med. Pul.

NITRICUM ACIDUM.

REGION.	WORSE.
MARGINS OF OUTLETS { Throat. Anus. Mouth.	**SLIGHT** { TOUCH. Jar. **Noise. Rattle of Wagons.**
GLANDS { **Liver.** Salivary.	COLD; **Air**; Bathing.
Blood.	**Motion.** Mercury.
Skin.	Change of Weather.
Bones.	BETTER.
	Mild Weather.
	Gliding Motions.

STICKING, LIKE A SPLINTER (Hep.) **or ulcerative gnawing.** HEMORRHAGE; bright. **Acrid, foul, thin, dirty or brown discharges;** cause redness, destroy the hair (Lyc. Merc. Rhus-t. Sil.), etc. Malignancy. **Exhausted, yet sensitive.** Sweats easily, then takes cold. Cracking joints (Thu.). Sense of a band. Brunettes.——**So angry he trembles;** hateful or profane. Head aches as if in a vise; < pressure of hat (Calc-ph.). Deafness (Grap.). Nasal diphtheria. **Yellow sickly face.** Corners of mouth ulcerated and scabby (Grap. Merc. Rhus-t.). Flabby gums. Moist fissured tongue (Flu-ac. Psor.). Salivation. Craves fat. Infantile hernia (Lyc. Nux-v.). Stools tear anus (Mez.); even if soft; then prolonged pain (Rat.). Moist anus. Fissure ani. **Painful piles.** URINE SMELLS STRONG, LIKE A HORSE'S (Ben-ac.) or seems cold. As of a hot wire in urethra. Bloody water from vagina (Calc-c. Mang.). Shattering cough starts from a spot in larynx; with stitches in small of back (Aco.); > cold. Cutting in larynx (Manc. Merc-c.). Orgasms to chest with palpitation and fear. Swelled finger joints. Warts on backs of hands. Weak ankles, (Carb-a. Mez. Nat-c.). Soft figwarts (Stap. Thu.). Copper colored spots. Dry skin; cracks in every angle. **Raw, ragged or rapid ulceration** (Ars. Dulc. Merc-c.); in mouth, on tonsils, genitals, etc.; with proud flesh. Syphilis. Broken chilblains. Sore bones, < tibiæ. Pulse drops each fourth beat. Jagged warts. **Icy, coldness, of soles.** Exhausting morning sweat (urinous). **Acrid, foul, axillary or footsweat.**
Complementary: Calc-c. Thu. Related: Ars. Kali-c. Merc.

NUX MOSCHATA.

REGION.
SENSORIUM.
Mind. Nerves.
FEMALE ORGANS.
Digestion.

WORSE.
Cold {**Damp.** Drafts. **Wind.** Feet.}
EMOTIONS. **Pregnancy.**
MENSTRUATION.
Mental {Exertion. Shock. Jar. Bruises.}

BETTER.
Warm Room. Dry Weather.

Scrawny, flatulent women; faint easily; laugh or cry by turns with small breasts. Hysteria. SLEEPY AND COLD. Complaints that cause sleepiness. Narcotic effects. EXTREME DRYNESS; < **mucous surfaces,** eyes. **Heaviness;** eyes, tongue, etc. **Dark hemorrhages.——Dreamy, clairvoyant state** (Aco.). Slow thought and perception. Dazed; objects seem changed. Levitation. Sudden loss of ideas; uses wrong words. Automatic acts. Cerebral exhaustion. Apoplexy. Pale face. Retracted lips. DRY MOUTH AND THROAT, WITHOUT THIRST (Bry. Pul. Saba. Sep.). **Weak digestion. Enormous bloating;** all food turns to gas (Iod. Carb-v. Nux-v.). **Flatulent colic.** As of a piece of wood across lower abdomen. Inactive rectum. **Stool difficult, altho soft** or putrid, yellow and undigested. Strangury from alcohol. **Thick, dark, irregular menses.** Deficient labor pains. Cough from heat of bed. **Hoarseness from walking against wind. Dry, cold skin. Palpitation.** Weak, irregular pulse.

Complementary: Lyc. Related: Cann. Mos. Op.

NUX VOMICA.

REGION.

Cerebro-Spinal Axis.

NERVES.

DIGESTIVE ORGANS { **STOMACH.** LIVER. **Bowels.**

RESPIRATORY ORGANS.

Male Brunettes.

WORSE.

EARLY MORNING.

COLD { **OPEN AIR** (dry). **Drafts.** UNCOVERING. **Wind.**

HIGH LIVING DEBAUCHERY { **COFFEE.** Condiments. LIQUOR. **Drugs.**

Sedentary Habits.

Mental Exertion.

SLIGHT CAUSES { **Anger. Noise. Odors.** Light. **Touch. Pressure of Clothes.**

BETTER.

FREE DISCHARGES. **Nap.**

Wrapping Head. Lying Down.

Hot Drinks. **Milk, Moist Air.**

Violent, spasmodic but irregular and inefficient action. Jerks. Drawing pains. Bruised feeling; brain, abdomen, etc. Takes cold easily. Internal rawness (Ars. Bar-c. Sang.). Bilious attacks.——**Active, intense, nervous; supersensitive or zealous.** Violent (suicidal) impulses. ANGRY; **so mad** he cries (Ant-t.). EXCITABLE. IMPATIENT; CAN'T STAND PAIN (Cham.). Nagging. Spiteful. **Sullen.** VERTIGO; with momentary unconsciousness. Dullness. Sensitive scalp. Lachrymation on affected side (Lach. Pul.). Migraine. Bloodshot eyes. Sore nostrils. Acute smell. Stuffy coryza; scanty secretion; fluent in open air (Cep.). **Red, turgid** or yellowish face. Jaws snap shut. BAD BREATH, **BAD, BITTER OR SOUR TASTE.** Itching palate (Ran-b. Saba. Wye.); eustachian tube (Petr. Sil.). **Rough, scratchy throat.** Putrid taste in throat on coughing (Sang.). Craves stimulants. HICCOUGH. HARD RETCHING (Phyt.); < when hawking (Cocc-c.). ERUCTATIONS. WATERBRASH. NAUSEA; **> if he can only vomit.** VIOLENT VOMITING; **bilious; sour.** FOOD LIES HEAVY. **As of a knot in stomach (Sep.).** Clothes oppress the waist. Pain from stomach to chest or back (Bell. Bism. Con. Cup.). INDIGESTION. **Colic.** Sore or enlarged liver (Mag-m. Sep. Sil.). Gall stones. **Bowels sore; < stepping or cough. UNEASY URGING, AS IF BOWELS WOULD ACT.** Hernia. Strains hard at stool (Alu. Chin. Nat-m. Sil.); **> STOOL. Flatus is retained in rectum** (Calc-c. Lach.). Inactive peristalsis (Bry. Op. Thu.). Constipation. Dysentery. Itching piles, > cold bathing. Sexual erethism. **Intermittent, early, profuse or prolonged menses. Violent cough.** Painfully stiff neck. Breaking back-ache; SITS UP TO TURN OVER. Shooting from toes to hips (Thal.) < after stool. Crawling along spine. Tense cramps in calves and soles. Sleepy in evening or sleepless from rushing ideas. **Awakes too early; can't sleep again, finally sleeps but on awaking feels miserable. Jaundice.** EASILY CHILLED; < UNCOVERING (Hep. Pho. Rhus-t.) OR MOTION; **even during the heat.** Sour sweat.

Complementary: Sul. Related: Ign. Lyc.

OCIMUM CANUM.

REGION.	WORSE.
Ureters (r).	Scanty Urine.

Sore pains in ureters (Berb.). Renal colic with hæmaturia and violent vomiting. Red sand in the urine. Swelled inguinal and mammary glands.

Related: Canth. Lyc. Urt-ur.

ŒNANTHE CROCATA.

REGION.	WORSE.
CEREBRO-SPINAL AXIS.	Sexual Disturbances. Injury.

Mania. Swelled, twitching face. Rosy red blotches on face and chest. Burning heat, < head and throat. Epilepsy with priapism. Status epilepticus (Aco.).

Related: Bell. Cic.

OLEANDER.

REGION.	WORSE.
Digestive Tract.	After Suckling. Rubbing.
Skin. Scalp.	Undressing.
Nerves.	BETTER.
	Looking Sidewise.

Numbing, paretic effects. Tremulous weakness. Emptiness in stomach and chest; after eating; > brandy.——Distraction. Slow comprehension. Vertigo. Thin stool escapes with the flatus; passes food eaten the day before. Crampy contraction of upper limbs. Sensitive skin; chafes and oozes or bleeds. Eruptions with itching biting, as of lice. Milk crust, < occiput. **Heat from mental exertion.**

Related: Anac. Chin.

OLEUM ANIMALE.

REGION.
NERVES. Digestive Organs. Excretions.

WORSE.
Eating. In Room. Suppressions.
BETTER.
Rubbing.

White of egg seems dried on lips (Phos-ac.). Mouth feels greasy. Toothache > biting. Snowy saliva. Acrid vapor in throat, causing cough. Hot or urinous eructations. As of water in stomach. **Profuse, pale urine smelling like fish brine** (Grap. Sanic. Tell.). Testes feel pulled up. Outward darting in breasts. Flesh feels torn from bones. Foul footsweat; on heels.

Related: Sul.

OLEM JECORIS.

REGION.
Chest. Liver.

WORSE.
Cold Damp.

Faulty nutrition. **Atrophic infants.**——Yellow tongue, leucorrhœa, sputum, skin, etc. Cough with palpitation. **Soreness or stitches in chest.** Burning spots. Milk crust. Ringworm. Always taking cold. Chilly up the back. **Heat in palms,** toward evening. Hectic.

Related: Pho.

ONOSMODIUM.

REGION.
MUSCLES AND Nerves { **Eyes.** **Occiput.** FEMALE PELVIC ORGANS.
Spine.

WORSE.
Sprains { EYE STRAIN. **Sexual Excesses.**
Darkness. Tight Clothes.
BETTER.
Rest. Sleep. Eating.

Aching, sore and stiff.——Confused. Forgetful. Slow thought. Nervous exhaustion. Aphasia. Vertigo < lying on left side. Headache from eyestrain. Pains up and down from (1) occiput (Sep.). **Eyes aching, heavy, tired and stiff.** Misjudges distances. Mushy yellow stool. Aromatic urine (Eupat.). Sexual desire gone. **Sore ovaries** and uterus. Acrid leucorrhœa. Sticky, white expectoration. Swelled, tender mammæ. Tired, numb legs and popliteæ. Seems to tread on cotton. Staggering.

Related: Cimic. Hyper. Lil-t. Rhus-t.

OPIUM.

REGION.
MIND.
SENSES.
Respiration.
Digestive Tract.

WORSE.
EMOTIONS. FEAR. **Fright.**
ALCOHOL. Sleep.
Suppressed Discharges.
Receding Eruptions. If Heated.
BETTER.
Cold.

Negative, torpid states; little pain (Old.), **secretion or reaction.** Twitchings, jerkings, tremblings. Internal dryness.——**Dull placidity** or **delirium** with terror. As if not at home or seems nothing ails him. **Lying. Intercurrent.** apoplectic congestion (Aco.). Painless paralysis (**Alu. Pho.** Plb.). Heavy occiput. Visual hallucinations. Inactive pupils. **Red, bulging,** staring eyes. Dark, turgid, sweating face (Bap.) or alternately **pale** and red. **Old look** (Sul.); after cholera infantum. Mouth twitches or hangs open. Paralysis of tongue (Dulc.). Craving, without appetite. **Vomiting;** in peritonitis. As of a heavy weight in abdomen (Alu. Lyc. (l.) Rhus-t.). Bowels feel obstructed. Paralytic atony of bowels and bladder (Con.). Hard tympany. Lead colic. **Stools of hard, black balls** (Thu.). Constipation. Retained urine. Lively foetal motions. Rattling, unequal breathing. Sighing. Stertor. **General itching.** Painless ulcers. **Tired,** but can't sleep. SOMNOLENT STATES (Ant-t. Nux-m.). Heavy, stupid sleep. **Bed feels too hot. Hot, sweaty and drowsy;** with cold limbs. Full, slow pulse.

Complementary: Alu. **Bar-c.** Bry. Pho. Plb. Related: **Nux-m.**

OSMIUM.

REGION.
Respiratory Tract. Trachea.

WORSE.
Coughing. Talking.

Foul secretions.——Greenish, rainbow colors about light. Fluent coryza with a sense of stoppage. Spasmodic cough with torn loose feeling and tenacious sputum. Sensitive air passages. Foul axillary sweat.

Related: Iod.

OXALIC ACID.

REGION.
Digestive Tract.
Nerves {Cord. Heart.

WORSE.
Thinking of it. Cold. Touch. Shaving.
BETTER.
After Stool.

Cold, livid, numb and weak. **Violent pains;** in streaks like lightning; burning; in spots, etc. Neuralgia.——Swimming vertigo. Numb, prickling in occiput and back. **Sour taste.** Gnawing emptiness. Colicky urging or involuntary, muddy-brown stools (Ars. Fer-p.), < lying. Testes feel crushed. Low voice. Paroxysmal, jerking breathing. Pain from lower chest (1) into epigastrium. **Back feels too weak to hold body.** Palpitation < lying. Angina pectoris. Fixed chest (Stry.). Cold creeps up spine (Chel.). **Weak, trembling hands and feet.**

Related: Ars.

PÆONIA.

REGION.
Anus. Skin.

WORSE.
STOOL. **Touch.** Motion.

Sensitiveness. Shooting or splinter like pains.——**Excessive pain or foul moisture at anus** (Nit-ac.). Anus covered with crusts. Fissure ani. Large, inflamed or ulcerated piles. Terrifying nightmare.

Related: Rat.

PALLADIUM.

REGION.
Uterus.
Right Ovary.
Mind.

WORSE.
Emotions; Lively. Chagrin.
Social Functions. Standing.
BETTER.
Touch. Pressure. Diversion.

Fleeting pains.——Loves praise. Easily offended. Headache from ear to ear across vertex (Nit-ac. Sabal.). Shooting from navel into breasts or pelvis. Bearing down, > rubbing. Cutting in uterus. Menses flow when nursing. Glairy leucorrhœa, before and after menses. Leaden heaviness in pelvis.

Related: Asaf. Plat.

PAREIRA BRAVA.

REGION.
Genito-Urinary Organs.
Left Side.

BETTER.
On Hands and Knees (Eupat. Euphorb. Sep.).

Must get on hands and knees to urinate; pains go into glans and thighs. Bursting feeling in bladder. Dysuria. Urine contains thick, stringy white mucus or red sand. Renal colic. Enlarged prostate.

Related: Berb. Med.

PARIS QUOD.

REGION.
Head.
Spine. Eyes.
One Side.

WORSE.
Thinking. Eyestrain. Touch.
BETTER.
Pressure.

Heaviness. Numbness (l.). Joints feel broken. **Parts feel too big or drawn together.**——Loquacity. Weight in nape (Nux-v. Rhus-t.). **Eyeballs seem pulled back** (Hep. Lach. Nic-s. Old. Pho. Pul.) **or feel too large.** Face seems drawn into root of nose. Imaginary bad smells. Hawks up tough, green mucus. As of a ball in throat. Periodical painless hoarseness. Painful skin; objects feel rough. Unilateral coldness or heat.

Related: Bell. Nux-v.

PETROLEUM.

REGION.
OCCIPUT.
SKIN { **Folds.** Scalp. Face. Genitals.
Mucous Membranes.
Stomach.

WORSE.
MOTION { CARS. CARRIAGE. BOAT.
Weather { **Cold; Winter.** Changing. **Thunderstorms.**
Eating. Vexation. Cabbage.
BETTER.
Warm Air.

Weak and tremulous; feels sick internally. **Internal itching. Emaciation;** < chest. Dreads open air.——Death seems near. Bewildered. **Beclouded.** VERTIGO; in occiput. **Occipital ache; heaviness** (Calc-c. Chel. Merc-i-r. Mur-ac. Op. Pic-ac.). Inflamed tarsi. Moist spots behind ears (Grap. Old.). Dryness in ears, nose, throat, etc. Foul mucus in throat. Gastric symptoms > eating. Hunger after stool. NAUSEA. **Sea or train sick-**

ness (Tab.). Inflated abdomen. Diarrhœa by day only; < cabbage; then miserable emptiness. Involuntary urine on rising. Cough at night only or < then. Cold air oppresses chest. Stiff or cracking joints. Limbs go to sleep. Ragged, chapped fingers (Nat-m.). Bleeding rhagades. **Fragile skin; it cracks deeply** (Sars.), < **in the angles** (Grap.), nipples, fingertips (Ran-b. Sars. Sil.) or palms. DIRTY, HARD, ROUGH, THICKENED SKIN; **it gets raw or festers, especially in the folds.** Thick, hard or moist, crusty eruptions; on occiput or genitals < cold. Eczema. Herpes. Vesicles. **Itching;** orifices (Amb. Caus.); with burning. Cold spots. Hot palms and soles. Sweat in spots; foul on feet or in axillæ.

Complementary: Sep. Related: Grap. Sul.

PHELLANDRIUM.

REGION.
Mucous Membranes.
Right Side { Chest. Mammæ.

WORSE.
Air; Cold; Open. Using Eyes.
BETTER.
While Nursing.

Catarrhal symptoms. Phthisis.——Everything tastes sweet. **Terribly foul expectoration.** Pain in milk ducts, > nursing. Pain from left border of right mammæ to between shoulders.

Related: Asaf.

PHOSPHORIC ACID.

REGION.
MIND.
Spine { **Sensory Nerves.** Muscles.
Bones.

WORSE.
DEBILITY FROM { LOSS OF FLUIDS. **Sexual Excesses. Fatigue.**
EMOTIONS { **Grief.** Chagrin. Unhappy Love. Homesickness.
Drafts. Cold. Music. Talking.
BETTER.
Warmth. Short Sleep. Stooling.

Relaxed, depressed states with free secretions and sensory illusions. Slowness. Pains go to side lain on (Pul.). Bruised soreness, like **growing pains.** Formication; along spine or limbs.——Weak, **apathetic,** obtuse or torpid. Dull despair. Averse to talking. Mild delirium; easily aroused. Poor memory. Difficult thinking (Dulc.); hunts his words (Arg. Lach. Thu.).

Brain fag (Pho.). Crushing weight in vertex (Men.). Sore skull bones. Crawling at roots of hair. Falling hair. **Dull, sunken eyes, with blue circles.** Pale, sickly face; white of egg seems dried on it. Bleeding gums. Slimy tongue. Craves juicy things. Sour stomach. **PROFUSE, PAINLESS, DIRTY-WHITE** (watery or lienteric) **STOOL, WITH LITTLE DEBILITY** (Calc-c.). **MILKY URINE** (Cina. Viol-o. Visc-a.). POLYURIA. Diabetes (Uran-n.). Weak, relaxed genitals; suddenly during coition (Nux-v.). Pollutions. Shaking cough. A draft on the chest gives him cold (Calc-p. Petr. Ran-b.). Paralytic weakness along the spine. Scraping bone pains at night (Saba.). Clammy, wrinkled skin. SLEEPINESS. Cold parts; one side of face, abdomen, etc. Burning along spine or below waist. Heat with sweat. **Profuse sweats;** < night. **Sluggish, painless fevers.**

Complementary: Chin. Related: Gel.

PHOSPHORUS.

REGION.

- **MUCOUS MEMBRANES**: **STOMACH.** BOWELS. **LUNGS** (Lower).
- **CIRCULATION**: HEART. BLOODVESSELS. Blood.
- **NERVES**: Brain. Cord.
- Bones: Jaw. Shin. Spine.
- Liver.

WORSE.

- **LYING**: **LEFT** or Painful **Side.** BACK.
- **SLIGHT CAUSES**: EMOTIONS. Talking. Odors. Light. Touch.
- **COLD**: HANDS (in Water). Open Air.
- **WARM INGESTA.**
- **Weather**: **Sudden Changes.** Windy. Cold. Thunderstorms.
- EVENING. **Mental Exertion.**

BETTER.

- **Eating.** **Sleep.** Cold: Food. Water.
- **Rubbing** (Magnetic). Sitting Up.

Active metabolism. Insidious onset ending in severe or **rapid disease** (Taren.), then paralytic debility. **Gracile, sensitive, nervous and delicate.** Weak spells; in joints. **Hemorrhage;** bloody discharges (Sul.).——Amative. **Anxious;** fear of being alone, twilight, ghosts, thunder (**Nat-c.**), etc. Excitable. Quickly prostrated by unpleasant impressions. **VERTIGO; with** levitation (Glo. Pho-ac. Sil. Stap.); as if sinking thro' bed (**Kali-c.**). Aching over one eye; with hunger (Bry. Psor.); < **lying on right side;**

> cold. Bald spots (Alu. Grap. Hep. Lyc. **Nat-m.**). Dandruff. **Flashes,** halos, red or black vision; > **twilight** (Con.). Deaf for human speech. **Nervous motion of alæ nasi.** Nose flows and stops. Pale about nose and mouth. Changing, sickly face; hollow eyed with blue rings. Numb teeth (Chin. Dulc. Plat. Rhus-t.). As of something hanging in throat (Alu. Lach. Plat. Saba. Val.). **CRAVES COLD DRINKS WHICH HELP, BUT ARE VOMITED WHEN WARM** (Pyro.), after chloroform. Waterbrash. RAVENOUS HUNGER; at night (Psor. Selen.). Regurgitation (Arg-n. Fer. Hyds.). Pressure above stomach (Nat-m.). EMPTY, GONE FEELING AT STOMACH; in bowels, as if hanging down (Ip. Pod.); < emotions (Calc-c. Dig. Kali-c. Lyc. Mez.). Stool contains grains like cooked sago. Involuntary diarrhœa; < coughing. Open anus. Slender, tough stools (Caus.). Pellicle on urine. Sexually erethistic, but weak. Prolonged menses. Leucorrhœa instead of menses. **Oppressed for breath.** Descending or relapsing colds, croup, hemorrhage, etc. Hard, dry, tight, tickling or hacking cough, with burning in air passages; < laughing, cold air. Rusty, salt or cold sputum. Pneumonia. Rough or raw in larynx. Hoarseness; painful; < evening. Violent palpitation. **Heavy or tight chest** (Sil.); stitches in left upper part. Mammary abscess. Cramp between scapulæ (Ip.) or pain from l. forward (Bar-c.). Spinal irritation; < **heat.** Tearing in shoulder (l), at night. Burning spot in lumbar region. Numb fingers (Calc-c. Lyc. Sec-c.) and toes (Sec-c.). Tottering; he stumbles easily. Periostitis (Asaf. Flu-ac. Merc. Mez. Pho-ac.); of tibia. Thin, foul pus. Pyæmia. Yellow spots; on abdomen. Jaundice, as a concomitant. Sleepless; from internal heat. Sleeps in short naps. Somnambulism. **CONGESTION; to lungs,** head, etc. Soft pulse. Coldness in cerebellum; **of knees, in bed** (Carb-v. Sep.). Burning heats; up back (Lyc. Sil.); face and hands, with anxiety. Sticky sweat. Painless fevers.

Complementary: Ars. Nux-v. Sang. Sep. Related: Caus. Con.

PHYSOSTIGMA.

REGION.	WORSE.
Spinal Motor Nerves. **Eyes.**	**Eyestrain.** Cold. Injury.

Weak; muscles fail to act. **Averse to bathing.** HORROR OF COLD WATER.——Active mind, even during sleep. **Twitching eye muscles.** Can't bear to raise eyelids. Affections of accommodation. Seems to have swallowed a lump. Torpid bowels. Numb womb. Heart seems to flutter in throat. **Sensitive spine.** Jerking limbs.

Related: Agar. Gel.

PHYTOLACCA.

REGION.	WORSE.
GLANDS { MAMMÆ. Tip of Tongue. **Tonsils. Throat.**	Heat { **Drinks.** Electric Changes. Bed.
Fibrous Tissues { NECK. **Back.** **Joints.**	**Swallowing. Raising Up. Motion.**
Right Side. **Bones.**	Cold { Damp. **Night.** Getting Wet.

Sore aching all over; < eyeballs, neck, back and limbs (Taren.). Restless. Hard glands.——**Faint on rising up.** Brain seems sore. **Frontal headache.** Jaws ache, as in mumps. Hot tears. Acrid coryza. Sickly, yellowish face. Everted lips. Grits the teeth. Yellow base of tongue; fiery red tip; it feels burnt or **pains** at root and **into ear on swallowing** (Kali-bi.). Increased, stringy saliva. Dark, rough (Arg-n.), raw, puffy throat. As of wash leather on tonsil. **Burning, like a hot ball in throat.** Very painful tonsilitis (Lach.). Diphtheria. Quinsy. Violent retching and vomiting; he would rather die. Continuous urging to stool; even during sleep. Dysentry. Dark red urine; chalky sediment. Sore spermatic cords (Ox-ac.). Menstruation with flow of saliva and tears. STONY HARD, HEAVY (Clem. Iod.), OR TENDER MAMMÆ; hard nodes in them (Carb-a.). Pains from nipple over whole body as child nurses. Cracked, sore nipples. Mastitis. Pain from heart toward the right. **Stiff neck.** Aching heels, > elevating them. Bone pains; in tibiæ. Syphilis.

Complementary: Bry. Related: Bry. Kali-bi. Merc. Rhus-t.

PICRIC ACID.

REGION.

Nerves { **Brain.** Occiput. Cord. **Lumbar Region.**

Sexual Organs.

WORSE.

Exertion; Mental or Physical.
Seminal Losses.

BETTER.

Rest. Cold. **Bandaging.**

TIRED AND HEAVY, in mind and body. Easily prostrated. Numb. Formication.——**Heavy occiput;** down spine (Pho.); **lower limbs.** Brain fag. Neurasthenia. Oily, burning stools (Asclep.). Priapism. Burning along spine. Aching legs (Helo.). Small, painful boils, < **nape** (Sul.).

Related: Gel. Ox-ac. Pho. Pho-ac.

PLANTAGO.

REGION.

Nerves { **Ears. Teeth.**

Kidneys and Bladder.

WORSE.

Night. Warm Room.

BETTER.

Sleep. Eating.

Sharp, shifting pains. Soreness. Neuralgia. As of a body between ears; in groins, etc.——As if brain turned over. As of a hair before (1) eye. **Pains center in ears and teeth** or alternate between them. Earache. **Saliva flows with the pains.** Toothache. **Dirty taste.** Bowels seem cold. Brown, frothy stools. **Polyuria.** Enuresis. Throbbing between scapulæ. Cold sweat on sacrum. Numb, tremulous legs. Sensitive skin. Gloomy dreams, exciting tears.

Related: Arn. Fer-p. Pul.

PLATINUM.

REGION.

FEMALE ORGANS.

Nerves { **Sensory.** Trifacial.

WORSE.

EMOTIONS { **Chagrin. Sexual.** TOUCH.

BETTER.

Sunshine. Walking in Cool Air.

Violent squeezing, cramping or numbing pains (Verb.), **irregular spasm;** or coldness in single parts, eyes, ears, muscles, etc. Tremor. Neuralgia. **Parts seem bandaged. Alternate mental and physical** (genital) **effects** (Arn. Cimi. Ign. Lil-t.). Hysteria.——**Disordered sense of proportion**

(Cann.); **objects look small** (Med. Stram. Thu.), strange, frightful, etc. HAUTEUR. **Arrogance.** Mental symptoms < in twilight (Pho.). **Clavus.** Scalp numb and tight. Sticky tears. Boring in jaws. **Hard, scant or soft, sticky, difficult stools;** of tourists. Dysmenorrhœa, with shrieks and jerks. Dark, thick, profuse menses, with dragging pain. **Painfully sensitive genitals** (Coff. Stap. Tarn. Zin.)——vulva; with crawling. Itching in uterus. Heat in ovaries. Ovarian irritation. Vaginismus. **Eroticism.** Onanism. Spasmodic yawning. Bruised backache, < pressure and bending backward. Knees drawn up and spread apart (Lyc.).

Related: Cup. Ign. Plb. Stan.

PLUMBUM.

REGION.

NERVES AND MUSCLES { **ABDOMEN.** Cord. Kidneys. }
Blood.

WORSE.

Exertion. Motion. Company.
Grasping Smooth Objects.

BETTER.

Rubbing. **Hard Pressure.**

Slow, insidious processes. Parts feel retracted. Cramps. Paralyses. Wasting of single (upper) parts, limbs (Calc-c.), etc. Sclerosis.——Timid, restless and anxious; fears assassins. Physical labor exhausts the mind. Melancholy. Delirium; nocturnal; alternating with colic or pains in limbs. Yellow sclerotic and inside of mouth. Trembling tongue. Sticky saliva. Sweet taste. Aphthæ. Dysphagia. **THE NAVEL SEEMS DRAWN TOWARD SPINE** (Pul. Stan. Ver-a. Zin.). **Colic;** accompanies many symptoms. Radiating abdominal pains; **boring** or as if forced through a narrow place (Bar-c.). Tense abdomen. Hernia at navel. **Anus feels drawn up or painfully contracted. Stools of hard, black balls, like sheep dung.** Constipation. Retracted testes. Bluish red spots. **Dry, sensitive skin** (Nat-m.). Dry, burning ulcers. Takes odd positions during sleep.

Complementary: Rhus-t. Related: Op.

PODOPHYLLUM.

REGION.
Liver { **Duodenum.** RECTUM.
Right Side { Ovary. Scapula. Throat.

WORSE
EARLY MORNING. **Eating.**
HOT WEATHER. **Dentition.**
Drinking. Motion. Mercury.
BETTER.
Stroking Liver.
Lying on Abdomen.

Biliousness.——Rolls head. Eyes half open. **Bad** breath. Burning, rough or flabby, indented tongue. **Bites gums together** (Lyc. Nux-v.); grinds teeth. Bitter taste. As of a lump in œsophagus (Chel.). **Painful liver. Weak, empty sinking or sick feeling in abdomen. GURGLING THRO BOWELS, THEN SUDDEN PROFUSE, PUTRID STOOLS, GUSH OUT PAINLESSLY** (Nat-p. Pho. Sec-c. Thu.). **White stools; like dirty water; with meal-like sediment** (Stro.); run right thro diaper (Benz-ac.); **then weakness.** Cholera morbus. Diarrhœa alternating with other symptoms. **Pale, hard stools.** Weak rectum; PROLAPSUS RECTI; before stool. Numb ache in ovaries; radiating to distant parts; $<$ stretching legs. Genitals threaten to prolapse during stool. Jaundice. Moaning and whining in sleep.

Complementary: Nat-m. Related: Alo. Merc.

POLYGONUM.

REGION.
Genito Urinary Organs.
Intestines.

WORSE.
Cold.
Dampness.

Pulsative pain; in prostate, wandering about, etc. Smarting discharges. ——Tongue seems swelled. Nausea in abdomen. **Griping, grinding belly-ache;** with diarrhœa, or kidney symptoms (Sars.). Itching pimples within anus. Hips feel drawn together. Aching of lower limbs (Solan.).

Related: Colo.

PRUNUS SPINOSA.

REGION.

- **Nerves**
  - **RESPIRATORY.**
  - Orbital.
- Bladder.

WORSE.

- Stooping.
- Ascending.

Pains cause shortness of breath or shoot outward. Crampings. Lightning like pains. Neuralgia. Nerve paralysis.——Pain from **forehead (r)** to occiput (Caus. Sep.). **Bursting in eyeball** (Sul.). **Teeth feel pulled out** (Calc-c.). **Cramp in bladder; he doubles up to urinate (Canth.) (reverse** Alu.). Strangury. **Dropsy; of feet.** Air hunger. **As of a lump below left** scapula. Heart disease.

Related: **Laur.**

PSORINUM.

REGION.

- **SKIN**
  - FOLDS OF.
  - **Sebacious Glands.**
- EARS.
- BOWELS.
- **Respiration.**
- Right Side.

WORSE.

- COLD
  - **Open Air.** Winter.
  - **Washing.**
- **Weather;** Stormy; Changing.
- **Heat**
  - Of Bed. Exertion.
  - Woolens.
- SUPPRESSIONS. **Yearly.**
- Contact of His Own Limbs.

BETTER.

- **Lying With Head Low;** Quietly.
- **Nosebleed.** Hard Pressure.

FOUL DISCHARGES; **bad odor of body** (Bapt. Nit-ac. Sil. Thu.). **Weak and tender;** easily chilled; takes cold; quickly exhausted; clothing seems large or he feels pushed down (Lyc.). Joints seem loose. **Hungry or** unusually well before an attack (Bry. Nux-v. Pho.), but **reacts badly and chronicity threatens.**——ANXIETY. Forebodings. DESPAIR; of recovery (Ars. Calc-c.). Horrid thoughts. Averse to work. Headache alternating with other troubles. Dull, dry hair. **Sensitive to drafts about head;** wants it covered (Sil.). Gummy, everted eyelids. Humid sores behind ears (Lyc.). PUTRID OTORRHŒA (Ars. Carb-v. Hep. Kali-p. Merc. **Sul.** Tell. Tub.). Hay fever. Pale, sickly, dirty or fuzzy face. Loose teeth. Tip of tongue feels burnt (Ign.). Hawks out foul, cheesy masses (Mag-c.). **Filthy taste.** Anorexia, with great thirst. Flatus like bad eggs. DARK, GUSHING, HORRIBLY PUTRID STOOLS (Stram.), < night. Cholera infantum. Bed wetting at full moon. Offensive genitals (Sars. **Thu.**).

Chronic gonorrhœa (Alu. Sep. Sul.). **Breathes > lying down or spreading arms apart** (Nux-v.). **Gurgling at heart. Panaris. Hot, itching soles. Skin breaks out; < flexures; is rough or scabby** (Bov.). **Condylomata on edges of skin. Intolerable itching; < heat (of bed); he scratches it raw or until it bleeds** (Lyc.). **Heat with steaming sweat. Profuse, easy sweating; < night; on palms; cold.**

Complementary: Sep. Sul. Tub. Related: Mang. Sul.

PULSATILLA.

REGION.

MIND.

VEINS.

MUCOUS MEMBRANES { TONGUE. **STOMACH.** BOWELS. **FEMALE. ORGANS. Eyes.**

One Side.

Right Heart.

WORSE.

WARMTH { **AIR. ROOM. BED. Clothes.**

Getting Feet Wet.

EVENING. REST.

BEGINNING MOTION.

LYING; **one Side.** (LEFT. **Painful**).

EATING { **RICH. FOOD. FATS.** Ices.

PUBERTY. PREGNANCY.

Before Menses. Iron and Quinine.

BETTER.

COLD; FRESH AIR; Applications. ERECT POSTURE.

Gentle Motion. After a Good Cry.

CHANGEFUL, SHIFTING SYMPTOMS; THIRSTLESS, SHORT OF BREATH AND CHILLY; WITH DIGESTIVE OR MENSTRUAL DISORDERS. SUPPRESSIONS; **of menses,** lochia, milk, etc. **Metastases.** Unilateral symptoms (Bell. Cocel. Rhus-t.). PROFUSE. THICK, BLAND, YELLOW-GREEN DISCHARGES. **Jerking or ulcerative pain. Numbness.**——MILD, PLEASANT, TIMID OR TENDER. EMOTIONAL; **sad; easily discouraged** (Stan.); **weeps easily.** Whining. **Craves sympathy.** Vertigo. **Eyes itch, fill with tears (acrid) or seem covered; < in wind. Cold attack eyes. Blind attacks; during menses** (Cyc. Grap. Sep.). **Sticky eyelids. Ophthalmia; infantile** (Arg-n. Cham. Kali-s. Nat-s. Thu.). **Blepharitis.** Styes (Stap. Thu.). **Nightly earache. Otitis. Pale face. Chlorosis. Bad odor** (Sul.) **or foul discharge from nose. Licks the lips;** (Ars. Lyc. Nat-c. Stram.). **Crack in center of lower lip** (Cham. Chin. Hep. Nat-m.). **FOUL BREATH. Drawing toothache > cold** (Coff.). **TASTE**

BAD; IN A. M., altered, bloody. Slimy mucus on tongue. Food leaves an after taste or lodges in throat (Chin. Lact-ac. Nat-m.). **Averse to fats** (Petr.). Craves what disagrees. Heartburn. Nausea. HEAVY OR DERANGED STOMACH. As of a heavy stone in bowels (Cup. Op. Nux-v. Rhus-t. Spig. Sul.). Indigestion. Pains radiate into groins. Two or three stools a day. Green mucous or bilious stools (Cham. Merc. Ver-a.); < night. Piles or urging to urinate, < lying (Kre. Lach.). Heavy pressure on bladder. **Nocturnal enuresis. Enlarged prostate** (Dig. Thu.). Feels like menstruating (Carb-a. Lil-t. Mos. Pho. Vib.). DARK, SCANTY, LATE, IRREGULAR OR ABSENT MENSES. Dysmenorrhœa. Weak labor pains. Retained placenta. **CRAVES FRESH AIR** (Fer.). Loose morning, then dry evening cough; from tickling at epigastrium (Kali-bi. Nit-ac.); 'it **pains the occiput;** must sit up (Hyos.). As of a weight on chest (Spig.). Soreness or stitches beneath clavicles. Palpitation. Milk in virgin breasts (Cycl. Merc.). Swelling of joints; of backs of feet. Numb elbows. Measles. **Veins full;** painful; varicose. Sleeps with hands over head; **awakes confused** (Aesc. Bov. Chin. Petr.) or tired. **CHILLY, YET AVERSE TO HEAT;** IN A WARM ROOM; **with the pain.** One hand cold (Chin. Dig. Lyc. Rhus-t. Sul.). **Partial sweats.**

Complementary: **Ars.** Lyc. **Sil.** Related: Ap. Cimi. Grap. Ham. Nat-s.

PYROGEN.

REGION.

BLOOD. Heart.
Circulation.
Muscles.

BETTER.

Motion { Change of Position. Rocking.
Heat. Pressure.

Aching, bruised, sore and prostrate; yet restless; bed seems hard. Bone pains. **Foul** taste, secretions, odor of body, etc. Sepsis.——Loquacious. Excited. Sense of duality. Violent throbbing headache. Fiery red, smooth tongue. Sweet taste. Adhesive urinary sediment. Feels the heart; as if tired (Rhus-t.), big and full. PULSE QUICK OUT OF ALL PROPORTION TO THE TEMPERATURE. Quickly oscillating temperature. Toe nails threaten to fly off. Chills start between scapulæ; **felt in bones** (Eupat.); at night. Fever at menstrual period (Rhod.). Puerperal sepsis. Slowly advancing hectic.

Related: Bap.

RADIUM.

REGION.

Skin. Nerves.
Muscles and Joints { Lumbo Sacral. Great Toe.
Shifting Sides.

WORSE.

Motion. Shaving. Washing.

BETTER.

Open Air. Hot Bath. Eating.
Cool Drinks. Continued Motion.

Dry, burning heat as if afire; **craves cool air. Sudden shifting** or electric pains. **Dull, hard ache; deep in joints** (Cimi.). Rheumatism. Gout. Arthritis deformans. Weak muscles.——Pain over eyes (l), backward. Red, smarting eyes, < reading. Rushing in ears > lying on face. Raw throat. Craves pork. Averse to sweets. Abdominal, alternating with ear or chest pains. Sore, prolapsed rectum. Dysuria, then erections. **Itching genitals.** Cough, < smoking. Tightness at heart. Weak between scapulæ. Ascending **lumbar pain. Irritable, thick, burning, itching skin;** moist if scratched; < face and genitals. Branny scales. Scabby; on ears. Eczema. **Psoriasis.** Naevi. Callosities. Vivid dreams; of fire; awakes, panting, with pounding of heart; seeming true.

Related: Pul. Rhus-rad.

RANUNCULUS BULBOSUS.

REGION.

NERVES. **Muscles.**
Serous Membranes.
THORAX. SKIN.
Left Side.

WORSE.

Evening. Alcohol. Touch.
AIR; **Drafts; Open; Cold; Damp.**
Changing Temperature.
Motion of Arms. Breathing.

STITCHING, SHOOTING PAIN. **Pains extort tears.** Burning, biting, **bruised soreness or as of deep ulceration. Sore spots.** Neuralgia. Trembling. Distended feeling.——Quarrelsome. Smarting in eyes. Crawling on palate, wants to scratch it (Ars. Carb-v. Pho. Sil.). Increased saliva. Scraping-burning down throat. Bruised hypochondria (Bry. Carb-v. **Chin.**). Tender abdomen. Pinching colic, alternating with chest pains. Anxious, oppressed breathing. STITCHES IN CHEST. Pleurodynia. Pleurisy. Chest is sensitive to air. Pain along inner edge of scapulæ. **BLUISH VESICLES.** Shingles. Pemphigus. Corrosive ichor. Horny scabs. Vesicles or herpes on palms.

Related: Rhus-t.

RANUNCULUS SCELERATUS.

REGION.
CHEST. SKIN.
Vertex.
Right Side.

WORSE.
Evening. Motion. Deep Breathing.
BETTER.
After Midnight.

Acridity, rawness or **burning-smarting. Eating, gnawing or boring pains;** causing faintness or short breath.——Sneezing coryza, with burning urine. Mapped tongue. **Stitches in chest muscles;** it is sensitive externally. As of a **plug forced between ribs** (Anac. Aur. Caus. Cocel. Lyc.), under navel, etc. Gout of small joints. **Yellow vesicles. Bullæ;** with acrid contents.

Related: Ars.

RATANHIA.

REGION.
Rectum. Anus.
Nipples.
Teeth.

WORSE.
Anxiety. Heat. Exertion. Touch.
BETTER.
Cool Bathing. Walking in open Air.

Sense of constriction. Fissure.——Bursting headache when straining at stool (Cob.). Nightly toothache, < lying, must walk about. Violent painful hiccough. **Constriction or as of sharp splinters** (of glass) **in rectum** (Sanic. Thu.); stool is forced out with great straining and followed by long aching-burning. Itching at anus. Ascarides. Fissure ani. Cracked nipples.

Related: Nit-ac. Pæon.

RHEUM.

REGION.

Muscles of { **Bile Ducts.** Duodenum. **Intestines.** }

Liver.

WORSE.

Dentition. Eating. Summer.

Nursing Women.

BETTER.

Warmth. **Wrapping Up.**

Sour, impatient, colicky children who scream and cry for everything.—— **Difficult teething.** Repugnance after the first bite. Colic with cries, then **sour, brown, fermented, slimy or acrid stools;** < evening, motion and eating; with shivering. **Burning in** bladder. Restless sleep with whining, cries and twitches of face and fingers. **Sweat on scalp** or about nose and mouth.

Complementary: Mag-c. Related: Cham.

RHODODENDRON.

REGION.

NERVES.

FIBROUS TISSUES.

Small Joints.

Mind.

Single Parts.

WORSE.

WEATHER { APPROACH OF STORMY. **Windy.** Cold. Damp. **Rough.** }

Rest. Night.

BETTER.

Continued Motion.

Heat; Wrapping Head; Dry.

Rapidly changing, descending, **tearing** or boring pains. Neuralgia. **Gouty-rheumatic subjects. SENSITIVE TO STORMS AND CHANGES OF WEATHER.**——Giddy and stupid; forgets his subject (Bar-c. Merc.). Tearing, jerking faceache or toothache; > food or warmth. Cool drinks lie heavy. Colic at navel. Pain from rectum to genitals. Diarrhœa. Profuse, foul urine. Testes and glans feel crushed. Hard testes. Itching, sweaty, wrinkled scrotum. Hydrocele (of boys). Menses with fever. As of a weight hanging to feet. Wants to cross legs. Drawing tearing in periosteum of long bones and under scalp. Rheumatism of hot weather (Reverse Rhus-t.). Sweat with formication.

Related: Rhus-t.

RHUS TOX.

REGION.

SKIN { **Face.** Scalp. **Genitals.**

Cellular Tissues.

BLOOD.

MUCOUS MEMBRANES.

GLANDS { PYERS. Parotid.

NERVES { CORD. SCIATIC.

Fibrous Tissues { Ligaments. Joints. Tendons. Spine.

Left Side or Left then Right.

WORSE.

EXPOSURE TO COLD { **WATER.** Drafts. **WASHING. Air. DAMPNESS.** CHILLED WHEN HOT OR SWEATING. **Uncovering; hands.**

BEGINNING MOTION.

AFTER MIDNIGHT. REST.

OVEREXERTION.

BETTER.

CHANGE OF POSITION.

CONTINUED MOTION.

HEAT { Hot Bathing. Warm Wraps. Becoming Heated.

Rubbing. Holding Abdomen.

An infective irritant causing **RHEUMATIC, TYPHOID OR PARETIC EFFECTS. Burning, swelling and lividity,** Cellulitis. Crawling. Numbness. Trembling. **Sore, bruised or stiff** (Ap. Nux-v.). **Torn loose feeling** (Calc-c. Plb. Stan.). **TEARING PAINS; CAN'T REST IN ANY POSITION.** Grippe. Variola. **Acrid, rusty-red, meat-water or musty secretions;** causing eruptions.——**Sad,** abstracted, confused, **depressed or beclouded.** Slow replies. Whirling vertigo; then headache. **Pressure (board-like) on forehead or shattering in head** (Calc-c.); < jar. **Painful,** stiff scalp > lying on it. **Pain behind eyes** (Chel. Cimi. Pod.); < motion. **Photophobia.** Adherent, **stiff** (Ap. Nat-m.), dry (Ver-a.) or firmly closed **eyelids.** Saccular conjunctiva. **Profuse, hot, gushing tears.** Red, sensitive tip of nose; it drips water (Ars. Sul.). Nosebleed; at night. Jaw cracks (Lac-c. Nit-ac.) or is easily dislocated. Faceache. Red spot on left cheek (Nat-m.). **Swelled, stiff face.** Acne rosaceæ (Kali-i.). Dry, cracked, crusty lips. **Sordes** (Hyo. Stram.). Teeth feel loose. Toothache. **RED TRIANGLE AT TIP OF TONGUE.** Diagonal coat on tongue. Dry, red (center) or cracked tongue. Bloody saliva flows during sleep. **Coppery or straw-like taste.** Red, puffy, itching fauces (Phyt.). Sore throat (1) in A. M. (Cimi.): with **swelled glands. Craves cold drinks (Ars.);** altho they < chill, cough, etc. Vomits from coughing, lying on back, etc.

As of a heavy lump in abdomen. Gelatinous, bloody, slimy or watery stools; involuntary or with tenesmus. Itching genitals. Œdema of prepuce (Flu-ac.). Nephritis. Metritis. Dry, hoarse, tormenting, tearing cough, from tickling behind upper sternum (Merc. Pho-ac. Rum.); with a bloody taste. Palpitation; when still. Heart feels tired (Pyro.); hypertrophy. Stiff neck. **Interscapular pain;** < swallowing (Kali-c.). Contractive or breaking backache; > hard pressure, lying on it or bending back (Sabi.). Rhagades on back of hands. **Pain down back of thigh;** < during stool. Sciatica. Itching below knees (Nat-s.). SKIN STIFF, THICK; dry, hot, itching < warmth; **painful to cold air.** FINE VESICULAR, ECZEMATOUS OR ERYSIPELATOUS ERUPTIONS; < **genitals** (Petr.). Shingles. Milk crust (Dulc. Sep.). Bakers itch. Weeping ulcers (Nat-s.). **LABORIOUS DREAMS;** awakes tired. Weak, rapid, sharp, tremulous or irregular pulse. EASILY CHILLED, < LEAST UNCOVERING OR MOTION; **with pains in limbs,** < of cough, etc. Chill, as if dashed with cold water; preceded by cough (Ap. Eupat.); alternating with heat; in single parts. Heat with busy delirium. Sweat < during pain.

Complementary: Calc-c. Calc-flu. Phyt. Related: Arn. Bry. Dulc.

ROBINIA.

REGION.
Secretions. Stomach.

WORSE.
Eating. Night. Fats.

Acidity; sour stomach; acid belching; **vomitus so sour it sets the teeth on edge** (Iris. Lyc. Sul-ac.). **Burning** in stomach and between scapulæ. **Squeezing** in stomach. Sick headache.

Related: Iris. Mag-c.

RUMEX.

REGION.	WORSE.
Mucous Membranes { **Larynx.** TRACHEA. Bowels.	COOL AIR { INHALING. **Open.** **Raw Changes.**
Nerves. Skin.	Uncovering. **Night.**
Left Side.	BETTER.
	Covering Mouth. **Wrapping Up.**

Dry, sensitive mucous membranes. Every cold affects joints (Calc-p.). Sharp pains; neuralgias.——**Dry posterior nares** (Sep.). **Hawks out much** tenacious mucus. **Sudden profuse, foul, early morning diarrhœa (5-9 A. M.);** after catarrh; in phthisis. EVERY BREATH OF AIR CAUSES TICKLING IN THROAT-PIT (Sep.) AND COUGH; > covering mouth (Ip. Kali-bi.). **Profuse, frothy expectoration. Suffocative feeling. Pain,** rawness or **burning under clavicle** (1), **as if the air penetrated there** (Chlor.). **Pain under left nipple** (Nat-s.). **Heart seems impeded then** heavy **pulsations thro chest.** Skin **itches** when **exposed to air.**
Complementary: Calc-c. Related: Seneg.

RUTA.

REGION.	WORSE.
Fibrous Tissues { EYES. **Flexor Tendons.** **Joints. Wrists.** Ankles. Back (Lumbar).	**Overexertion** { EYESTRAIN. Injury. Sprains.
Cartilages. Periosteum. Uterus.	COLD { **Air.** Wind. **Damp.** Wet.
Skin.	LYING. **Pressure on an Edge.**
	BETTER.
	Motion. Warmth.

BRUISED, ACHING AND RESTLESS. **Painful weariness. As of a rough, blunt plug in part;** head, nose (Kali-bi. Nat-c. Psor.), etc. Nodes. **Paralytic rigidity.** Rheumatism. **Gnawing-burning.** Neuralgia.——Itching inner canthi. Eyes burn. Lachrymation. **Dim vision.** Woody taste. Urging to stool, but only **rectum prolapses;** < after labor, stooping, etc. Corrosive leucorrhœa. Weak, bruised feeling in small of back, hips or lower limbs in A. M. Stumbles easily (Con. Nat-c. Plat.). Lumbago. **Thighs feel broken.** Nodes in palms (Caus.). Bursæ (Sil. Stict. Sul.). Erosive itching. **Chafing.** Flat warts. Glowing heat of face, skin, etc.
Complementary: Calc-p. Related: Phyt. Ran-sc. Symp.

SABADILLA.

REGION.

MUCOUS MEMBRANES { **NOSE.** ANUS. Digestive Tract.

NERVES.

Lachrymal Glands.

Throat.

WORSE.

COLD; Air; Drinks.

PERIODICALLY { **Same Hour.** Forenoon. **New and Full Moon.**

Odors. Undeveloped Exanthems.

BETTER.

Heat. Eating. Swallowing.

Weak, nervous; easily startled. Miserable. Twitches. **Trembling.** Worms. Alternate nerve and bodily symptoms.——**Erroneous (fixed) ideas about himself.** Anger. **Pain alternates sides in forehead. Unilateral** headache. Itching scalp. **Lachrymation;** with the pains (Chel. Nat-m. Ran-b.); < open air. Red, itching tarsi. **Sensitive smell.** VIOLENT SNEEZING. Influenza. Hay fever. Itching of soft palate. Sore **throat,** first (l) then (r), < empty swallowing, > hot drinks. As of a lump, thread or skin (Pho.) in throat. Canine hunger. No thirst or **craves hot** or **sweet things or milk** (Rhus-t. Stap.). Bowels feel twisted into a knot. Brown, frothy, floating stools. **Crawling, itching at anus; alternating** with tickling in nose or ears. Pinworms (Sinap.). Violent coughing attacks. Upward jerking of arms. Cracks under toes. **Shivers; attend** the other symptoms. Thirst after the chill only.

Related: Pul.

SABAL.

REGION.

Genito-Urinary Organs { **Prostate. Ovaries.** Mammæ. **Bladder.** Urethra.

WORSE.

Women and Old Men.

Weather; Cold Damp; Cloudy.

Sympathy.

Sharp, stinging pains. Debility.——Voices seem distant. **Irritable bladder** (Buchu.) and urethra. Strangury. Enuresis. **Limy urinary sediment.** Testes drawn up. **Enlarged prostate.** Painful emission of semen. **Ovarian** pains. Vulva feels open (Bap.). Absent sexual passion. **Mammæ sore,** tender and full, < cold bath. Backache from coition.

Related: Sep.

SABINA.

REGION.		WORSE.	
PELVIC ORGANS	UTERUS. Rectum. **Nerves.**	HEAT	**Of Room.** Exercise. **Of Bed.**
		Foggy Weather. Pregnancy.	
Serous and **Fibrous Tissues**	**Small Joints.** Heels.	BETTER.	
		Cold. Cool, **Open Air.**	

Gouty, rheumatic females. Violent pulsations. Fulness. Red, shiny swelling (Mang.). HEMORRHAGE (Erig.).——Music is unbearable. Craves lemonade. Quivering, as if alive, in abdomen. Piles alternate with pains in limbs. **Itching, excited genitals.** PAIN FROM LUMBAR REGION TO PUBES (Pho. Vib.) or reverse **or shooting up vagina** (Rhus-t. Sep.). GUSHES OF FLUID, HOT OR WATERY BLOOD MIXED WITH CLOTS (dark) FROM UTERUS; < motion (Sec-c.); with joint pains. Abortion at third month (Bell. Sec-c. Sep. Thu.). Bleeding between periods. Foul, acrid leucorrhœa. Crawling in nipple. Gout of right big toe. Hot, moist figwarts. Intolerable, burning heat.

Complementary: Thu. Related: Caul. Puls.

SAMBUCUS.

REGION.	WORSE.
Respiratory Organs.	Head Low.
Kidneys.	Cold Drinks While Heated.
Skin.	Pressure over a Sharp Edge.
	BETTER.
	Motion. Wrapping Up.

Tendency to sweat; with short breath; with many symptoms. Nephritis. Dropsy.——Fretful. Half open eyes. Sniffles. Bluish, puffy face. SUDDEN SUFFOCATION or **strangling cough, awaking him after midnight** (Aral-r. Lach.). Respiratory spasm. Laryngismus stridulus. Croup. **Dry, burning heat while asleep, but copious sweat on awaking;** < coughing.

Related: Bell. Brom.

SANGUINARIA.

REGION.

Vaso-Motors Circulation { HEAD. LIVER. **Chest.**

Mucous Membranes.
Deltoids.
RIGHT SIDE.

WORSE.

Periodically { WITH THE SUN. **Weekly.** Night.

Climaxis. Odors. Raising Arms.
Looking Up. **Jar.** Light.

BETTER.

SLEEP. **Vomiting.** Cool Air.
Passing Flatus.

Burning sensations, upward congestion, migraine and colds. Internal rawness. **Checked catarrh, then diarrhœa.** Offensive, acrid discharges. **Lies on back, with head elevated** (Gel.).——PAIN ASCENDS FROM OCCIPUT AND SETTLES OVER EYE (r) > free urination. Swollen temporal veins (Ars.). Sun pain. Pain at root of nose. Sensitive to odors. Red, burning cheeks. **Hectic flush** (spot) (Pho.). Full and tender behind angle of jaw. Palate feels scalded (Sanic.). Craves spices. Nausea, > eating. Coughs, belches foul air (Lach.) and passes flatus. Burning under sternum. Expectoration; tough and bloody (Cob.); purulent or a plug. Pneumonia (Typhoid). Phthisis. **Weak heart;** feeble, intermittent pulse. Omodynia < night (Fer.). Dry skin. Jaundice. Polypi. **Flushes of heat rising into face and head** (Kali-bi.) HOT PALMS AND SOLES.

Complementary: Ant-t. Pho. Related: Sul.

SANICULA AQUA.

REGION.

NUTRITION.
Female Organs.
Rectum. Skin.

WORSE.

Motion { Downward. **Of Hands Behind Him.**

Cold Wind on Occiput or Neck.

Thin and old looking. Dirty brownish skin, < neck. Thick, yellow, acrid pus.——Stubborn and touchy. Can't bear cold air on occiput and neck (Pso. Sil.). Craves bacon (Calc-c. Mez.) or ice cold milk. Stool of large, heavy masses; impacted (Calc-c. Sele. Sep. Sil.). Briny urine or leucorrhœa; < during stool. **Pain in back, < putting hands behind him** or raising arms. Coldness in lumbar region. Lumbago. Cold, clammy hands and feet. Cramps in feet. Burning soles. Profuse sweat on occiput and neck (Calc-c.). Foul foot-sweat, chafing toes, stiffening hose or destroying the shoes.

Related: Psor. Sul.

SARSAPARILLA.

REGION.
Genito-Urinary Organs.
Skin.
Right Side.

WORSE.
At Close of Micturation. Spring.
Cold Wet. Mercury. Night.
Suppressed Gonorrhœa.
BETTER.
Standing.

Thin, frail, shrivelled and old looking. Marasmus. Tendency to gravel and eruptions. Nightly bone pains. Very sore, gouty nodes.——Pain depresses him. Pain from occiput to root of nose, which is swelled. **Painful urination extorts screams,** > standing; passes drops of blood or white acrid material at its close. Urine dribbles while sitting. Renal colic (r) (Parei.). Gassy urine. **Crusty urinary sediment** (flaky Mez.). Sand in the stools (Lyc.). Moist, foul genitals. Bloody semen. Retracted nipples (Sil.). Deep cracks on fingers and toes, < sides. Ulcerated finger-tips. **Blotchy,** hard or shrivelled skin < about neck. Itching, scaly spots. Irritating pus. Chill from bladder to back.
Complementary: Sep. Related: Calc-c. Petr.

SCOPARIUS.

REGION.
Heart. Kidneys.
Cord.
Muscles.
Left Side.

WORSE.
Turning on Left Side.
BETTER.
Cool Air. Rapid Motion.
Passing Flatus.

Heavy ache; stomach and bowels seem filled with stones (Ant-t. Calc-c. Nux-m.) or a firm mass. **Flatulency.** Colic, then bright, acrid, foamy stools followed by burning at anus (Colo.). **Very profuse,** bright, foaming urine, then burning pudendum. **Intercurrent congestion of kidneys** (Solid.). Anxious oppression at heart radiating to left shoulder and neck. Palpitation, with congestion to head. Deadness of right arm and fingers.
Related: **Pho.**

SECALE.

REGION.

Muscles { **BLOODVESSELS.** **UTERUS.**

BLOOD.

Nerves.

Cord.

WORSE.

WARMTH. During Menses.

Pregnancy. Loss of Fluids.

BETTER.

Cold. Uncovering.

Forcible Extension.

Dusky, scrawny and **hemorrhagic.** **Dark, thin, foul or exhausting discharges.** Decomposition. Fetor. Petechiæ. Varicoses. **Burnings.** Numbness or insufferable **tingling formication** (Coca.); starting in back; in fingertips (Rhus-t.); after the pains. **Twitching or cramps;** in single parts; starting in face or spine (Nux-v.).——Mania, with fear. Sparks before eyes. Distorted or sunken countenance; blue rings about eyes. **Thirst;** craves acids. Empty retching. Gushing, painless, watery, olive-green or bloody stool, with collapse. Everything seems loose and open (Bov.). Inertia of uterus or **bearing down with coldness** (Castor. Sil.). Hour-glass contraction. Miscarriage. Green lochia (Lac-c.). Metritis. **Brown leucorrhœa.** Pains thro chest on pressing spine. **Fingers spread apart** (Lac-c. Lyc.) or bent backward; look water soaked. **Leg cramps.** Boils with green pus (Syp. Tub.). Blood blisters. **Cold, dry, bluish skin,** < over affected part. EXTERNALLY ICY COLD, YET BURNING HOT INTERNALLY; OBJECTS TO BEING COVERED (Cam. Med.). Heat as of sparks on skin. Erysipelas. **Cold or foul sweat.**

Complementary: Ars. Cann. Related: Nux-m. Ust.

SELENIUM.

REGION.

Nerves { **GENITO-URINARY ORGANS.** Supra Orbital (1).

LARYNX.

Liver.

WORSE.

Debilitating Causes { **Hot Days.** Sexual Excesses. Loss of Sleep.

Singing. Drafts.

After Sleep. Tea.

BETTER.

After Sunset. Inhaling Cool Air.

Debility; senile. Emaciation of single parts.——Loquacity. **Sadness.** **Forgetful** when awake but dreams of it as he falls asleep. **Falling hair.** Don't want the hair touched. Craves stimulants. Rash over liver. **Abdominal pulsation;** hinders sleep. Very large stools. Coarse **sand in**

urine. **Lascivious but impotent. Easy loss of semen; at** stool, etc. Watery semen (Sul.). **Hoarseness;** of singers (Arg-n.). **Hawks up clear** mucus. Oily skin; itching in its folds or about ankles. Acne. Burning spots. **Sweat leaves a salty deposit.**

Related: Sul.

SENECIO.

REGION.	WORSE.
Mucous Membranes { **Female Organs.** / **Genito-** / Kidneys.	**Puberty.** Getting Wet. Open Air.

Profuse catarrhs. Hemorrhage.——Sharp pain over (l) eye to temple. **Sneezing.** Averse to sweets. **Nausea and backache; in renal affections** (Samb. Scop.). Globus. **Heat in neck of bladder, with pain in kidneys. Dysuria. Pain from ovaries into breasts. Amenorrhœa. Thick yellow** leucorrhœa; **after or instead of menses; flows down thighs. Lumbar backache** (Solid.). **Many vivid or erotic dreams. Feet cold in bed.**

Related: Pul.

SENEGA.

REGION.	WORSE.
MUCOUS MEMBRANES and Muscles { CHEST. / **Eyes.** / Bladder.	**Rest. Air** { **Inhaling Cold.** / Wind. Open.
	Looking Fixedly. Old Persons.
	BETTER.
	Motion. **Bending head back.**

Catarrhal, paretic states.——**Headaches go into eyes > cool air (Pul.).** Eyeballs feel distended (Sul.). **Diplopia > looking backward. Dry mouth and throat.** Coppery taste. **Shreddy urine. Hoarse, unsteady** voice. **Incessant strangling, choking cough, ends in sneezing, < lying on** right side. **Loose rattle in chest but expectoration is tough and slips back. Chest feels sore** (in spots), **as if bruised. As of a weight on or weakness starting from chest. Pleuro-pneumonia.**

Related: Caus. Hep.

SEPIA.

REGION.
VENOUS CIRCULATION.
Nerves.
Connective Tissue.
FEMALE PELVIC ORGANS.
Digestive Tract.
SKIN.
Liver.

WORSE.
COLD { AIR. North Wind. Snowy or Wet Weather.
SEXUAL EXCESSES.
PREGNANCY. Abortion.
Morning and Evening. **Rest.**
11 A. M. and 4 P. M.
BETTER.
VIOLENT MOTION. **Warmth.**

Sluggish, **relaxed** or lithemic. **Portal and uterine troubles. Symptoms alternate with uterine affections. Pains settle in back, shoot upward,** < in vagina, or cause shuddering. AS OF A LUMP **or a rolling over internally.** Hollow feeling. Wants to lie down. **Easy dislocation.** Milky discharges.——Anxious fear. Averse to company, yet dreads solitude. Sad and indifferent or frets and scolds. **Irritability alternating with indifference.** Antipathy to loved ones (Lyc.). **Poor memory.** Shocks thro head. Weight on vertex. Hemicrania. Jerks head back and forth. **Drooping eyelids.** Red, itching tarsi. Motes before vision. **Odors are repulsive.** Foul plugs in nose; thick green discharge. **YELLOW SADDLE ACROSS NOSE** (Carb-a. Sul.). Chloasma (Gaul.). Lower lip swells and cracks. Hawks much mucus in A. M. Morning nausea. Milky vomiting. FAINT SINKING AT EPIGASTRIUM (Ign. Kali-c.); **not** > **eating** (Carb-a.). Gnawing hunger. Pot belly (Calc-c. Colch. Pod.). Stools followed by gelatinous mucus. Oozing from anus. Diarrhœa from boiled milk. **As of a ball in anus** (Cann. Lach. Lil-t. Plat. Sul-ac). Cutting before micturition. Enuresis during first sleep (Benz-ac. Caus. Cina. Kre. Pho-ac.); when coughing, sneezing, etc. FOUL URINE; ADHERENT, RED SEDIMENT (Colo. Pul.). Menses absent at puberty, after weaning. etc. Sticking in os uteri. Subinvolution (Caul. Helo.). Tendency to abortion. **DRAGGING WEAKNESS OR BEARING DOWN FEELING; must sit close.** Abscess of labia (Hep.). Stinging, burning leucorrhœa; gonorrhœal (Sabi.). Stomach cough (Bry. Pho. Pho-ac.); with foul sputum. LUMBAR BACKACHE; **as if weak.** Weak knees. **Skin blotched,** raw, rough, hard or cracked, < flexures. Herpes. Ringworm (Ol-jec. Tub.). Itching vesicles. Boils in axillæ. Thick crust on elbows. Ulcers on small joints (Mez. Psor.). Epithelioma of eyelids, lips, etc. Loud talking in sleep. Dreams when lying on left side. **Ebullitions;** at night.

Full veins. Easily chilled. **Cold vertex; between scapulæ** (Ars.); **feet in bed** (Calc-c. Fer. Grap. Kali-c. Men. Nit-ac. Psor. Sil. Zin.). **Anxious hot** flushes. Warm hands with cold feet, or vice versa. Easy sweating. Irregular fevers.

Complementary: Pho. Related: Caus. Gel. Lil-t. Nat-m. Pul.

SILICA.

REGION.

NUTRITION. NERVES.
CELLULAR TISSUES.
GLANDS.
Tubular Tracts { Tear Ducts. Eustachian Tube, etc.
Bones.
Cartilage.
Skin.

CHILDREN.

WORSE.

COLD { **AIR.** DRAFTS. DAMP. **UNCOVERING. Bathing.**
Changing Temperature.
CHECKED SWEAT, < **OF FEET** (Merc.). Alcohol.
Nervous Excitement. Jarring.
Pressure on Spine.
Change of Moon. Night.

BETTER.

WARMTH { WRAPS; to Head. From Active Motion.
Profuse Urination.

Malnutrition; with keen senses. **Oversensitive to pain and cold.** Exaggerated reflexes. Constriction of sphincters. Spasms. Late in learning to walk. Arrested development. Slow processes that end in induration (Grap.), **suppuration,** fistulæ (Nit-ac. Petr.), abscess, etc. Hard cicatrices. Swollen diseased glands. Scrofulo-rachitic diathesis. Oedema in morning (Ap. Aur. Jus. Pho. Sep.). **Sticking pains.** Parts lain on go to sleep. Extrudes foreign bodies.——Fidgety. Lacks grit. Sullen and stubborn. **Ascending vertigo or headache; from occiput; to over (1) eye** (Lac-c. Par. Petr. Spig.); > pressure. Migraine. Throbbing in vertex (Lach. Sul.). Lumps in scalp. Inflamed eyes. Dark or spotted vision. Deafness; hears again with a snap. Waxy paleness. Enlarged parotids. Sticking in tonsil. Hawks down foul lumps (Mag-c. Psor.). **Averse to hot food.** Hard, hot abdomen. Pain from rectum to testes. **Receding stools** (Op. Sanic. Thu.); < at menses. Foul urethral discharge. Itching, moist spots on scrotum. Hydrocele. Nursing causes a flow from uterus. Biting, gushing leucorrhœa (Calc-c. Grap. Lyc.). Itching vulva. Retching, gagging cough < cold drinks. Profuse, foul, lumpy sputum. Sore, retracted nipples. Dry fingertips. Distorted or ingrown nails (Grap. Mag-p-aus. Pho-ac.). Panaris. Soreness thro' arch of foot. Weak ankles.

FOUL, EROSIVE FOOTSWEAT. EVERY INJURY FESTERS AND IS SLOW TO HEAL. **Carbuncle** (Anthr. Ars.). **Bunions. Osteitis. Foul,** spongy ulcers. Somnambulism. CHILLINESS; < **lying in bed, during** exertion, etc. **Coldness of painful part. Icy chills.** Hectic. PROFUSE SWEAT; **on upper parts, head, or affected parts; at night.**

Complementary: Flu-ac. Thu. Related: Calc-c. Kali-p.

SOLIDAGO.

REGION.

KIDNEYS. Digestive Tract.
Lower Limbs.
Blood.

WORSE.

Pressure.

BETTER.

Profuse Urine.

Weak and easily takes cold. Hemorrhage. Bitter taste. Difficult, **dark and scanty** or clear, stinking **urine.** Pain from kidneys to bladder (Oci.) and down thighs. VERY TENDER OVER KIDNEYS (Fer.); they ache or feel distended (Helo.). Lumbago. Nephritis. Dropsy. Cystitis. Prostatitis. **Petechiæ on lower limbs.** Diabetic gangrene.

SPIGELIA.

REGION.

NERVES OF { **TRIFACIAL. HEART. Neck.**
Eyes.
LEFT SIDE.

WORSE.

TOUCH. MOTION. **Jar.**
Tobacco. Coition. Washing.

BETTER.

Lying on Right Side with Head High.

Pain extends to eyes. VIOLENT, RADIATING NEURALGIA, **mostly left-sided or ascending from occiput to left eye** (Chel. Sabi).——Stammering. Fear of pointed things. Eyes feel sore and too large. Squint. Lachrymation on affected side. Yellow rings about eyes. Post nasal dropping (Hyds. Kali-bi. Lach. Nat-m. Nux-v. Sep. Sul.). Toothache. **Pains about navel;** in children. Lumps of mucus in stools. Worms. **Audible or visible palpitation;** alternating with other symptoms. Purring or compression at heart. Pain from heart to left shoulder and arm. Rheumatic metastasis. Numbness of left arm. Tremulous pulse. Pulsation in patellæ. **Shudders** when touched or bruised.

Related: Cact.

SPONGIA.

REGION.

LARYNX. HEART.

GLANDS.

Trachea.

WORSE.

COLD, DRY WIND.

AWAKING. **Exertion.**

Inspiration. **Before Midnight.**

BETTER.

Lying. Warm Food or Drinks.

Flabby. Weak and heavy; he feels stuffed full (Coc-c.). Orgasms. Hard swelling; of glands (ductless).——**Terrified, anxious look.** Protruding eyes. Sore throat < sweets. Painful, swelled spermatic cord and testes. Squeezing in testes. Dry air passages. TIGHT, CROUPY, RINGING, CROWING, SAWING OR BARKING COUGH; wakes child from sleep (Lach.); then burning in chest (Coc-c. Seneg.); < cold drinks or excitement. HOARSE. Larynx pains when singing, talking or swallowing; he must grasp it. Diphtheria. **Suffocation;** a plug, leaf or valve (Ant-t. Bar-c. Ign. Pho.) in larynx awakes him, < lying, > leaning forward. **Fulness in chest.** SURGINGS TO CHEST AND FACE. **Palpitation.** Goitre. Numb fingertips or lower half of body. Heat; with cold, numb thighs < thinking of it; with anxiety.

Related: Iod. Led.

SQUILLA.

REGION.

MEMBRANES { MUCOUS. **Serous.**

Kidneys. Heart.

WORSE.

Early Morning. Motion.

Uncovering.

Old People.

PROFUSE SECRETIONS. Dropsy with profuse urine. Gurglings.——Acrid coryza. Wants to rub eyes (Caus. Gym. Pul.). **Black spots on teeth.** Sweet taste; of food, expectoration, etc. Dark, brown, frothy stools. Sudden urging; passes much urine. **Spurting urine. Spasmodic,** RATTLING COUGH **with sneezing,** coryza, **watery eyes, spurting urine** or heat; < cold drinks and inspiration. **Stitches in chest** (1). Pleurisy. Broncho-pneumonia. Heat with aversion to uncovering. Absence of sweat.

Related: Ars.

STANNUM.

REGION.

NERVES.
MUCOUS MEMBRANES.
CHEST.
FEMALE ORGANS.

WORSE.

Using Voice. Cold.
MOTION { **After.** Gentle. / **Lying on Right Side.**

BETTER.

Rapid Motion. Hard Pressure.
Expectoration.

Repeated short attacks. EXTREME WEAKNESS; FELT MOST IN THE CHEST (Pho-ac.); **in throat, stomach, upper arms and thighs; drops into** a chair; **can't even talk** (Pho. Sul.); trembles on moving. **Paralytic heaviness. Profuse, muco-purulent secretions.** Emaciation. PAINS INCREASE GRADUALLY, THEN AS GRADUALLY SUBSIDE. **Pressive drawing.** Neuralgias. Cramps. Spasms. Hysteria.——**Anxious, nervous and sad;** < before menses. Pressive stupefying headache. Pale face with sunken eyes. Faceache. Malar neuralgia (Cimi. Colo. Kali-bi. Mag-c. Mez. Verb.). Violent vomiting. Burning in liver (Aur-m.) Painful pinching colic, > hard pressure and stool which exhausts. Worms. Atony of bladder. Easy sexual orgasms. Pollutions. Prolapsus uteri, < during stool (Pod.). Gushes of debilitating leucorrhœa. Much mucus in trachea. Deep, hollow voice. **Short of breath from every effort; must** loosen clothes. **Cough; easily expectorates quantities,** of sweet pus or balls of mucus. Catarrhal phthisis. Rawness in chest. Limbs give away on the act of sitting down. Swelled hands and ankles. Chill at 10 A. M. with numb fingertips. Hectic. Debilitating, musty sweat at 4 A. M.

Complementary: Pul. Related: **Lach.**

STAPHYSAGRIA.

REGION.

NERVES. TEETH.
Genito-Urinary Organs.
Fibrous Tissues { **Eyelids.** / **Skin.**
Glands.

WORSE.

Emotions { **Chagrin. Vexation.** / **Indignation.** Quarrels.
Sexual Excesses. Onanism.
Touch. Cold Drinks. Incision.
Mercury.

BETTER.

Warmth. Rest. **Breakfast.**

Sensitive widows and brides. **Nervous trembling. Squeezing or stinging-smarting, as if cut.** Pains move into teeth (Chin. Fer. Kali-bi. Merc. Mez.).

Figwarts.——**Morbidly sensitive;** easily offended. **Angry. Petulant;** he throws things (Colo. Tub.). Bad memory. Compressive, stupefying headache. As of heavy load in forehead. Moist, foul, eroding milk crust. Dryness in eyes. Nodes in lids. Blepharitis. **Sickly, hollow-eyed.** Ulcerating coryza. Swelled submaxillary glands. Pale, bleeding gums. **Loose, aching, black, crumbling teeth** (Plan.), < eating and during menses, > **hard pressure.** Pyorrhœa. **Hungry;** craves milk. Painful flatulence. Colic. Dysentery. Irritable bladder. Trickling along or burning in urethra. Dysuria; of brides; in pregnancy (Pop-t.). Sensitive vulva. Sexual erethism. Prostatitis. Pain from ovaries into thighs (Xan.). Salpingitis. Crural neuralgia. Tight chest at close of coition (Amb.). Cough from cleaning teeth or alternating with sciatica. Violent yawning; after headache; brings tears. Backache; in morning in bed. Fine tearing in (Bism.). or numb fingertips. Nodes on finger joints. Weak knees. Biting-itching as of vermin (Saba.), changing place on scratching. LACERATED WOUNDS; pains in stitches. Amorous dreams, with pollutions. Sweat and flatus smell like bad eggs.

Complementary: Colo. Related: Cham. Merc.

STICTA.

REGION.

Nerves.

Membranes: **Nose.** Chest. Bronchi. Joints.

WORSE.

Night. Lying Down. Motion. Change of Temperature.

BETTER.

Free Discharges. Open Air.

Nervous, rheumatic subjects; that develop catarrhs. Painful, dry mucous membranes. Diagonal pains.——Must talk. Seems to be floating. Burning eyelids. **Pressure and stuffy fulness at root of nose** (Par.); **blows it without relief** (Kali-bi. Lach. Mar. Naja. Psor.). Coryza. Hay fever, **Incessant, dry, hacking cough, preventing sleep** < coughing and inspiration; after measles (Dros.). Numbness in air passages. Bronchitis. Sore, stiff neck; pains to shoulder (Guai. Lachn.). Rheumatism. Red spot over affected joint. Bursitis.

Related: Cetrar. Guai. Lach.

STRAMONIUM.

REGION.	WORSE.
BRAIN.	**Glistening Objects.**
Circulation { Throat. Skin.	AFTER SLEEP. **Fright.**
Spinal Nerves { Arms. Genitals.	**Suppression.** Intemperance.
	BETTER.
	LIGHT. **Company.** Warmth.

Absence of pain with suppressed excretions, especially urine. Very mobile states. **Nervous tremor. Disorderly, graceful or rhythmic actions** (Elap.), **more of head and arms.** Chorea. Spasms.——DREADS THE DARK (Med.), **wants light and company** (Val.), **yet has a horror of bright objects. Very active, variable delirium;** talks incessantly; sees great numbers of, or vividly hideous phantoms, more to one side (Lac-c.); gets wildly excited and full of fear, desiring to escape, as in night terrors or delirium tremens (Cimi.), or does all sorts of crazy things. Raving mania with cold sweat, cursing and praying. Religious insanity (Ver-a.). **Loss of reason.** Stupid. Imbecile. Jerks head up and drops it again. Fixed sparkling stare. Squint. Diplopia. Night blindness (Lyc. Ver-a.). Crowding visual hallucinations (Op.). Delusions, as to size and distance. Red, bloated or rapidly changing face, now flushed now pale; a sardonic grin, then expressing **terror.** Wrinkled forehead. **Fine red dots on tongue.** Stammering. Dry throat with great thirst, yet DREADS WATER, it chokes him (Bell. Canth. Hyos.). Hydrophobia. Putrid (dark), painless diarrhœa. Excessive menses preceded by sexual excitement. Grasps the genitals (Canth. Zin.). Nymphomania. Nervous asthma. Drawing in back. Sensitive spine. Violent pain in hip (Thu.). Unilateral paralysis with twitchings. Non-appearing exanthems. Fiery scarlatinous rash. Sopor. **Awakes in fear** (Cina. Nat-p. Sul. Zin.) or screaming. Night terrors (Bell. Thu.).

Related: Bell. Hyo. Op.

STRONTIUM.

REGION.	WORSE.
Circulation { **Heart. Kidneys.**	**Walking. Sprains** (old).
	After Hemorrhages.
Ankles. Marrow.	**Least Uncovering. Evening.**
Right Side.	BETTER.
	Heat of { Sun. Wraps. Bright Light. **Baths.**

Congestive tension. FLEETING PAINS, HARD TO LOCATE; SEEMING

IN BONES. Rheumatism. Burning. **Gnawing.** Oedema. Violent starts. **Immobility of part;** of one side. **Sense of paralytic weakness.** Emaciation.——**Headaches** into upper jaw; with vertigo and nausea. **Numb mouth.** Pressure in stomach during digestion. Cramp about navel. **Hard,** knotty, difficult stool, then burning at anus. Nightly diarrhœa of yellow water. Pale, ammoniacal urine. As of a load on chest. **Heart feels smothered.** Numb hands. **Sprained or puffed ankles.** Cramp in calves and soles. Surgical shock (Cam.). **Flushes of heat, yet averse to uncovering.** Nightsweats. Climacteric.

Related: **Calc-c. Rhus-t.**

STROPHANTHUS.

REGION.
HEART. Circulation.
Kidneys.

WORSE.
Exertion. Alcohol. Tobacco.
Tea.

Stitches. Twitchings. Increased secretions. Throbbings or undulations.——Feels lifted up (Pho.), during siesta. Very mobile pupils. Red spots on face. Throat seems constricted. Vomiting. Rumbling, colicky diarrhœa; with burning at anus. **Sense of lively heart action.** Anguish at heart. Cardiac dyspnœa. Atheroma. Heavy forearms and fingers. Itching feet. Hives; receding.

Related: Spig.

SULPHUR.

REGION.
VENOUS CIRCULATION.
NUTRITIVE ORGANS { **ABDOMEN. Liver.**
Chest.
Rectum.
SKIN; **folds of.**
VERTEX. SOLES.
Chest. Joints.

WORSE.
SUPPRESSION. BATHING.
EXERTION. STANDING.
WHEN HEATED { IN BED, from woolens, etc.
Periodically { **11 A. M. Climacteric.**
Speaking. Atmospheric Changes.
BETTER.
Motion. Warm Application.

DEFICIENT REACTION (Ars. Carb-v. Psor. Ver-a.). Empty, overful, rough (Nat-m.) or asleep feeling. **Local burning or congestion.** Effusion. Deposits. **Foul, acrid or blood streaked discharges. RED ORIFICES;** tarsi, lips, ears, etc. (Alo.). **Weak, faint spells.** STOOPED, LANK, UNCURED AND UNWASHED. **Emaciation.** Psora. Scrofula. Rheumatism.——**Slow, lazy and always tired.** Hopeful. **Dreamers;** ecstatic, religious, philosophic, etc. Peevish, mean and prying or easily excited. Melancholy. Sunday headaches; preceded by photopsies (Nat-m. Psor.). **Heavy or sensitive vertex.** Band about forehead. Dry, cold hair. Cutting under eyelids. Bursting in eyeballs. Halo about light. Photophobia. Ophthalmia. Nose swells, drips or turns red if cold. Sensitive smell; imaginary odors. OLD LOOK. Spotted face. **Tongue dry;** red edges and tip (Ap.). Nursing sore mouth. Sensitive dental fangs (Gel.). As of a swelling in throat. **Drinks much, eats little.** Vapor rises in throat (Ap. Fer.). EMPTY SINKING AT EPIGASTRIUM; AT 11 A. M. (Pho.). Distended or **sore abdomen;** > pressure. Borborygmi. Colicky babies. Urging in rectum. Holds stool back from pain (Nit-ac. Thu.). HURRIED, EARLY MORNING DIARRHŒA (Nat-s. Pod. Rum. Tub.). Diarrhœa from milk (Lyc. Nat-c. Sep.). **Changing, mushy, stinking stools.** Constipation alternating with diarrhœa. Itching at anus. Piles. Burning, itching, sore vulva; < sitting (Berb. Kre. Stap.). Puerperal sepsis (Lyc. Pho. Pul. Pyro.). SUFFOCATIVE ATTACKS. **Air hunger.** Violent cough. Rattling or heat in chest; in A. M. As of a load on chest or shoulders. **Pain from left nipple to back.** Pneumonia. Heart feels too big (Glo.). Palpitation; < lying (Nux-v. Pul.). Nipples crack at base (Carb-a.). Red or brown spots on chest. Weak neck. Walks bent from lumbar pain. **Jerks one limb on falling to sleep.** DRY, ROUGH, SCALY OR ITCHING SKIN; DISPOSED TO BREAK OUT OR FESTERS AND WON'T HEAL; burning when scratched. Crops of boils (Echi.). Itch. Skin is painfully sensitive to air, wind (Hep. Kali-c. Psor.), washing, etc. **Eruptions alternate with other complaints, asthma** (Hep.), etc. Creeping erysipelas. Eczema. Rhagades. Ulcers. Sleeps, cat naps. Singing during sleep. FEELS TOO HOT; **HOT BURNING SOLES AT NIGHT;** uncovers feet; burning in vertex (Lach. Pho.), between scapulæ, **flashes of heat,** etc.

Complementary: Alo. Calc-c. Related: Psor. Syph.

SULPHURIC ACID.

REGION.

DIGESTIVE TRACT.
Blood.
Bloodvessels.
Left Side.

WORSE.

Open Air. Cold. Liquors.
Injuries. ODOR OF COFFEE.
Climacteric. Morning.

BETTER.

Hot Drinks. Hands near Head.
Moderate Temperature.

Suited to old age, old topers, etc. **DISPROPORTIONATE WEAKNESS.**

SENSE OF INTERNAL, TREMBLING (Hep); wants to be held. **Sourness.** Erosions. **Profuse, acrid, stringy discharges. Hemorrhage** (dark, thin). Parts feel stiff and tight. **Pains come on slowly, but** CEASE SUDDENLY (Bell.). **Great painfulness or as of a blunt pressure.——Hurried,** morose, irascible and vascillating. Brain feels loose. Deathly pale or wrinkled face; white of egg seems dried on it (Alu.). Aphthæ. Craves liquors. Pyrosis. Hiccough. Sour belching; it sets teeth on edge. **Nausea.** Vomiting; < lying on left side. Weak sinking at stomach, < after stool. Drinks chill the stomach. Very foul, green, black or **hacked diarrhœa.** Oozing piles. Cough, then belching; bloody expectoration. Fingers jerk when writing (Caus. Cyc. Stan.). Weak knees. Black and blue spots. Petechiæ. Hot flashes, then trembling or cold sweat, < on upper part of body, > motion.

Complementary: Pul. Related: **Sep.**

SUMBUL.

REGION.
Nerves.
Heart.
Left Side.

WORSE.
Motion. Inspiration. Music.
Climacteric.

BETTER.
Gentle Motion.

Nervousness. As of hot water flowing thro part. Yellow, tenacious discharges.——As of a cobweb on face. **Choking constriction in throat.** Hysteria. Burning pyrosis. Bloated abdomen. Oppressive tightness in left chest. Asthma. Nervous palpitation. Trickling along spine. Pale, cold skin. Internal itching. Dreams of falling.

Complementary: Lactuca. Related: **Mos.**

SYMPHYTUM.

REGION.
CARTILAGE. PERIOSTEUM.

WORSE.
INJURIES. FRACTURES.

Injuries to the cartilages and periosteum with excessive pain. Comminuted fractures. Eye injuries. **Prickling,** stitching pains. Non-union (Calc-p.). Coldness.

Related: **Calc-p.**

SYPHILINUM.

REGION.
Mucous Membranes.
Nerves.
Bones.

WORSE.
NIGHT; Sundown to Sunrise.
Gradual $<$ then slow $>$.
Extreme Heat or Cold.
During Thunderstorms. Damp.
BETTER.
Changing Position. Slow Motion.

Syphilitic taint. Poor reaction. **Weakness;** $<$ awaking. **Ulceration.** Bald head; pouting lips and big belly. Dwarfish. Foul odor of body. Violent or linear pains Knots in muscles.——**Horrid depression.** Rush of ideas. Feels as if going insane. Crossness. **Impulse to wash hands** (Coca Lac-c.). Imbecility. Nightly delirium. **Deep, crushing headaches; across base.** Beats head against wall (Tub.). Head feels pulled back (Cimi.). Inflamed cornea. Ophthalmia. Ozœna. Abscess of middle ear. Wrinkled face. **Teeth feel sticky** (Psor.). As of a worm in teeth. Caries at edge of gums (Thu.). Putrid taste. Crack along center of tongue (Mez. Nit-ac.). Capricious appetite. Craves liquors. Rectal stricture. Voids urine $>$ standing. **Profuse, acrid leucorrhœa;** with itching; running to heels (Alu. Onos. Senec. Tub.). Coughs $<$ lying on right side (Carb-a. Merc. Stan.). Pain from base to apex of heart. Backache $<$ urinating. Cold pain in legs. Bones pain as if sawed. Bilateral exostoses. Biting as from bugs. **Succession of abscesses. Foul or green pus (Tub.).** Conical crusts (Sil.). Bullæ. **White cicatrices.** Distorted nails. **Sleeplessness.** As of hot water in veins.

Related: Merc.

TABACUM.

REGION.
Nerves { Cerebro-Spinal / **Vagus.** / **HEART.** }
GLANDS.
SECRETIONS.

WORSE.
MOTION; **of Riding.**
Lying on Left Side.
BETTER.
Cold; Fresh Air. Twilight.
Uncovering. Abdomen.

RELAXING IRRITATION **which prostrates, causes free secretions and excites the muscles of hollow organs.** Paroxysmal effects. Jerky movements. Pains $<$ heat.——Morose, despairing and wretched. Mental fag. **Excessive vertigo** $<$ opening eyes. Sudden faintness. Deathly pale, pinched look.

Retracted lips. Spasm of lower jaw. Tetanus. **Clutching about throat. Deathly nausea and violent vomiting; < least motion;** with much spitting (Aut-t.). Pregnancy. Seasickness. Acidity. **Sinking at epigastrium. Wants abdomen uncovered.** Colic. Involuntary choleraic or thick, curdled, watery stool, like sour milk. Dribbling urine. Renal colic. Emissions. Impotency. Constriction of chest. Asthma. Twisting about heart. Angina pectoris. Palpitation with interscapular pain. Unsteady heartbeat. Fuzzy fingertips. Nightmare. **Icy cold skin.** Cold legs. Heat; of one cheek; or down spine; internal. Sudden cold sweats; with chills.

Complementary: Op. Related: Ars. Gel.

TARAXACUM.

REGION.
Liver.
Stomach.

WORSE.
Rest; Sitting; Standing.
BETTER.
Walking. Touch.

Bilious, sick feeling. Stitching.——Depression. Heavy pressure in occiput. **Coated tongue with raw patches** (Tereb.), i. e., **mapped.** Sour taste or hawks sour mucus. White stools. Jaundice. Restless limbs with tearing pains. Chilly after eating. Cold fingertips. Burning toes. **Nightsweats.**

Related: Nux-v.

TARENTULA.

REGION.
NERVES. **Spine.**
Heart.
Respiration.
Genitals (Female).

WORSE.
TOUCH. **Cold.** Noise.
Periodically; Yearly; Evening.
BETTER.
RELAXATION { **Rubbing.** Smoking. **Sweating.** }
Music. Open Air.

NERVOUSLY SENSITIVE. **Excessively restless, hurried and fidgety; in incessant motion** (Ars.) though walking <; **rolls from side to side** (Lach.). **Twitching. Jerking.** Chorea. **Sexual synalgias** (Ap.).——Suddenly changing moods. Hysteria. Angry despair. **Hateful, devilish,** sly. Destructive impulses. Malingering. Kleptomania. As of needles pricking brain. Rubs head on pillow. Headache accompanies many symptoms. Bloated face. Heaviness in pelvis. Very sensitive genitals. Sexual erethism. Hot semen. Dry, hot, itching vulva and vagina. Motions or burning in uterus. Suffocative shortness of breath. **Painfully sensitive spine; touching it excites pain in chest, heart, etc.** (Bell.). **Heart seems to twist and turn around. Must keep her hands busy; picks** the **fingers** (Ars. Kali-bro.). **Purplish discoloration. Swelling.**

Related: **Myg. Plat.**

TARENTULA CUBENSIS.

REGION.
Cellular Tissue.

WORSE.
Cold Drinks. Exertion.

Slow incubation then **rapid onset, with alarming prostration, atrocious burning-stinging pains, board like hardness of part and copious sweat.** Intense diphtheric fever. Malignancy, Sepsis. Carbuncle. Felon. Bluish abscess. **Death agony.** Paralysis followed by convulsions.—Tendency to vomit. Pruritus vulvæ. Trembling hands. **Fidgety feet.** Purple discoloration. Gangrene. Pungent heat of surface.

Related: Anthx. Lat-m.

TELLURIUM.

REGION.
Spine. Nerves.
Skin. Ears.

WORSE.
Touch. Lying on Part.
Cold. Empty Swallowing.

Offensiveness; like putrid fish brine (Ol-an.). Acrid **discharges; cause itching** or vesicles. Otitis. Periostitis. **Numbness. Sharp,** quick pains, then soreness. Sense of retention.——Vertigo on dropping to sleep (Arg-n. Nat-m.). Linear head pains. Thickened tarsi. **Inflamed, bluish, puffy ears.** Fluent coryza, **hoarseness** and watery eyes (Cep.). **Twitching face** pains jerk angle (1) of mouth up. Retching ends in yawning. **Very sensitive spine** (Chin-s. Nux-v.). Deep sciatic pain; < coughing, sneezing or straining. Itching pricking as from bugs. Circular **eruptions. Ringworm.**

Related: **Cepa.**

TEREBINTHINA.

REGION.
Mucous Membranes {KIDNEYS. Bladder.
Respiration. Heart.
Blood.

WORSE.
Dampness. Cold.
Lying. Pressure.
BETTER.
Motion.

BURNING. **Congestion.** PASSIVE HEMORRHAGE.——**Smooth, sore, glossy tongue** (Pyro.). Pains excite urination (Thu.). **Bruised soreness; of abdomen or bladder** (Equi. Thu.). **Flatulence. Tympanites.** Ascites. Profuse mucus stools. **Smoky urine;** with coffee grounds sediment (Ap. Lach.) or odor of violets. Nephritis. Strangury. Cystitis. Hæmaturia. Metritis. Bronchial asthma. Advancing purpuric spots. **Drowsiness.** Rapid pulse. Cold sweat on legs.

Related: Canth. Erig. Pho.

THERIDION.

REGION.
NERVES.
Bones.

WORSE.
NOISE. **Touch. CLOSING EYES.**
Least Motion. Riding. Jar.
BETTER.
Rest. Warmth.

HYPERSENSITIVE: **Noise is too penetrating** (Asar. Coccl. Lil-t. Plan.), **affects the teeth** (Plan.), causes nausea, etc. Water feels too cold.——Fruitless activity. Sense of duality. Hysteria. **Vertigo, with nausea on closing eyes.** Luminosities, then blurred vision. Too much air seems to enter passages (Chlor.). Yellow-green, thick, foul nasal discharge, Ozœna. **Nausea from least motion.** Seasickness. Burning in liver (Aur-m.). Bounding internally. Cough jerking the body together. Stitch back thro apex of left lung (Myrt.). Phthisis florida. Cardiac anxiety. Spine is sensitive to pressure or jar. Bones seem broken. Necrosis. Scrofula. **Stinging thrusts** in skin. Cold sweat is easily excited.

Related: Sil.

THUJA.

REGION.

Mind. **Nerves.**

Mucous Membranes { **GENITO-URINARY ORGANS.** Intestines.

SKIN.

Glands.

Left Side.

WORSE.

COLD DAMP. **Warm Bed.**

Gonorrhœa. Vaccination (Sil.).

Urinating. TEA.

Periodically { **Night.** 3 A. M. Yearly. Increasing Moon. During Menses.

BETTER.

Warmth { **Moist.** Air. Wrapping Head.

Turning from Left to Right.

Sneezing. Touch.

Exuberant, warty or fungoid tissues (Nit-ac. Pho.). Condylomata. polypi, etc. **Sycosis.** **Foul, acrid, greasy or sweetish odor;** of body, sweat, genitals, etc. Parts emaciate rapidly or look dead. Flesh feels beaten from bones. **Tricklings.** Burning-sticking, numbing pain, < warmth. Exhaustion.——**Illusions ending in fixed ideas;** as of being frail (Bell. Calc-c. Rad-b.), **of a live thing internally,** etc. Anxious dwelling on trifles. Split hair. Tearing in brow (1). **Photopsies, just beyond the field of** vision. Sclerotitis. Scabs or briny odor in nose. Waxy face. **Boring in** zygoma (Stro.). Gnawing toothache < cold. Ranula (Merc.). Mucus in choanæ. Rancid or noisy belching or flatus. Pushings in abdomen (Lyc.). Cutting squeezing in lower bowels, groins, bladder or urethra. Ileus. Stools gurgle out like water from a bung hole (Alo. Gam.); < breakfast. Moisture at anus or perineum. Trickling along urethra (Kali-bi. Petros.). Diabetes. Burning or dribbling urine. Bruised feeling in testes. Sloughing foreskin. Chordee. Tearing in ovaries (1). **Sensitive vagina.** **Short, difficult breath.** Anxious palpitation. Pressure over kidneys. Pulsation in back. Limbs feel paralysed; hips give away. Crawling in or inflamed tips of fingers and toes. **Painful soles** (Ant-c. Kali-c. Lyc. Med.). **Dirty, brown spotted or hairy skin** (Med.). Eruption on covered parts—elbows,—itching from cold water. Bloodboils on back. Bluish white ulcers. Naevi (Sul.). Brittle, distorted nails. SLEEPLESS; when on left side. Dreams of the dead. Shaking chill with yawning; < urinating; not > heat. Heat rises into chest, with icy cold hands, nosebleed or cough. **Sweat on bare parts,** with dry heat under covers; cold on hands; > awaking; **profuse on genitals.**

Complementary: Nit-ac. Sabi. Related: Merc. Nit-ac. Sabi.

TILIA.

REGION.
Muscles. Female Genitals.
Urinary Organs.

WORSE.
SWEATING. Drafts.
After Sleep.

Dragging pains.——**Soreness; about uterus,** abdomen, etc.; the bed feels too hard. **Profuse sweat without relief;** THE MORE HE SWEATS THE GREATER THE PAIN. Rheumatism. Heavy dragging in urethra (Saba.). Scanty urine. Cough from tickling in left side of throat (Hep.). Neuralgia. **Sleepiness.**

Related: Ap. Calc-c. Lil-t.

TRILLIUM.

REGION.
FEMALE SEXUAL ORGANS.

WORSE.
Motion.
BETTER.
Tight Bandage.

Hemorrhage.——Feeling as if the bones of the hips and back were being separated (Calc-c. Sabi.); with **faintness** and **sinking** at the stomach. Menses every two weeks (Calc-p. Lyc. Mag-c. Pho.). **Bleeding fibroids** (Calc-c. Nit-ac. Pho. Sul-ac.). Menorrhagia.

Complementary: Calc-p.

Related: Sabi.

TUBERCULINUM.

REGION.
LUNGS.
Mind.
Head.
Glands.
Larynx.

WORSE.
CLOSE ROOM. **Motion.**
Weather; DAMP (cold); **Changing.**
Awaking. Noise. Mental Excitement. Thinking of it.
Pressure of Waistband.
BETTER.
Cool Wind; Open Air. Motion.

Constantly changing indications. Low vitality; increasing debility and susceptibility. **Poor reaction.** Rapid breakdown (Lyc.). **Takes cold easily.** CONSUMPTIVE TAINT (Pho.). Quiverings.——**Sensitive and irritated by every trifle;** < awaking. Fits of temper. **Dissatisfied and** reckless; always wanting a change (Sep.). FEAR; **of dogs** (Chin.). **Deep,**

head pains; tears her hair or beats her head (Aco.); < motion. Brain seems loose. Eczema tarsi. Old, dingy look. Teeth feel jammed (Lach. Merc-i-f.); are sensitive to air. Dryness in choanæ (Sep.). Hawks mucus after eating (Sil.). Adenoids. Craves cold milk (Chel. Pho-ac.), sweets or hot water. Drum belly. Tearing in rectum on coughing. Sticky urinary sediment (Pyro.). Menses return soon after childbearing. Frightful dysmenorrhœa. AIR HUNGER. Sore spot in chest (Ol-jec.). Heaviness at heart. Sensitive skin; easily tanned; itching in cool air. Brown fingertips. Branny scales. Frightful or vivid dreams; of shame; awakes in horror. Cough with chill and red face; < evening. Cold feet; < left; in bed (Ars.). Heat; on cheek of affected side; in flushes; in spots burning; on genitals; < eating. **Easy sweating;** cold; clammy; on upper parts; on hands (Thu.). **Clothes feel damp** (Guai. Lac-d. Pho. Ran-b. Ver-v. Vis-a.). Wants covers in all stages.

Complementary: Calc-c. Sep. Related: Sep.

URTICA URENS.

REGION.

MAMMÆ.

Genito-Urinary Organs.

Liver. Spleen.

WORSE.

Cool { Moist Air. / Bathing. } Yearly.

Burns. Stings. Snow Air (Sep.).

Stinging-burning (Ap.). Hemorrhage. Urinous odor of body.——White stool. Pinworms. Acrid urine, causing itching. Lithiasis. ABSENCE OF MILK. **Fever at night;** with vertigo and general pulsation. Acute gout (Colch.). Itching skin. Uric acid intoxication. Vesicles. Nettlerash (Dulc.). Prickly heat (Ant-c.). Urticaria with rheumatism.

Related: Form. Nat-m. Ocim.

USTILAGO

REGION.

Female Sexual Organs. Skin.

WORSE.

Touch. Motion. Climacteric.

Tumid tissues tending to slow bleeding. Hemorrhage.——Depression. **Loss of hair and nails.** Milk crust. Masturbation. Menses half liquid, half clots or stringy; vicarious. The uterus seeps dark, clotted blood. Metrorrhagia. Acute ovarian pain. Burning in right ovary; soreness in left and of uterus. Pains shoot down thighs. Foul yellow or brown leucorrhœa. Pain under left breast (Cimi.). Dry, hot skin.

Related: Bov. Sec-c.

VALERIANA.

REGION.

NERVES { **Spinal.** Genito-Urinary.

Mind.

Muscles, etc. { Calf. Heels. Tendo Achilles.

WORSE.

REST. STANDING.

Excitement. Evening.

BETTER.

Changing Position.

Walking About. Rubbing.

Changeable disposition and symptoms; alternations and **want of reaction. Pains move outward** (Pru-sp. Zin.), are here and there, or come and go. **Illusions;** of smell, taste or hearing. Sense of floating (Asar.). **Impulse to move. Jerks. Weak parts;** eyes, arms, popliteæ, etc.——**Nervous,** excitable and weak or inclined to faint. **Anger.** Very mobile ideas, suddenly going from one extreme to another. Hysteria. Coldness in upper head. Luminosity before eyes in the dark. Objects seem too near the eyes. Greasy or rancid taste. **As of a thread in throat.** Eructations like bad eggs. Hunger with nausea, as if from navel. **Flatulence.** Colic. Polyuria. Heels pain when sitting. Strangling on falling to sleep. Fever composed of disagreeable, great heat only. Gushes of sweat.

Related: Ign. Pul.

VARIOLINUM.

REGION.

BLOOD. **Spine.** Muscles.

WORSE.

Motion. **Vaccination.**

General aching, < in back, occiput and legs.——Green vision on rising. Every odor nauseates. Putrid, coppery taste. Tongue protrudes during sleep. Food seems to want to regurgitate. Tympanites, pouting upward; she looks pregnant. **Breaking backache. Pustular eruptions;** foul. Smallpox. Shingles. Ulcers look scooped out. As of cold water trickling down back. Violent chill. Intense burning fever. Foul sweat.

Related: Ant-t. Cimi.

VERATRUM ALBUM.

REGION.	WORSE.
MIND.	EXERTION. DRINKING.
NERVES { **ABDOMINAL.** / **Heart.**	**During Pain.** Wet Cold.
	BETTER.
Vertex. Blood.	Walking About. Covering.

VIOLENT EFFECTS, WITH PROSTRATION, COLD SWEAT ON THE FOREHEAD, FAINTNESS OR COLLAPSE (Colch. Sec-c.). SUDDEN, EXCESSIVE EVACUATIONS. **Progressive weakness and emaciation; during** acute diseases; **eg, whooping cough, ague, etc. Cramps with rigidity.**——**Delirium**; with violence, loquacity or lewdness; during pain. **Prays**, curses and howls in turn. Acute manias, insanities, etc. Sits in silence. Melancholia. Overpowering headaches. Bristling hair (Laur.). **Face turns deathly pale on rising up. Bluish**, sunken, pinched or distorted countenance. Jaws cramp when chewing. Heaviness in teeth. **Thirst for ice cold water.** Painful epigastrium. EXCESSIVE VOMITING WITH PURGING. **retching, cutting colic, cramps in limbs and rapid prostration. Cholera;** morbus, infantum, etc. Watery green, almost odorless or colorless stool (Cam.). The air seems too hot (Ast-r.). Tickling down throat into lungs (Cham.). Continuous violent cough with retching. **Aphonia.** Visible palpitation. Weak heart. Thready pulse. **Cramps in calves;** between scapulæ, in fingers, toes, etc.; > motion. GENERAL COLDNESS (icy): **of vertex** (Calc-c. Calc-p.), in mouth (Tell.), waterbrash, limbs, sweat, etc. The blood seems to run cold or internal heat with cold, (wrinkled) surface (Sec-c.). Fevers that show external coldness only. Congestive chills (Aco.).

Complementary: Carb-v. Related: Ars. Cup. Tab.

VERATRUM VIRIDE.

REGION.	WORSE.
VASO-MOTORS { MEDULLA. / CHEST. / **Heart.**	RAISING UP. **Lying on Back.**
	Motion. Cold.
	BETTER.
	Rubbing.

SUDDEN, VIOLENT CONGESTION (Glon.); especially basilar or pulmonary. General pulsation. Erratic convulsive motions. **Spasms;** with shrieks. Eclampsia (Stry.). Muscular prostration.——Head thrown back or nodding motions (Chin. Ign.). BLOATED, LIVID FACE, YET HE

BECOMES FAINT ON ATTEMPTING TO SIT UP. Apoplexy. Heat stroke, etc. Chewing motions. DRY, RED STREAK ALONG CENTER OF TONGUE (Ant-t. Arn. Pho. Rhus-t.). Violent vomiting. **Burning in pharynx and gullet.** Hiccough. Oesophagitis. Gastritis. **Stomach seems** to press against spine. **Slow, heavy breathing.** Pneumonia. **Aching neck and shoulders.** Dreams of water. Rapidly oscillating temperature (Pyro. Sal-ac.) or hyperpyrexia with sweat. **Full, soft pulse;** slow. **Cold, clammy sweat.** Cerebro-spinal fever.

Related: Gel.

VERBASCUM.

REGION.

Nerves (facial) { Ears. Zygoma.

Respiratory Tract. Bladder.

Left Side.

WORSE.

Change of Temperature. **Drafts**

Talking. **9 A. M. to 4 P. M.**

BETTER.

Deep Inspiration (Osm.).

Spasmodic catarrhal and neuralgic effects. Earache. **Cramping, crushing, squeezing faceache;** in malar bones. Piles. Enuresis. Deep, hollow, **barking** or trumpet toned cough. Nervous cough. **Hoarseness.**

Related: Aco. Sep.

VIBURNUM.

REGION.

FEMALE ORGANS.

Nerves.

WORSE.

BEFORE MENSES.

Lying on Left Side.

BETTER.

Rest. Open Air.

Cramping. Faint on sitting up. Heavy ache or excruciating cramps in pelvis; > menses starting. **Frequent, profuse urination;** during headache, menses, hemorrhage, etc. (Sars. Sul.). Pain in **back which ends in a** cramp in uterus or **goes down face of thighs.** Excruciating dysmenorrhœa (Med. Plat. Sep. Sul. Tub.). UTERINE HEMORRHAGE. Nervous metorrhagia. Miscarriage. After pains. False labor pains. **Polyuria.** Cramps in calves before menses.

Related: Caul. Pul. Sep.

VIOLA ODORATA.

REGION.

Nerves { **Eyes.** **Ears.**

Wrists (r). **Skin.**

WORSE.

Cloudy Weather.

Cool Air. Music. **Puberty.**

Tension. Nervous activity, then sudden exhaustion. Combined eye, ear and worm symptoms.——Pain over brows. Cramp in eyes. Otorrhœa. Craves meat. Itching at anus. Milky urine (Vis-a.). Enuresis. Weight on chest. **Dry skin with moist palms.** Cold shudders.

Related: Pul.

VIOLA TRICOLOR.

REGION.

Skin. Scalp.

Urinary Organs.

WORSE.

Pressing on Opposite Side.

Suppressed Eczema.

Cracked, gummy crusts on scalp, exuding tenacious yellow fluid, matting hair together (Ant-c.); with swelled cervical glands (Lyc.). Milk crust. Eczema. Urine smells like cat's urine. Emissions with vivid dreams.

Related: Rhus-t.

VIPERA.

REGION.

VEINS.

Blood.

WORSE.

LETTING LIMB HANG DOWN.

Cold. Yearly. Touch.

Bursting feeling. Hemorrhagic tendency.——Epistaxis. **Excruciatingly severe pain in epigastrium.** Enlarged liver. FULNESS AND UNBEARABLE PAIN AS IF LIMB WOULD BURST; must elevate parts. Varicose veins. Varicose ulcers. Phlebitis (Pul.). Goitre.

Complementary: Grap. Related: Elap.

XANTHOXYLUM.

REGION.

Nerves.

Female Sexual Organs.

Left Side.

WORSE.

Sleeping.

BETTER.

Vomiting.

Grinding pains.——Nervous feeling. The head threatens to fly off. Peppery taste. Grinding dismenorrhœal pains (Med.) that make her desperate; not relieved by any position. Leucorrhœa instead of menses.

Related: Lach.

ZINCUM.

REGION.

BRAIN; Occiput.
Spine. NERVES.
Root of Nose.
Inner Canthi.
Eyes.

WORSE.

EXHAUSTION. **Suppression.**
Wine. **Noise. Touch.**
After Being Heated.

BETTER.

Motion. Hard Pressure.
Warm Open Air. Free Discharges.

Ennervation. Depressed vitality; can't develop exanthems, discharges, etc. Brain exhaustion threatens. **Isolated effects;** one part numb, another sensitive; **formication;** pains in spots; between skin and flesh, etc. Automatic acts. **Tremor.** Jerkings. Spasm. Transverse pains. Descending paralysis. Disabling bone pains. Bloody discharges.——Fretful mood; cries if vexed. Easily startled, excited or intoxicated (Bov. Con.). Muddled. Forgetful; repeats the question then answers. Brain fag. **Screams;** if moved; during sleep; with the pain, etc. Pressure on vertex or root of nose. Head pains into eyes; < warmth. Crashing in head on falling to sleep (Glo.). Heat of occiput. Hair of vertex is painful. Weak vision with headache. Squint. Pterygium. Swelled nose. **Pale,** bluish, miserable **face.** Sticky lips. Bitter mouth. Voracity. As of a lump at navel. Itching at anus during stool. Violent urging but urinates only in certain positions, bending backward, crossing limbs, etc.; blood follows the urine. Pressive cutting about kidneys. Grasps genitals; with each cough, etc. Pain (boring) in left ovary. Profuse lumpy menses. Sexual excitement. Spasmodic dyspnœa < flatulency > expectoration (Ant-t. Grind. Lach. Sep.). Bursting, one hard throb at or a cap over heart. Nape tired by any exertion. Aching burning along spine < sitting (Kob. Sep.). Sensitive spine. Trembling hands. **RESTLESS LEGS OR FEET** (Agar. Ars. Carbo-v. Caus. Kali-c. Med. Rhs. Sul. Taren.). Sensitive soles. Sweaty feet with sore toes. Varicose; chronic; on genitals.

Related: Ign.

SUPPLEMENTAL REFERENCE TABLE

Dirty 17, 31.
Discharges 6, 23.
Disdain 32.
Disgust 45.
Dissipation 6.
Distending pain 16.
Distrustful 32.
Dogs, fear of 30.
Doubling up 10.
Downward over head or chest: Hyper.
Drafts of air 4, 28.
Drawing 19, 26.
    up of limbs 10.
Drawn inward 23.
Dread 30.
Dreaminess 32.
Drinking 13.
Drinks 7, 44.
Dwarfish: Bar-c.
Dysentery: Merc-c.

Ears, touching meatus <: Lach.
    moisture behind: Petr.
    and nose dry: Grap.
    open too: Mez.
    otorrhœa, putrid: Psor.
Eating, a little <: 6, Lyc.
Echoes: Caus.
Eclamptic: 18, Hyo.
Ecstasy: 32.
Eczema: 61.
Effusions: Bry.
Eggs, like bad: Cham.
Emaciation, descending: Nat-c.
    with hunger: Iod.
    of parts: Mez.
Emissions: 6.
    from mere contact: Con.
Ennervated easily: 18.
Epigastrium, lump in: Con.
    sensitive: Bry.
    sinking at: Sep.
    tickling in: Pul.
Epileptic: 18, Lach.
Erect posture: 11.
Erosion: 27.
Erotic: 29.
Erratic: 29.
Eructations, frothy: Kre.
Eruption, checked: 6.
Eustachian tube, itching: Nux-v.
Evil, fear of: 31.
Exacting: 30.
Exaltation: 29.
Excitement, mental: 6.
Excrescences: 61.
Exhale, can't: Chlor.
Expectorating <: Coc-c.
Expectoration: 23, 55.
    slips back again: Caus.
    suds, like: Kali-io.
Expiration: 5.
Extremities, lower, heavy: Alu.
Eyes, ascending into: Sang. (r), Spi. (l).
    behind, pains: Rhus-t.
    big, balls feel: Arg-n.
    blind, during menses: Pul.
    bloodshot: Arn.
    closing, sees visions: Bell.
    closure, spasmodic: Hyo.
    crossed, as if: Con.
    drawn back, as if: Par.
        together: Merc.
    drooping lids: Gel.
    hollow: 41.

Glowing: 17.
Gluttony: 44.
Gnawing: 20.
  under nails: Alu.
Goitre: 56.
Gone feeling: 47.
Gonorrhœa, chronic: Psor.
Gouty: 15.
Grasping: 5.
Gray: 17.
  early: Ars.
Greed: 29.
Greenish: 17.
Grinding: 15.
Groaning: 32.
Guilt, sense of: 32.
Gurgling: Berb.

Hacking: 22.
Hæmoptysis: Mill.
Hair, combing: Carb-ac.
  destroying the: Nit-ac.
  falling, in spots: Pho.
  letting it down >: Bell.
  on tongue: Kali-b.
Hands, coldness of one: Pul.
  eruption on dorsæ: Pul.
  sweaty, during heat: Fer-p.
  washes the: Syph.
  water, in: 5.
Hanging down, of part: 10. 47. 49.
Hangnails: 58.
Hardness: 24, 61.
Hatefulness, hatred: 31.
Head, ascending to: Sil.
  band about: Merc.
  big: Calc-c.
  bruised, as if: Chin.
  cap on, as of: Lach.
  cracking in: Kalm.
  hot, with cold limbs: Bell.
  jerking: 35.
  linear pain: Tell.
  looseness in: Chin.
  lump, in: Con.
  nodding: Caus.
  opens and shuts: Cocel.
  shocks thru': Glo.
  standing on: Glo.
Headache, basilar: Gel.
  blindness, before: Kali-b.
  < coughing: Bry.
  into nose: Lach.
  photopsies, before: Sul.
  < straining at stool: Bry.
  >wraps: 5.
Healing poor see Suppuration or Ulceration.
Heart to arms: Glo. Lat-m. (1).
  coldness at: Nat-m.
  floating: Buf.
  hands over: Laur.
  hard beating: Spo.
  metastasis to: Lach.
  soreness at: Nat-m.
  stopping, as if: Dig.
  tumultuous action: Lycops.
  turning over: Cact.
Heat of bed 5.
  flashes of: Lach.
  lack of vital 5.
  radiated 8.
Heats 28.
Hectic: Chin.
Hemiopia 38.
Hemorrhage, stringy: Croc.
Here and there 16, 56, 57.
Hernia, infantile: Nit-ac.

Liver, sore or enlarged: Nux-v.
Livid 17.
Load, as of a 20, 47, 57.
Loathing 45.
Location, loss of sense of 29.
Loose, as if 23, 35, 42.
Love, unhappy: Ign.
Lumbar region to pubes: Sabi.
Lump 21, 48, 56.
Lumpy 24, 50.
Lying 10, 30.

Madness 29.
Magnetism 9.
Malar bone, pain: Stan.
Mammæ, heavy: Phyt.
  infra (l): Cimi.
  < before menses: Lac-c.
  milk in virgin: Pul.
  stitches in: Con.
Maniacal 30.
Marasmus 19.
Marrow 15.
Mastoids 38.
Mealy 61.
Measly 60, Pul.
Melancholic 32.
Memory, sudden loss of: Laur.
Menses, coming, as if: Pul
  gushing: Bell.
  indelible: Mag-c.
  more flow more pain: Cimi.
  pain, excessive: Vib.
  two weeks, every: Trill.
  weakness, with: Iod.
Mental exhaustion 33.
  shock 30.
Metastasis: Abrot.
Migraine 41, Kali-bi.

Milk, craving: Tub.
Milkcrust: Rhus-t.
Milky 24.
Misfortune 31.
Moist parts 19.
Moody 29.
Mortification 7.
Mottled 17.
Mouldy, musty 24.
Mouse, like a 23.
Mouth, covering the >: Rum.
  dry without thirst: Nux-m.
  dry and hot: Bell.
  hangs open 43, Lyc.
  sticky: Kali-bi.
Move, impulse to 32.
Mucus 24.
  patches: Merc-p-r.
Muddled 30.
Musca volitantes 38.
Muscles obey feebly: Hell.

Nail 23, 35.
Nails, biting: Ars.
  ingrown: Sil.
Nares, mucus drops into posterior: Spig.
Narrow, as if 19, 43.
Neck, air on <: Sanic.
  emaciated: Nat-m.
  stiff on one side: Stict.
Necrosis 27.
Needles 26.
Nephritis: Canth.
Nervousness 30.
Neuralgia, orbital: Ced.
  shingles, after: Mez.